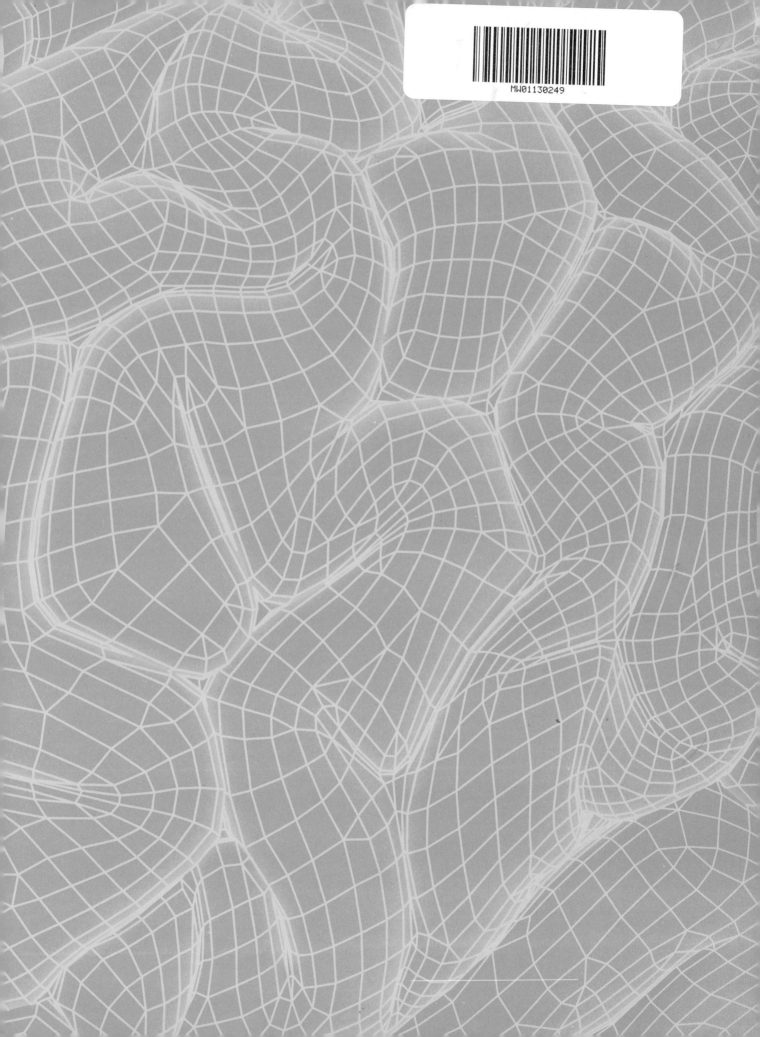

MW01130249

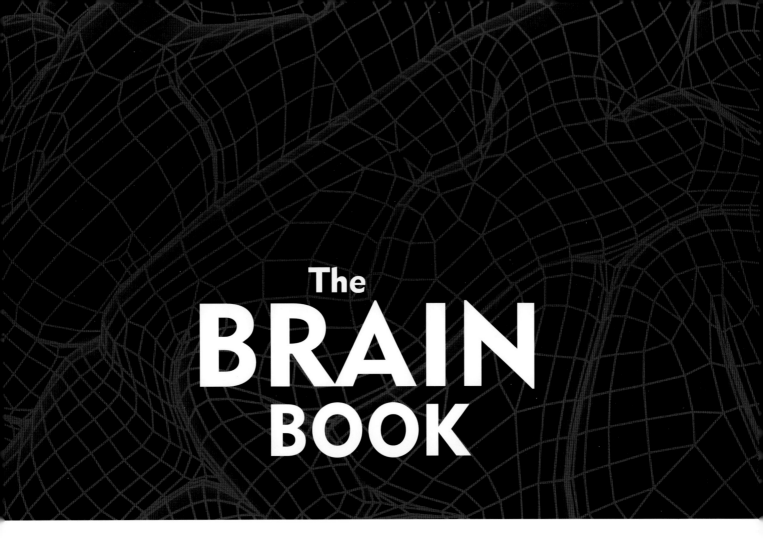

The
BRAIN
BOOK

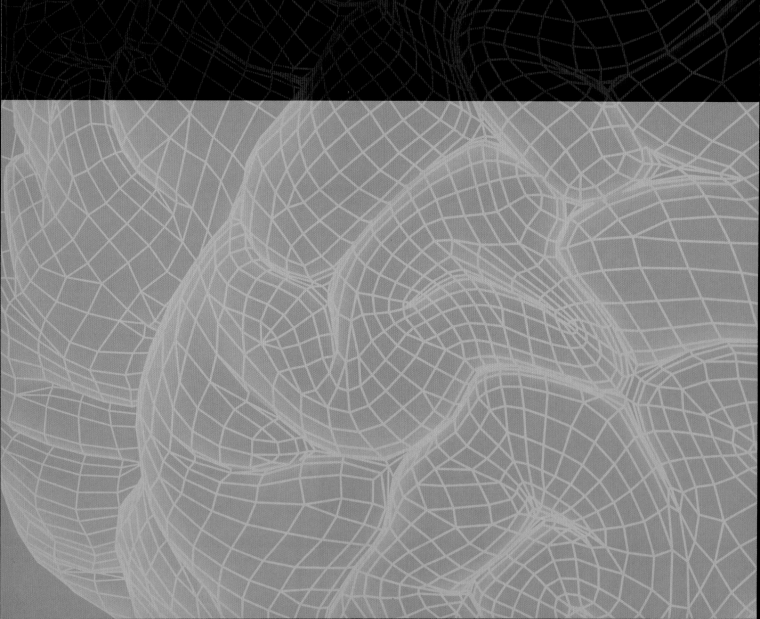

The
BRAIN
BOOK

Development • Function • Disorder • Health

Professor Ken Ashwell
Foreword by Professor Richard Restak, M.D.

FIREFLY BOOKS

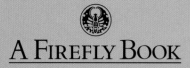

A FIREFLY BOOK

Published by Firefly Books Ltd. 2012

This publication, arrangement and text copyright © 2012 Global Book Publishing Pty Ltd
Illustrations copyright © 2012 Global Book Publishing Pty Ltd
All illustrations by Peter Bull Art Studio, except pages 23 (tl, tr) and 198 (bl), which are from the Global Book Publishing archive.

All rights reserved. No part of this publication may be reproduced, stored in a retrieval system, or transmitted in any form or by any means, electronic, mechanical, photocopying, recording or otherwise, without the prior written permission of the Publisher.

First printing

Publisher Cataloging-in-Publication Data (U.S.)

Ashwell, Ken.
   The brain book : development, function, disorder, health /
   Dr. Ken Ashwell ;
foreword by Richard Restak.
[352] p. : ill., photos. ; cm.
Includes index.
Summary: Covers diverse topics in brain science from development to disorders, the nature of consciousness through to aging and brain disease.
ISBN-13: 978-1-77085-126-9
1. Brain. I. Restak, Richard. II. Title.
612.82 dc23   QP376.A859 2012

Library and Archives Canada Cataloguing in Publication

Ashwell, Ken W. S.
   The brain book : development, function, disorder, health /
   Ken Ashwell ;
foreword by Richard Restak.
Includes index.
ISBN 978-1-77085-126-9
   1. Brain. I. Title.
QP376.A85 2012   612.8'2   C2012-901051-0

Published in the United States by
Firefly Books (U.S.) Inc.
P.O. Box 1338, Ellicott Station
Buffalo, New York 14205

Published in Canada by
Firefly Books Ltd.
66 Leek Crescent
Richmond Hill, Ontario L4B 1H1

Front cover: Corbis
Back cover: Global Book Publishing (2)

Color separation Splitting Image Colour Studio, Australia
Printed in China by i BOOK Printing Ltd

While every care has been taken in presenting this material, the medical information is not intended to replace professional medical advice; it should not be used as a guide for self-treatment or self-diagnosis. Neither the authors nor the publisher may be held responsible for any type of damage or harm caused by the use or misuse of information in this book.

This book was developed by:
Global Book Publishing Pty Ltd
181 Botany Road, Waterloo
NSW 2017, Australia

Publisher	James Mills-Hicks
Managing Editor	Barbara McClenahan
Project Manager	John Mapps
Project Editors	John Mapps
	Lachlan McLaine
Chief Consultant	Dr. Ken Ashwell B.Med.Sc., M.B. B.S., Ph.D.
Contributors	Dr. Ken Ashwell B.Med.Sc., M.B. B.S., Ph.D.
	Dr. Matthew Kirkcaldie B.Sc., Ph.D.
	Dr. Margaret Morris B.Sc., Ph.D.
	Dr. Richard Restak M.D.
Cover and internal design	Stan Lamond
Illustrators	Peter Bull
	Peter Chesterton
	Andrew Green
	John Francis
	Tony Randall
Illustrations Editor	Selena Quintrell
Assistant Illustrations Editor	Kylie Rees
Picture Researcher	Jodie Streckeisen
Indexer	Puddingburn Publishing Services
Proofreader	Crimson Lane Publishing Services
Production Manager	Karen Young
Editorial Coordinator	Kristen Donath

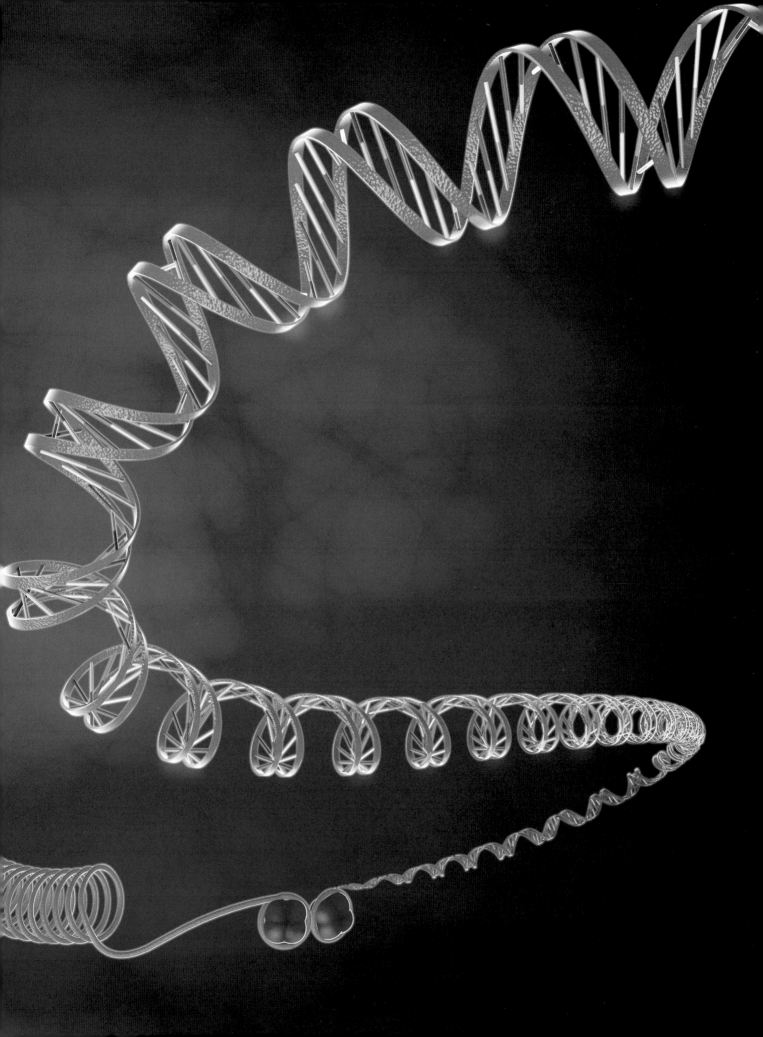

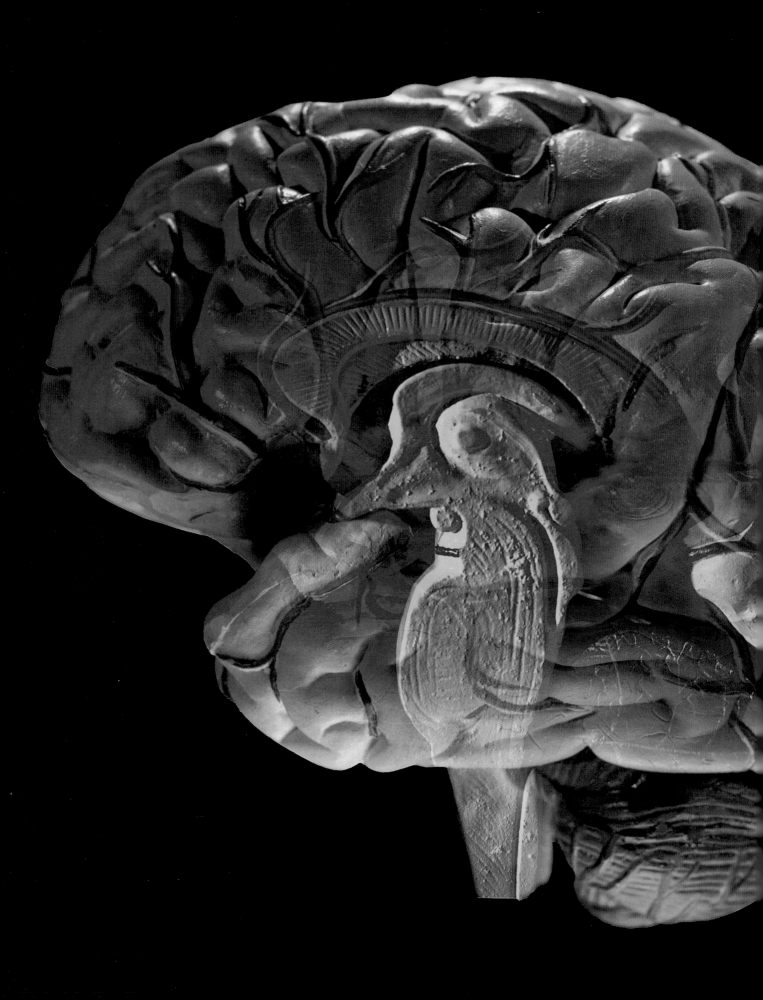

Contents

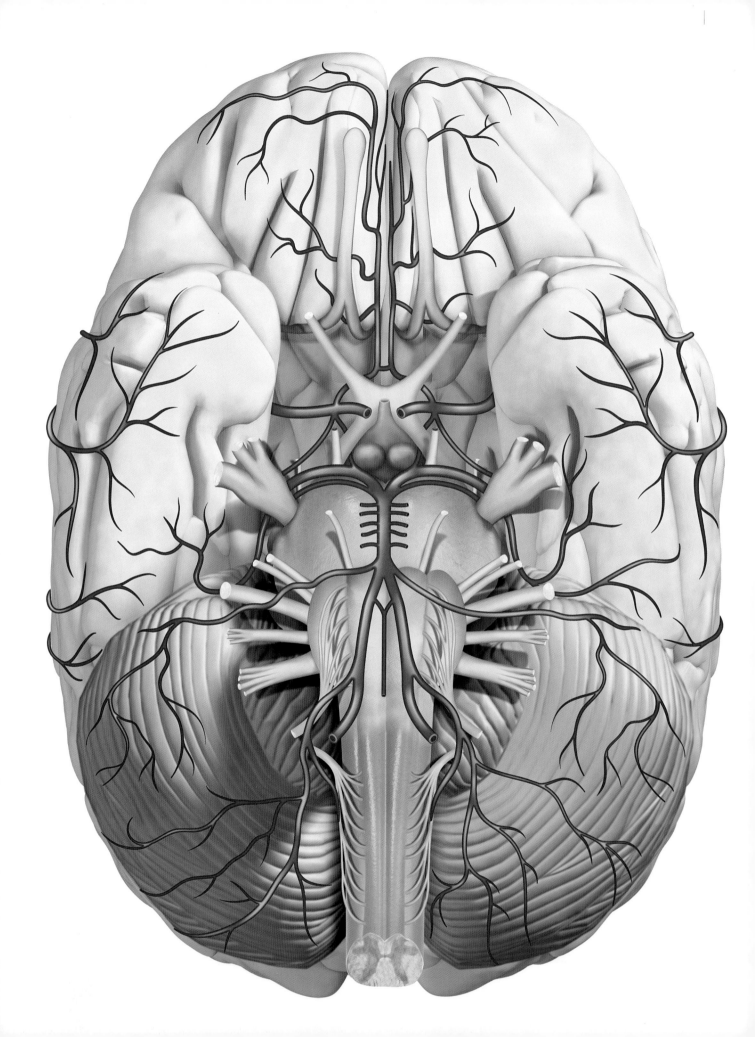

Foreword

The human brain is the most complex structure in the universe. Nothing—not even the most advanced computer—comes close to equaling its performance in carrying out feats of information processing. And no computer has anything like a sense of self, yet each one of us has a multifaceted sense of ourselves as a unique individual. Although our knowledge of its workings is still far from complete, we have much to gain from learning all that we can about the brain: the more we know about the brain, the more we know about ourselves. *The Brain Book* is a rich resource for advancing that goal.

The Brain Book provides a one-stop reference guide for understanding the brain in all of its aspects. It explains, among many other topics, how we interact with the world and respond to it; the workings of the basic functional unit of the brain—the nerve cell (neuron); the control of automatic functions like digestion and breathing; the nature of sleep; how alcohol and other drugs affect brain function; and the brain's ability to store and retrieve memories.

As explored in detailed sections of the book, the brain's organization and functioning underlie such disparate activities as reading and writing, appreciating music, planning, negotiating, and cooperating with others. This incredible versatility depends on plasticity: the brain's ability to remake itself in the light of experience. Plasticity explains the changes in thinking, experiencing, and acting that occur throughout our lives.

But the brain, as with any complex structure, can sometimes malfunction. Brain injury or disease can deprive us of abilities that we take for granted, such as speaking, coordinating our movements, and even controlling our tempers. *The Brain Book* clearly describes and explains brain dysfunctions, ranging from mild concussion and behavioral disorders to coma-inducing brain trauma and debilitating strokes.

Ordinarily, to learn about such a wide span of topics, a reader would have to consult multiple sources, including textbooks and professional journals, that presume familiarity with the subject. By contrast, *The Brain Book* provides a lucid overview of the brain that does not assume any previous knowledge. Thanks to meticulous research, the book includes recent scientific advances and break-throughs presented in easily understandable language. It simplifies without oversimplifying. Nearly 200 full-color digital illustrations make it easier to internalize a dynamic working model of brain function that will aid in understanding the brain at every level. Consulting these illustrations is like scanning the brain using a series of powerful lenses that provide dissected, detailed views of the brain, clearly showing internal structures.

Finally, *The Brain Book* fulfills an important niche in human understanding. In the near future, I believe that neuroscience will be an integral part of everyone's education. This effort will be justified by the benefits that will accrue from learning about the organ that is responsible for all that we are. *The Brain Book* is a wonderful companion to be consulted at every step along this fascinating journey.

Professor Richard Restak, M.D.

Clinical Professor of Neurology
George Washington University School of Medicine and Health Sciences, Washington, D.C.
Recipient of the Chicago Neurosurgical Center's "Decade of the Brain Award" and *New York Times* bestselling author

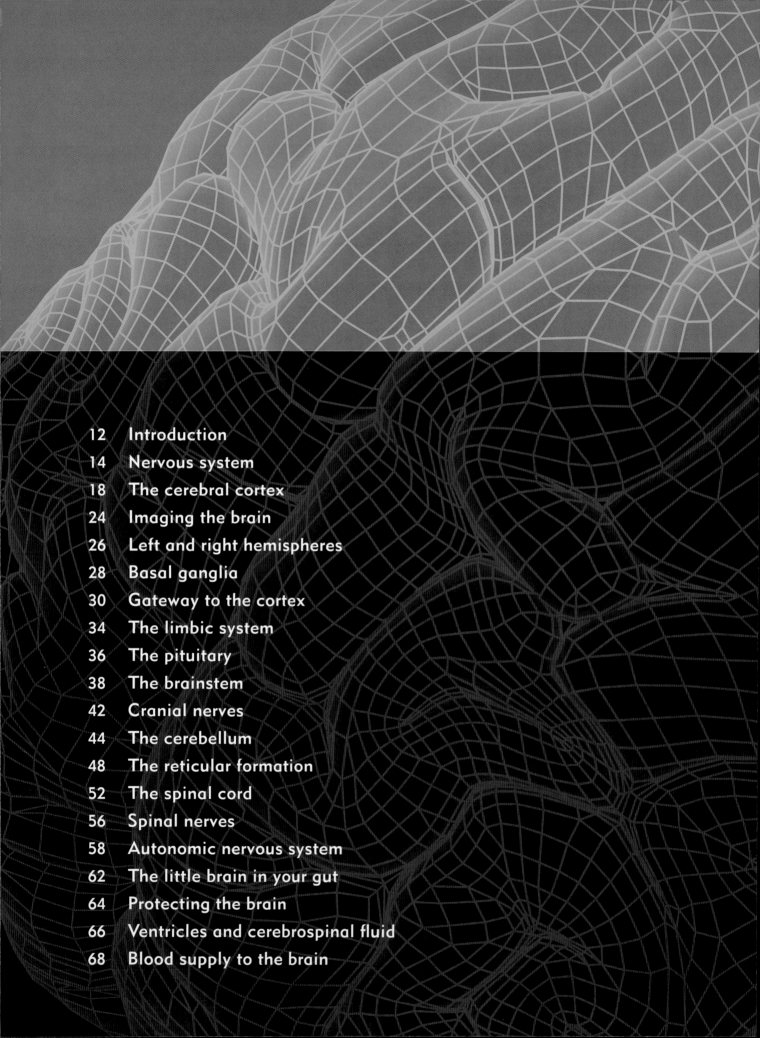

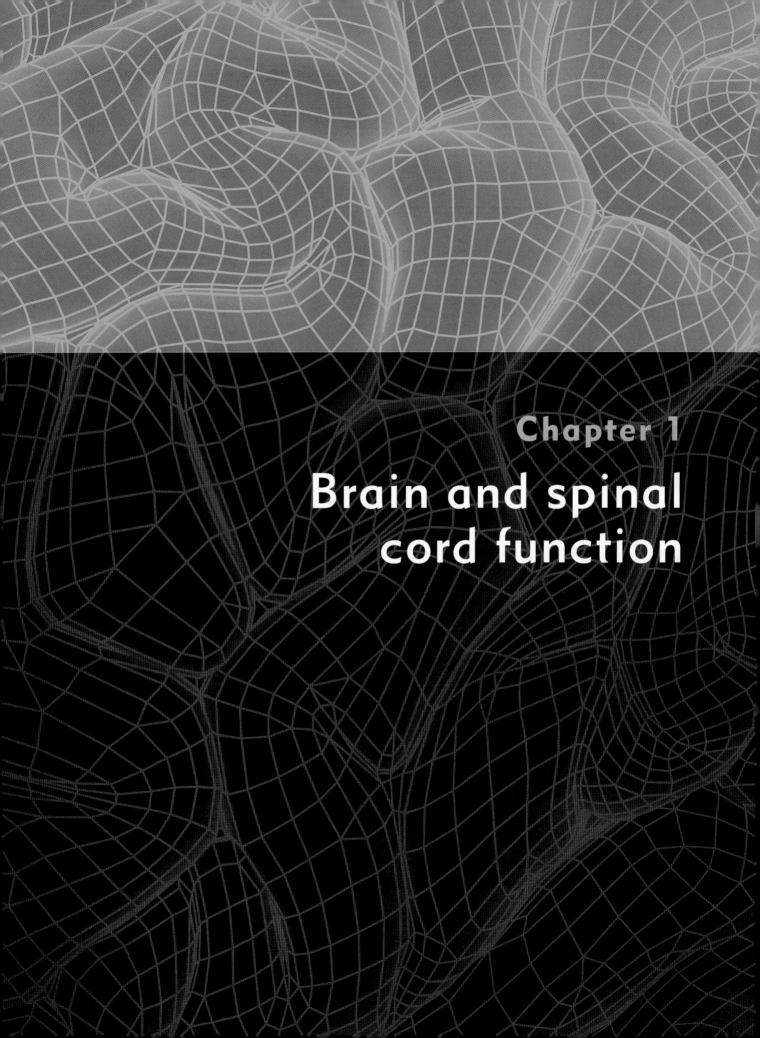

Chapter 1
Brain and spinal cord function

Introduction

The brain and spinal cord are the main components of a large and complex network that controls every aspect of human life, from digesting a meal to writing a novel.

The nervous system, with the brain at its center, processes sensory information about the world around us and the organs inside us, makes decisions about how to respond to that sensory information, and commands our muscles or glands to make changes that keep our body stable and healthy. Sensing the internal and external worlds requires the conversion of a stimulus (touch, odor, light, etc) into electrical signals.

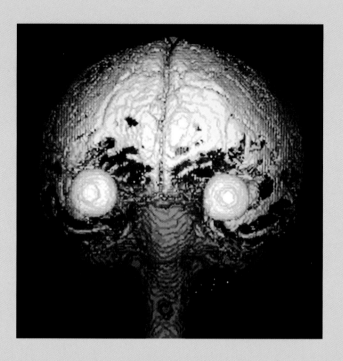

↑ **This MRI scan highlights the close coupling of the brain and the eyes. The brain continuously interprets the visual information gathered by the eyes to produce a detailed, accurate image of our environment.**

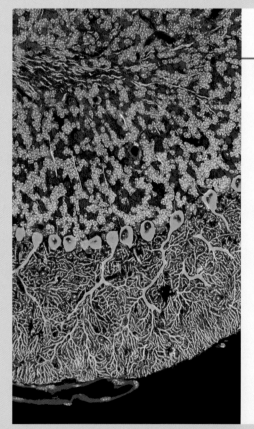

Nerve cells

The basic unit of the nervous system is the nerve cell, also called the neuron. A typical nerve cell has a cell body and a number of branching outgrowths (dendrites), which receive incoming information, and an outgoing fiber (the axon), which carries information away from the nerve cell body. Nerve impulses (action potentials) can be passed from one nerve cell to another through the junction (synapse) between the axon of one nerve cell and the dendrite or axon of another. A group of connected nerve cells is called a circuit. Some nerve cells connect to skin, muscle, or glands and are said to innervate those structures. When many axons are bundled together, they make up pathways that carry information in bulk between parts of the nervous system. Often, neuroscientists talk about the path that an axon follows as a projection, because it projects information to a distant site.

← **Purkinje cells, shown in green in this micrograph of part of the cerebellum, are one of several types of nerve cell.**

The sensory world

Among the main ways we sense the world are vision and hearing. To see and hear, our sense organs must be able to convert the information in the photons our eyes detect or sound waves our ears perceive into electrical changes that can be transmitted through the nervous system for processing and perception. Another category of external sense is the chemical senses (taste and smell). Sensations from the skin surface (touch, pain, temperature, and vibration) and from the joints and muscles are collectively called somatosensation.

Just as important as these external senses is viscerosensation, the detection and processing of sensory information from internal organs. This may not reach conscious awareness, but it is essential to regulate vital unconscious systems, such as those controlling blood pressure and body temperature.

Reflexes, decisions, and higher functions

Some responses to sensory information are stereotyped (i.e., consistent and unchangeable) and even "hard-wired" into the nervous system (e.g., spinal cord reflexes) and require no decisions. These responses are dealt with at the local level, in the spinal cord or brainstem. For more complex responses, information must be passed up the nervous system and into the brain. There, decisions are made in the light of basic drives to feed, drink, avoid predators, and produce children.

Some functions of the nervous system are much more than a simple response to the external environment or the satisfaction of basic drives. The human cerebral cortex has higher functions that are of an executive (overriding) nature, or allow very sophisticated processing of sensory information. These functions include planning, language, appreciation of music, working memory, long-term memory, and complex spatial perception. The ability to plan for years ahead, communicate complex ideas to other people, and conceive the shape and design of a new tool are all features that are highly advanced in our species, and which we regard as defining features of humankind. Our society depends on our ability to negotiate and cooperate with other people, an ability that largely resides in the prefrontal cortex.

The cerebral cortex is vitally dependent on nerve cell groups in the midbrain that maintain consciousness. Furthermore, most functions of the cerebral cortex involve not just the streaming of information between parts of the cortex, but also complex looped pathways involving structures deep inside the forebrain, as well as pathways that run down to the brainstem and cerebellum and back up to the cerebral cortex.

↓ **The brain weighs around 3 pounds (1.4 kg) and in its fresh state is extremely soft, making it vulnerable to injury from violent impacts to the head.**

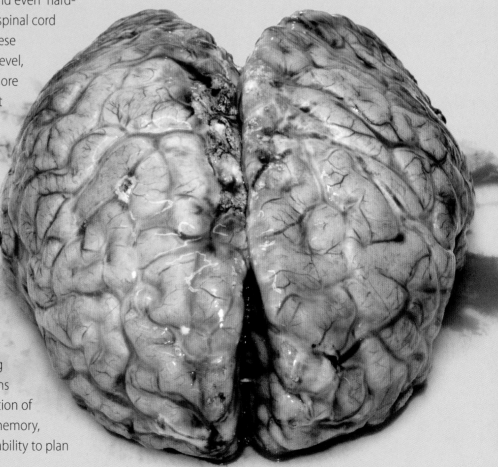

Nervous system

The nervous system processes information about the environment and the body's interior, and initiates movement of the limbs or changes in the body.

The nervous system consists of a central nervous system (CNS) and a peripheral nervous system (PNS). The brain and spinal cord together make up the CNS. Outside these areas is the PNS, which mainly contains sensory receptors and nerve fibers but also has some collections of nerve cell bodies in clusters called ganglia.

Peripheral nervous system

The PNS carries impulses to and from the brain and spinal cord. It links the CNS to sensory receptors in the skin, joints, muscles, and internal organs (the sensory division) and to those body organs (glands and voluntary and involuntary muscles) that can produce changes in the internal and external environment (the motor division).

The PNS can be further subdivided into a part concerned with the control of voluntary functions (the somatic nervous system) or the control of automatic functions (the autonomic nervous system), but in some cases the boundary between these two is blurred. For example, breathing is something we usually do without thought, but it can also be controlled deliberately.

Some PNS ganglia have a sensory function and are located alongside the spinal cord or near the brainstem. Other ganglia are part of the autonomic nervous system and may be found in the internal body cavities.

→ **The nervous system comprises all nerve tissue in the body, including that of the brain and spinal cord, as well as the peripheral nerves.**

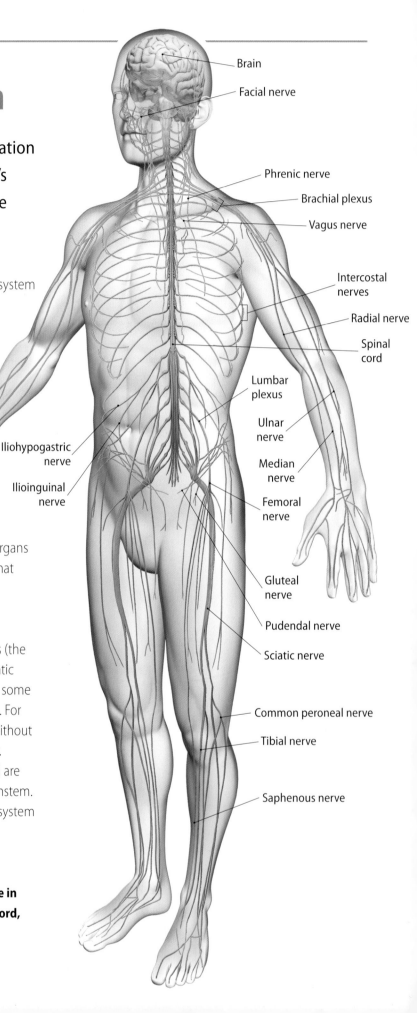

- Brain
- Facial nerve
- Phrenic nerve
- Brachial plexus
- Vagus nerve
- Intercostal nerves
- Radial nerve
- Spinal cord
- Lumbar plexus
- Ulnar nerve
- Median nerve
- Femoral nerve
- Gluteal nerve
- Pudendal nerve
- Sciatic nerve
- Common peroneal nerve
- Tibial nerve
- Saphenous nerve
- Iliohypogastric nerve
- Ilioinguinal nerve

Components of the central nervous system

The convention is to describe the brain as being that part of the CNS within the skull and to say that the spinal cord starts at the skull base. This is a convenient anatomical division, but it ignores the fact that some columns of nerve cells concerned with particular functions (e.g., the sense of touch from the head and neck) have an almost seamless continuity across this border. Certainly, the spinal cord is the part of the CNS that receives sensory information from the trunk and limbs and controls the muscles and glands of those regions. A bony framework (the vertebral column) protects the spinal cord, but the demands of flexibility of the trunk mean that this protection is not a complete shell like the protection for the brain. So the spinal cord is quite vulnerable to crushing or shifting of the bones of the vertebral column.

The cerebral cortex

The largest part of the brain, the forebrain, is capped by the cerebral cortex, a crinkled sheet of nerve cells and their processes that takes up about half the volume of the brain. Although the surface of one person's brain may differ slightly from another, there are consistent grooves on the surface of the cortex that mark out functional areas that are similar in all people.

The cerebral cortex is commonly called gray matter, because of its color, which is due to the numerous nerve cell bodies there. Beneath the cerebral cortex are large areas of white matter where axons—the fibers of nerve cells (neurons)—run between different parts of the cerebral cortex and between the cortex and deeper brain structures. These axons and their fatty myelin coat dominate—the myelin coating of nerve fibers increases the speed and reliability of nerve impulse conduction—giving these areas a whitish color.

→ **Most nerve cells, such as those making up this peripheral nerve, have axons (blue) surrounded by myelin coats (gold). The thicker the myelin coat, the faster the speed of nerve impulse transmission.**

How special is the human brain?

We like to think that the human brain is special. Although it has some special functional features (e.g., a facility for language, and long-term planning), the human brain is rather similar in internal structure not only to other primates' brains, but also to those of most other mammals. In terms of *absolute* size, our brain is not particularly large: the brains of whales, dolphins, and elephants are much larger. On the other hand, in terms of *relative* size (i.e., relative to what you would expect for a primate of our body weight), the human brain is about three and a half times larger than would be expected. This enlarged brain is achieved by a prolonged period of brain growth extending from late prenatal life into the first few years after birth. A large brain may have its advantages, but it also comes at a price: the big human brain consumes about one quarter of all the nutrients that the body takes in. It also requires a substantial nutritional investment to build during fetal life and early childhood.

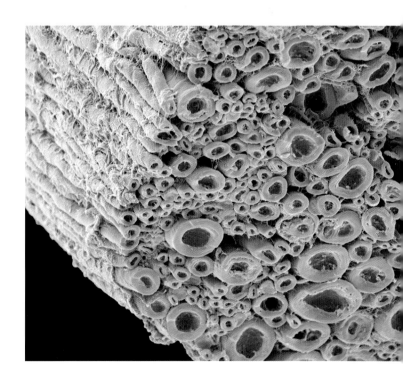

Deep structures of the forebrain

If you were to slice the human brain open, you would see that the surface of the cerebral cortex is gray in color, but that other areas of gray matter are located deeper inside the brain. These are the basal ganglia, which play key roles not just in the control of movement, but also in decisions and emotions. Other regions of gray matter inside the brain include the diencephalon, which includes a pair of large egg-shaped structures called the thalamus that relay information from lower parts of the brain and areas within the cortex. Below the thalamus is the hypothalamus, a region concerned with satisfying animal needs, such as eating and mating, and the control of the body's internal environment. The diencephalon and basal ganglia are arranged around a set of three fluid-filled spaces (two lateral ventricles and a midline third ventricle), which are part of the ventricular system of the brain.

CNS versus PNS

The two main divisions of the nervous system have important cellular differences, which are reflected in their response to injury. The nerve cells of the central nervous system have only a poor ability to repair themselves, and an injury to the CNS, such as a traumatic brain injury suffered in an automobile crash, typically results in permanent loss of function. By contrast, the peripheral nervous system has the ability to regrow nerve fibers after injury. For example, a severed nerve in a finger can heal, and normal function may return over time.

→ **The brain has gray matter areas on the outside (cerebral cortex) as well as deep inside (caudate nucleus, putamen, globus pallidus, thalamus). The corpus callosum connects the two sides of the brain.**

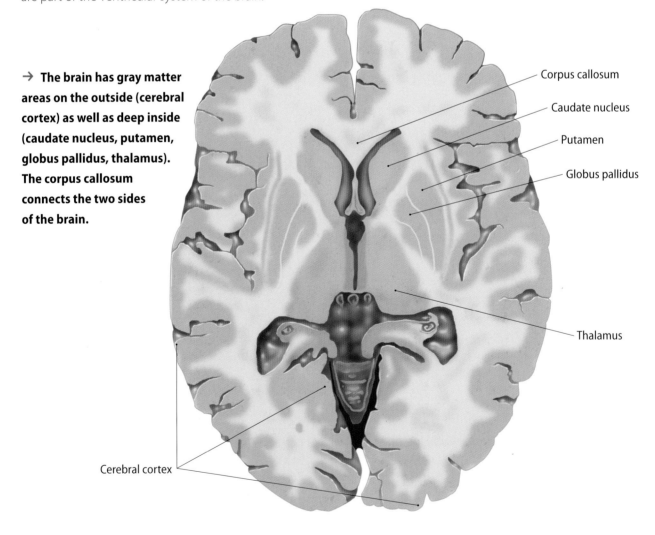

Corpus callosum

Caudate nucleus

Putamen

Globus pallidus

Thalamus

Cerebral cortex

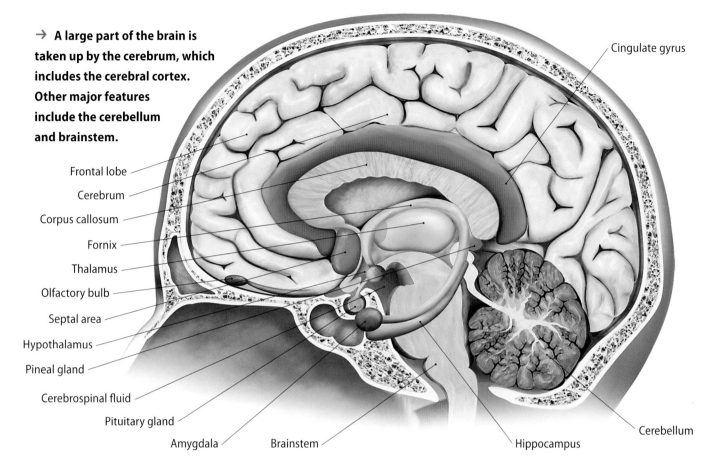

→ **A large part of the brain is taken up by the cerebrum, which includes the cerebral cortex. Other major features include the cerebellum and brainstem.**

Cingulate gyrus

Frontal lobe

Cerebrum

Corpus callosum

Fornix

Thalamus

Olfactory bulb

Septal area

Hypothalamus

Pineal gland

Cerebrospinal fluid

Pituitary gland

Amygdala

Brainstem

Hippocampus

Cerebellum

The brainstem and cerebellum

The part of the brain between the diencephalon and the spinal cord is called the brainstem, which has changed very little during evolution. In fact, the human brainstem is identical in structure to any other mammal's. It accommodates a collection of nerve pathways for information coming from the spinal cord to reach the higher parts of the brain, and for the higher parts of the brain to control the brainstem and spinal cord. It also houses groups of nerve cells concerned with controlling automatic functions such as heart rate, breathing, and blood pressure.

Attached to the brainstem is the final part of the brain, the cerebellum, a structure with a highly folded surface like the cerebral cortex. The cerebellum is connected to the brainstem by large bundles of fibers that carry information into and out of its interior. The main functions of the cerebellum are coordinating movement and planning motor activity.

→ **The cerebellum's folds give a large surface area, allowing high information-processing power. This part of the brain uses information about balance, muscle tension, and joint position to coordinate movement.**

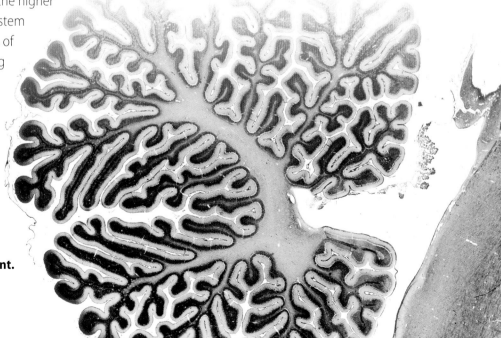

The cerebral cortex

The cerebral cortex is only about a fifth of an inch (a few millimeters) thick, yet it contains one third of all the nerve cells in the human brain. This is the site where the highest level of neural processing takes place, including language, memory, and cognitive function.

The cerebral cortex is the outer surface of the forebrain (the word "cortex" simply means outer layer). It can be broadly divided into frontal, parietal, temporal, and occipital lobes—each lobe corresponding to a bone of the skull that it lies beneath. A deep groove called the lateral fissure separates the frontal and temporal lobes. Open this groove and you can see an additional part of the cortex, the insula, deep inside.

Layers, columns, and nerve cells

About 90 percent of the cerebral cortex is known as isocortex. This has six horizontal layers either in adult life or at some stage during its development, but the layered structure may be modified to serve special functions in different parts of the cerebral cortex. Other parts of the cortex, such as the hippocampus or olfactory cortex, have fewer layers.

The cortex is also organized vertically: nerve cells are stacked on top of each other into columns. Analysis of the functional organization of the cortex suggests that the basic functional unit of the cortex is a minicolumn about 0.002 inches (0.05 mm) wide and containing around a hundred nerve cells. These minicolumns may be linked together to form larger functional columns up to 0.02 inches (0.5 mm) wide. The nerve cells in one of these columns are concerned with processing information of a similar nature. For example, nerve cells in a column of visual cortex will respond to bars or edges with the same orientation in the visual world. Given this columnar organization, one approach to increasing the processing power of the cerebral cortex would be to pack in as many cortical columns as possible. The columns must sit

Frontal lobe

Gyri

Sulci

Lateral fissure

Parietal lobe

Central sulcus

Occipital lobe

Temporal lobe

← **The surface of the brain is highly folded to form gyri (ridges) separated by sulci (grooves). The cerebral cortex is divided into four sections called lobes. The frontal and parietal lobes are separated by the central sulcus.**

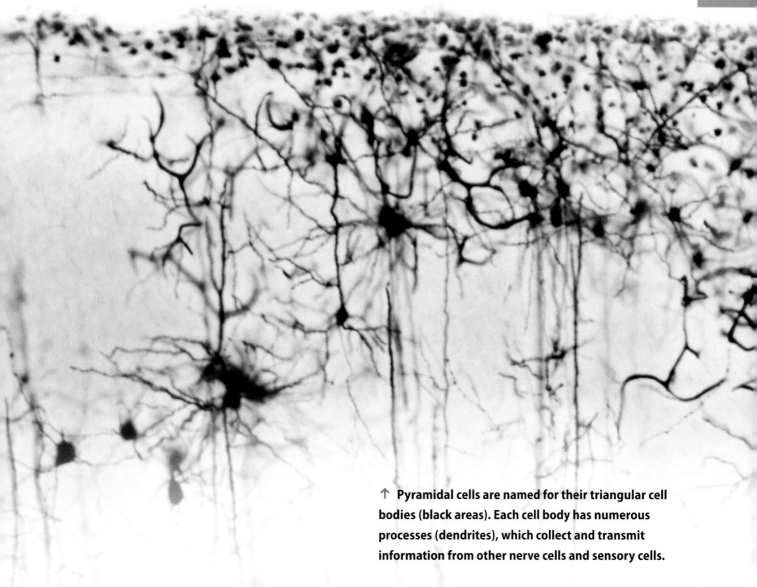

↑ **Pyramidal cells are named for their triangular cell bodies (black areas). Each cell body has numerous processes (dendrites), which collect and transmit information from other nerve cells and sensory cells.**

side by side, so increasing the number of columns will increase the surface area of the cortex. Accommodating this increased surface area inside the skull requires folding of the cortex into the bumps and grooves that we see on the surface of the human brain.

An estimated 30 billion nerve cells make up the cerebral cortex. The commonest type is the pyramidal nerve cell, which gets its name because of its pyramid-shaped cell body. Pyramidal nerve cells have large branching dendritic trees to receive a rich input of contacts from other nerve cells. Pyramidal cells also have axons that provide the output from the cortical columns. Other nerve cell types in the cortex include the star-shaped stellate cells that receive much of the incoming information to each region of cortex. Sensory areas of the cortex are particularly rich in stellate cells.

Damage to the cortex

Damage to the right parietal lobe causes a sensory neglect syndrome, in which the patient may ignore the left side of the body and objects in the left half of their environment. Damage to the parietal/temporal/occipital association cortex may result in agnosia: an inability to recognize everyday objects by a given sense such as touch, even though the basic sense of touch is intact. Damage to the left parietal lobe may cause apraxia: an inability to perform a complex action, even though the muscles required are normal and able to perform movement.

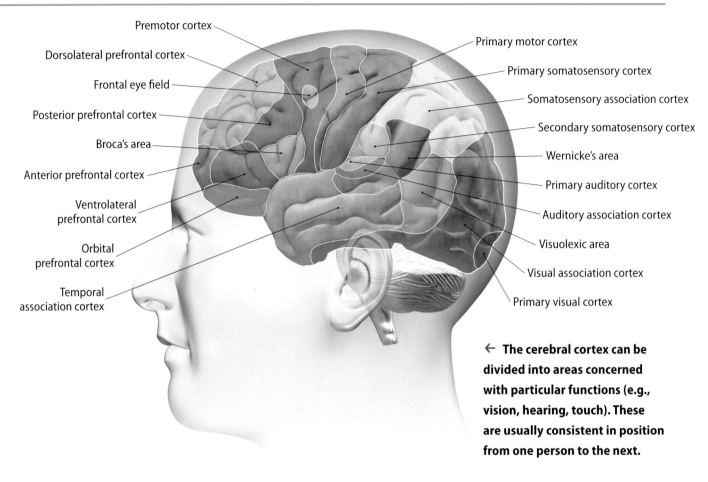

Premotor cortex

Dorsolateral prefrontal cortex

Frontal eye field

Posterior prefrontal cortex

Broca's area

Anterior prefrontal cortex

Ventrolateral prefrontal cortex

Orbital prefrontal cortex

Temporal association cortex

Primary motor cortex

Primary somatosensory cortex

Somatosensory association cortex

Secondary somatosensory cortex

Wernicke's area

Primary auditory cortex

Auditory association cortex

Visuolexic area

Visual association cortex

Primary visual cortex

← **The cerebral cortex can be divided into areas concerned with particular functions (e.g., vision, hearing, touch). These are usually consistent in position from one person to the next.**

Functional layout

Different parts of the cerebral cortex serve different functions. Beginning in the 19th century, studies of patients with brain injury to distinct parts of the brain have led to a good understanding of functional localization within the cortex. These lesion studies have been supplemented and extended by functional MRI and PET scanning that allows neuroscientists to detect increased activity in cortical regions while a living subject is performing different tasks.

We know of specific functional areas concerned with motor control (primary motor cortex and premotor cortex), perception of touch (primary somatosensory cortex), sound (primary auditory cortex), smell (primary olfactory cortex), and sight (primary visual cortex). Other areas include the vestibular area (concerned with the sense of balance), which is located in the parietal lobe, and the taste (gustatory) area, in the primary somatosensory cortex. Neuroscientists have also identified language areas, mainly in the left hemisphere.

Comparing mammal brains

The cerebral cortex has undergone enormous enlargement in the course of evolution. Mammals with particularly large and folded cerebral cortices include the primates and cetaceans (whales and dolphins). Humans have greatly expanded cerebral cortices, which are at least three times larger than those of our nearest relatives, the chimpanzees. A particularly important development in mammal brain evolution is the increasing proportion of the cerebral cortex devoted to higher functions (i.e., not simple sensory or motor function), such as planning and complex spatial perception.

OTHER

AUDITION
Temporal lobe

MEMORY
Medial temporal lobe,
posterior cingulate cortex

BODY SENSATION
Parietal lobe

EMOTION
Anterior cingulate
and orbital cortex

MOTOR AND PLANNING
Frontal lobe

GUSTATION
Insula

OLFACTION
Medial temporal
cortex

VISION
Occipital cortex and
temporal cortex

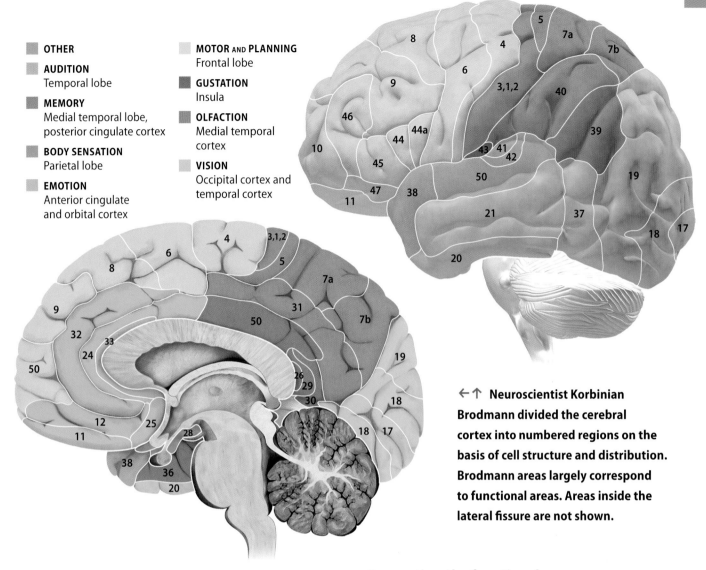

← ↑ **Neuroscientist Korbinian Brodmann divided the cerebral cortex into numbered regions on the basis of cell structure and distribution. Brodmann areas largely correspond to functional areas. Areas inside the lateral fissure are not shown.**

Connecting the functional areas

Information must be constantly transferred between the areas of the cerebral cortex and from one side of the brain to the other. The large mass of white matter beneath the gray matter of the cortex is like a richly interconnected array of data cables joining the cortical regions. Some of these axon cables run only about an inch (a few centimeters), others run the entire length of each half of the brain. A particularly important bundle is the arcuate fasciculus, which interconnects the language areas of the cerebral cortex. Damage to it causes a language problem where patients are unable to monitor the accuracy of their own speech.

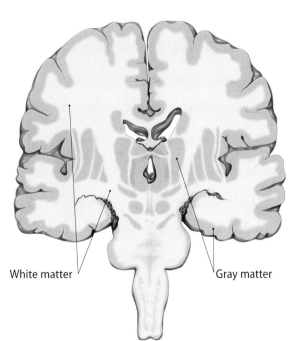

White matter

Gray matter

← **The cerebral cortex is a thin layer of gray matter over an expanse of largely white matter.**

Each hemisphere receives sensory information from the opposite half of the visual world and body. So, for example, the left visual cortex receives information from the right visual field. The two sides of the brain are in constant communication through the 250- to 300-million axon bundle called the corpus callosum, which allows the two halves of the brain to share this information and for each brain half to be aware of both sides of the body. Cutting the corpus callosum as a therapeutic measure (as used in the early to mid-20th century to control serious epilepsy) results in two independent hemispheres in the one skull.

The sensory and motor cortices

One way that the cerebral cortex deals with the vast amount of information streaming to it every second is to distribute the information in "maps" across the brain surface. The nature of these maps reflects the quality of the information that is most behaviorally important.

The primary motor and somatosensory cortices are organized somatotopically: different body parts are mapped onto the cortex in distinct but contiguous regions. The primary visual cortex, by contrast, is organized visuotopically. In other words, different parts of the visual world are mapped onto different parts of the visual cortex, although the areas concerned with central vision have by far the largest proportional area. Sound is represented rather differently. The primary auditory (hearing) cortex is located in the temporal lobe and is organized by the frequency (pitch) of sound.

The frontal cortex

The frontal lobe contains a group of areas that control movement (motor control) and appear to be organized in a hierarchy. The primary motor cortex has the most direct control on individual muscles on the opposite side of the body. It is influenced by the premotor cortex, located above and in front of the primary motor cortex, which plans motor movements involving large groups of muscles. A supplementary motor cortex is located near the midline in front of the primary motor area and is concerned with postures involving muscles on both sides of the body.

The somatosensory cortex

Neuroscientists often illustrate the relative size of the body part representations on the somatosensory (touch) cortex by maps called homunculi (from the Latin for "little man"). The primary somatosensory cortex has a large area devoted to representation of the face, and in particular the lips. This reflects the immense behavioral importance of the face in non-verbal communication. The rich sensory supply from the face allows us to precisely control our facial expressions to convey emotions.

The primary somatosensory cortex also has a large area devoted to the hands, in particular the fingertips and the thumb, reflecting the need for fine-scale sensory feedback from the skin and joints of the hands when controlling the digits during skilled movements.

The cerebral cortex by numbers

If the human cortex were unfolded it would have an area of about 2 square feet (0.18 sq m), but a thickness of about 0.2 inches (a few millimeters), and yet it contains about 30 billion nerve cells, about one in three of all the nerve cells in the human brain. These nerve cells are interconnected by over 60,000 miles (100,000 km) of axons and dendrites, with each nerve cell having as many as tens of thousands of contacts from other nerve cells. Neuroscientists estimate that there are as many as 100 trillion synaptic contacts between nerve cells in the cerebral cortex.

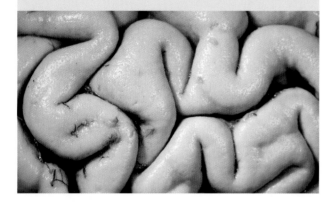

MOTOR ACTIVITY

SENSORY ACTIVITY

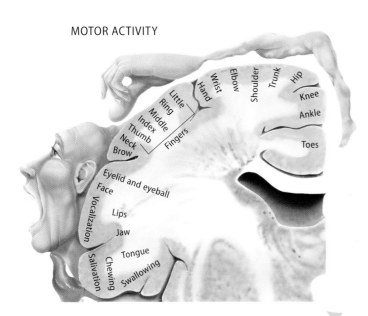

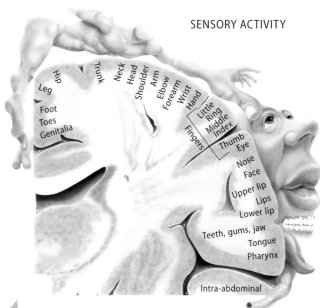

↑ **The size of the body part in this motor homunculus reflects the proportion of the precentral gyrus (location of the primary motor cortex) involved in motor activity in that specific area of the body.**

↑ **The size of the body part in this sensory homunculus reflects the proportion of the post-central gyrus (location of the somato-sensory cortex) involved in sensory activity in that specific area of the body.**

The visual and olfactory cortices

The primary visual cortex, in the occipital lobe, is concerned with initial analysis of visual information. Immediately surrounding the primary visual cortex are regions concerned with processing information about color and visual texture. From here, visual information is channeled either toward the posterior parietal lobe (dorsal stream) for analysis of the location of visual features in space, or down into the inferior temporal lobe (ventral stream) for the recognition of the visual form and texture of objects (including facial features).

The sense of smell is not strong in humans, but the human brain does contain areas in the cortex concerned with processing odor information. The sense of smell (primary olfactory area) is located in the inferior temporal lobe very close to parts of the limbic or emotional system (the amygdala and hippocampus), allowing smell to influence the emotional tagging of memories. This explains why a particular odor can sometimes transport us back to childhood.

The association cortex

Large areas of the cortex have neither sensory nor motor functions. These are the association areas, and they play important roles in the most complex analysis of sensory information and planning of behavior.

The prefrontal cortex is a type of association cortex that is particularly large in humans. It is concerned with social function, planning, and forethought. People with prefrontal cortex lesions tend to be tactless, impulsive, and unconcerned about the future or the consequences of their actions.

The parietal cortex lies between the somatosensory, auditory, and visual cortices. This region contains an association area that brings information from those key senses together to create a model in our mind of the world around us. Another association area, the parietal/temporal/occipital (PTO) association cortex, concerns itself with spatial orientation and perception, mainly of the opposite side of the body and world, but the right side seems to be most important in humans.

Imaging the brain

Modern neuroscience has an astonishing array of techniques for probing the living brain. These rely on a combination of advanced principles in physics and rapid computerized analysis of vast quantities of data.

Imaging is vital to diagnose illness, monitor treatment, and advance medical science. Since the discovery of X-rays in 1895, increasingly sophisticated imaging techniques have been developed to give ever more precise insights into the nervous system.

Computerized tomography (CT)

This imaging technique produces pictures of brain tissue based on differences in the absorption of X-rays between different types of tissue. A computer analyzes the X-rays to create "slices" of the scanned body part. CT scanning is good at detecting bone, areas of hemorrhage, and the shape of the ventricles. CT scan data can also be used to generate three-dimensional images that can be rotated in virtual space. Blood vessels can also be accentuated by injecting an X-ray-opaque contrast chemical into the circulation. Unfortunately, CT scanning is not so good at detecting fine details of internal brain structure, because differences in the X-ray absorption of different brain tissue (e.g., gray versus white matter) are subtle.

Magnetic resonance imaging (MRI)

MRI uses magnetic fields to induce resonance in atoms within the brain tissue. Atomic nuclei with an odd number of protons (e.g., hydrogen in water) behave like tiny magnets. Applying a magnetic field to the head causes the hydrogen nuclei to align with the field. Once this has happened, the nuclei preferentially absorb and emit electromagnetic energy at a particular frequency. Computer analysis of MRI produces images of the brain that reflect the water content of the tissue, allowing the clinician to see clear differences between "watery" gray matter and "fatty" white matter. The technique also allows mapping of changes in blood flow during brain activity (functional MRI, or fMRI).

↓ **A patient enters a CT scanner. An image is generated by computer analysis of many passes of X-rays through the head. Information about X-ray absorption is turned into pictures of head "slices."**

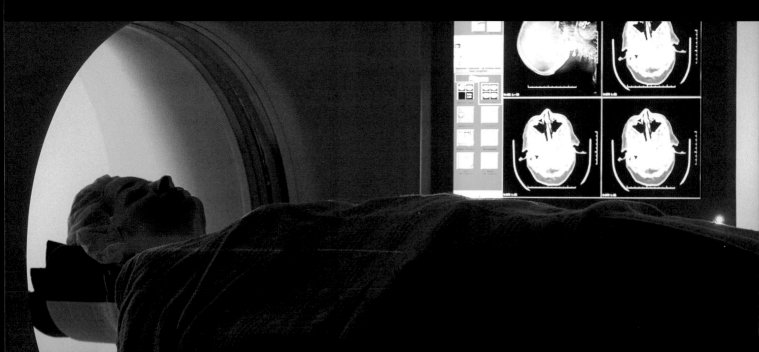

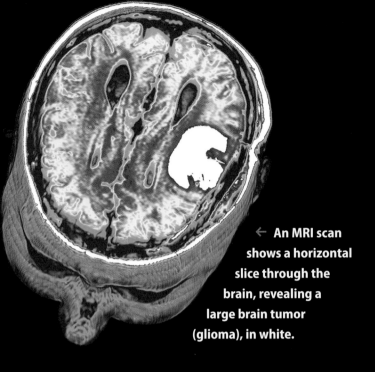

← **An MRI scan shows a horizontal slice through the brain, revealing a large brain tumor (glioma), in white.**

How safe are brain scans?

Having one or two CT scans is very safe, although having regular CT scans represents a significant radiation exposure. PET scans also involve some exposure to radiation, but this does not exceed safe levels if the patient has only an occasional scan. Although safe for most people, MRI scans involve the use of very strong magnetic fields, which pose a major hazard for some people: any surgical steel in the patient's body will experience strong forces when the magnetic fields are activated, with potentially disastrous effects.

Positron emission tomography (PET)

This technique relies on mapping the emission of subatomic particles called positrons (the antimatter equivalent of electrons). The patient receives an injection of a type of glucose (deoxyglucose), which has been labeled with radioactive fluorine that releases positrons. Glucose is incorporated into the brain's metabolic pathways, so the most active brain regions take up more and are highlighted by strong positron emission. Alternatively, a positron-emitting isotope of oxygen can be incorporated into water to follow changes in blood flow. These techniques are very expensive but, when combined with MRI for anatomical resolution, provide extraordinary images showing the functional activity of the brain while the patient performs different tasks.

Endoscopy of cerebrospinal fluid pathways

The CSF-filled spaces inside and around the brain provide neurosurgeons with pathways for reaching deep-seated abnormalities. Flexible endoscopes can be carefully threaded through the complex shape of the CSF pathways to see the internal or external surfaces of the brain in astonishing clarity. If the ends of these are equipped with fine tools, surgery can be performed to remove tumors and repair abnormal blood vessels.

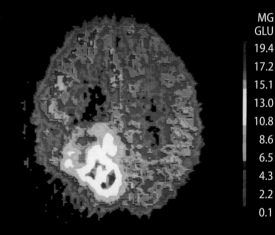

MG GLU

| 19.4 |
| 17.2 |
| 15.1 |
| 13.0 |
| 10.8 |
| 8.6 |
| 6.5 |
| 4.3 |
| 2.2 |
| 0.1 |

↑ **A PET scan detects differing levels of uptake of radioactive glucose (MG GLU), in this case highlighting a brain tumor (yellow and red regions).**

Electroencephalography (EEG)

In this technique, electrodes fitted to the scalp detect regional changes in brain electrical activity. Its advantage is that it can follow changes in electrical activity with a time resolution measured in thousandths of a second. Its disadvantage is that it has very poor anatomical resolution. A type of EEG is used to detect changes in the speed of conduction along visual pathways (visual evoked response) as may occur in multiple sclerosis. It is also useful in diagnosing epilepsy.

Left and right hemispheres

Many brain functions are shared more or less equally between the two cerebral hemispheres. Two vital functions, however, are located in one hemisphere rather than the other.

Some parts of the cerebral cortex are the same on each side; both hemispheres have areas that control motor function and process sensory information from the opposite side of the body. In contrast to these functions, language and spatial perception are located exclusively or preferentially in one hemisphere.

Language: Broca's and Wernicke's areas

Many insights into brain function have come from studies of people with damage to the brain. During the late 19th century, careful analysis of the brains of people who had suffered localized brain damage allowed neurologists such as Paul Broca and Karl

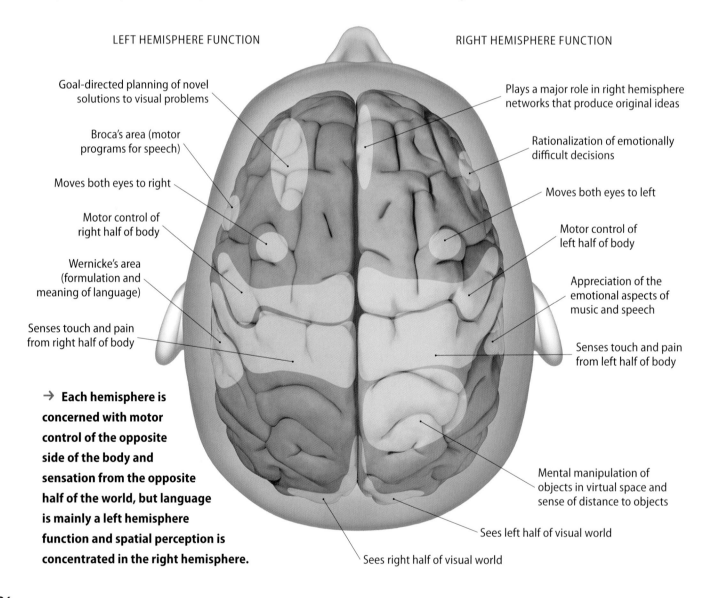

LEFT HEMISPHERE FUNCTION

Goal-directed planning of novel solutions to visual problems

Broca's area (motor programs for speech)

Moves both eyes to right

Motor control of right half of body

Wernicke's area (formulation and meaning of language)

Senses touch and pain from right half of body

RIGHT HEMISPHERE FUNCTION

Plays a major role in right hemisphere networks that produce original ideas

Rationalization of emotionally difficult decisions

Moves both eyes to left

Motor control of left half of body

Appreciation of the emotional aspects of music and speech

Senses touch and pain from left half of body

Mental manipulation of objects in virtual space and sense of distance to objects

Sees left half of visual world

Sees right half of visual world

→ **Each hemisphere is concerned with motor control of the opposite side of the body and sensation from the opposite half of the world, but language is mainly a left hemisphere function and spatial perception is concentrated in the right hemisphere.**

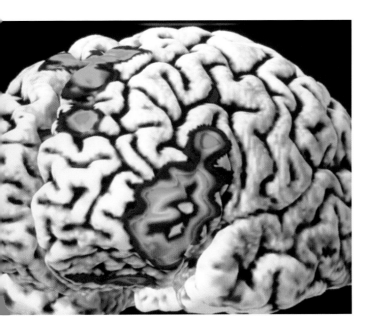

↑ **Areas involved in speech are highlighted in this MRI scan of brain activity made while a person was speaking. The front of the brain is at left.**

Wernicke to determine that there are specialized regions of the brain concerned with language. In both right- and left-handed people these areas are usually located in the left cerebral hemisphere, but about 15 percent of left-handed people have their language areas in the right hemisphere. The hemisphere that is more important for production and comprehension of language is called the dominant hemisphere.

Broca's area is in the frontal lobe near the face area of the primary motor cortex. Damage to Broca's area causes a type of language disorder (Broca's aphasia) where the patient has great difficulty producing words, either written or spoken, and will often use emphatic stock phrases (e.g., "Oh boy!", "You bet!", "Forget it!") in response to questions. If they can speak at all, they will tend to leave out all but the most meaningful words in the sentence. On the other hand, Broca's aphasic patients are able to comprehend language quite well.

Wernicke's area is located on the upper surface of the temporal lobe and extending back into the lower parietal lobe. Patients with damage to Wernicke's area (Wernicke's aphasia) will be able to produce written and spoken words, but the information content of their language is poor. They will often substitute one word for another, insert new and meaningless words, and string together words and phrases in a way that conveys no meaning. This suggests that patients with Wernicke's aphasia are poor at formulating language and unable to understand their own speech to correct themselves.

A fiber bundle, the arcuate fasciculus, joins the areas, allowing continuous feedback from Wernicke's to Broca's areas so an individual can monitor their own speech. Damage to this bundle is called conduction aphasia: the patient can understand language but is unable to repeat phrases and speaks fluently, but with poor meaning.

Spatial perception: the right parietal lobe

The posterior parietal cortex is an important brain area when it comes to thinking about tasks that involve the manipulation of objects in space—e.g., when we think about the design of a solid object, such as furniture, a tool, or pottery, and how it would appear from different angles. The area is also important for our sense of distance to objects. These functions seem to be better developed in the right hemisphere than the left. Damage to the right parietal lobe causes a neglect syndrome, where the patient will ignore the left side both of their own body and objects around them.

Adding emotion: the right hemisphere's role in speech

Not all aspects of language are concentrated in the left hemisphere. Evidence suggests that the right cerebral hemisphere controls the emotional content of spoken language, as conveyed by the rhythm and musical aspects of speech. This aspect of language is known as prosody and is almost as important as word choice and syntax in conveying meaning. For example, you can say the words "I'm finished" in a variety of ways that could convey jubilation, resignation, anger, or a simple statement of fact.

Basal ganglia

Deep within the brain are interconnected collections of nerve cells called the basal ganglia. While most parts are concerned with the control of movement, some units of the basal ganglia may also be involved in language, thought, emotion, or motivation.

The basal ganglia are a group of nerve cell clusters (nuclei) in the forebrain and midbrain. The largest components are found inside the cerebral hemispheres: the putamen, caudate nucleus, nucleus accumbens, and globus pallidus. Two other basal ganglia nuclei are outside the cerebral hemispheres: the subthalamic nucleus in the diencephalon, and the substantia nigra

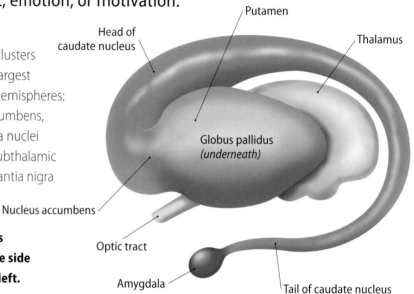

→ **The basal ganglia and nearby structures (thalamus and optic tract) are seen from the side in this view. The front of the brain is to the left.**

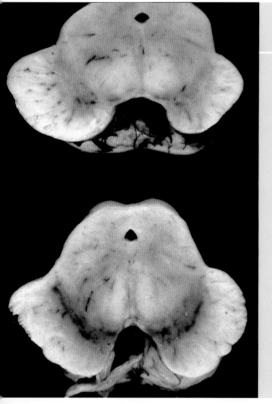

Movement disorders and the basal ganglia

Two types of movement disorders follow damage to the basal ganglia and their connections: those that increase involuntary movement (hyperkinetic disorders) and those that decrease all movement (hypokinetic disorders).

Hyperkinetic disorders may involve slow, writhing, sinuous, and aimless movements (known as athetosis) due to damage to the striatum; or brisk, purposeless, dancelike movements (chorea) usually due to damage to the caudate nucleus. Damage to the subthalamic nucleus causes violent flailing movements on the opposite side of the body (hemiballismus).

Parkinson's disease is a good example to illustrate the hypokinetic disorders. Degeneration of the dopamine-using nerve cells of the substantia nigra in this disorder causes an impassive, masklike face; rigid limbs; a slow, shuffling gait; problems starting movements; and a tremor at rest.

← **A section through a normal midbrain (bottom) shows the blue-black dopamine-secreting cells of the substantia nigra. These cells have been lost from the midbrain of a person with Parkinson's disease (top).**

→ **The main basal ganglia circuit (red lines) starts from the cerebral cortex and passes through the striatum, globus pallidus, and thalamus before returning to the cerebral cortex. Other circuits (blue and green lines) provide input from structures outside this loop, such as the subthalamic nucleus and substantia nigra.**

Motor part of cerebral cortex

Caudate (part of striatum)

Motor thalamic nuclei of thalamus

Globus pallidus

Claustrum

Putamen (part of striatum)

Subthalamic nucleus

Substantia nigra

in the midbrain. All of these groups of nerve cells are linked together in circuits concerned with ensuring that movements are smoothly performed. Together, the caudate, putamen, and nucleus accumbens are called the striatum.

What the basal ganglia do

The basal ganglia are crucial to performing smooth, controlled movements. Damage results in characteristic movement disorders, involving either decreased or increased motor activity (see "Movement disorders and the basal ganglia," opposite).

The basal ganglia are also thought to play a key role in language, thought, emotional behavior, and motivation. One suggestion is that the basal ganglia selects and reinforces appropriate actions or behaviors, while extinguishing or inhibiting unwanted or inappropriate actions or behaviors.

The circuitry of the basal ganglia

The basal ganglia are involved in a number of circuits. The most obvious one begins with a pathway from the cerebral cortex to the striatum and subthalamic nucleus. Nerve cells in the striatum in turn project to the globus pallidus or substantia nigra. The globus pallidus projects to parts of the thalamus concerned with motor activity, which in turn project to the cerebral cortex.

This simple description belies the complexity of the pathways: within this pathway there are at least three circuits running in parallel. For example, the part of the

cerebral cortex that controls movements projects to the putamen, the part of the striatum that is also involved in movements; whereas association parts of the cortex concerned with thought project to the caudate; and areas of the cortex concerned with emotions and motivated behavior project to the nucleus accumbens. Each of these three zones of the striatum feeds back to the corresponding parts of the cerebral cortex: the putamen feeds back to motor areas of the cortex, the caudate to the prefrontal cortex (for thought and planning), and the nucleus accumbens to the limbic areas (for emotions). These observations suggest that the basal ganglia circuits can be divided into motor, thought, and emotional loops.

The subthalamic nucleus and substantia nigra play key roles in regulating activity in the basal ganglia circuits. The subthalamic nucleus, which receives axons from nerve cells in the cortex and sends axons to the globus pallidus, is divided into different regions dealing with motor, thought, and emotional functions. The substantia nigra receives input from the putamen and globus pallidus and sends axons back to the striatum. An important part of the substantia nigra does this by a pathway that uses the neurotransmitter dopamine.

Gateway to the cortex

The diencephalon is a group of structures in the core of the brain. Its main components, the thalamus and hypothalamus, are involved in many vital sensory, endocrine, cognitive, and motor functions.

The diencephalon comprises four parts: the thalamus, hypothalamus, subthalamus, and epithalamus (including the pineal gland). These four are involved in a range of functions, including processing sensory information (the thalamus), controlling automatic functions and the neuroendocrine system (the hypothalamus and epithalamus), and motor circuits (the subthalamus).

The thalamus

The largest structure in the diencephalon is the thalamus, an egg-shaped region on each side of the third ventricle. Sometimes called the gateway to the cerebral cortex, it primarily acts as a relay station, receiving information from many senses (all except

smell), processing the information, and passing the resulting data up to the cerebral cortex. It is also a key element in many of the looped circuits running between the cortex and deeper parts of the brain that are concerned with motor function, in particular those involving the cerebellum and the basal ganglia. These function as feedback loops, allowing the cerebral cortex to request and retrieve motor programs (instructions on how to activate muscles for particular movements) from the basal ganglia and cerebellum. Neuroscientists divide the thalamus according to the different types of information that different regions receive.

The thalamus: a relay system

The thalamus is made up of several nerve cell clusters (nuclei). Some of these, called relay thalamic nuclei, get very specific types of information that they then pass on to a specific part of the cerebral cortex. Their role is to deliver information from particular functional systems to the cerebral cortex. Some of this information may be about the senses, some may be about movement, and some is concerned with emotions (limbic relay).

Sensory relay nuclei include the ventral posterior nucleus of the thalamus that receives information about touch, precisely localized pain, and joint position (proprioception) in the head and body. This type of sensory information is called somatosensory, because it is about the body (*soma*) rather than the external environment. The ventral posterior nucleus then passes this information (with processing) on to the part of the cerebral cortex that is concerned with these senses. Similarly, visual information from the retina in the eye is received by the lateral geniculate nucleus, processed, and passed to the primary visual cortex.

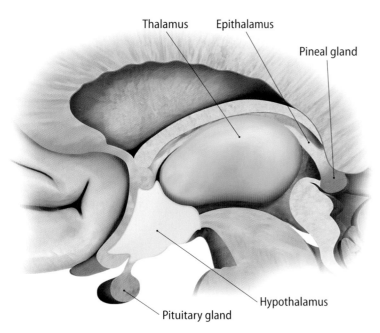

Thalamus   Epithalamus

Pineal gland

Hypothalamus

Pituitary gland

↑ **The main components of the diencephalon are the thalamus and hypothalamus. Another part, the epithalamus, includes the pineal gland.**

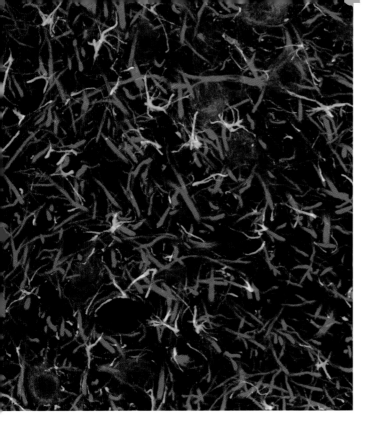

↑ These nerve cells and their processes are in the thalamus. Many nerve cells in the thalamus convey information to the cerebral cortex.

Motor relay nuclei are the ventral anterior and ventral lateral thalamic nuclei that relay motor information from the basal ganglia or cerebellum to the motor parts of the cerebral cortex. These nuclei are key parts of the loops that allow us to perform smooth movements.

The anterior thalamic nucleus is the main relay nucleus for the limbic system, a set of brain structures involved in the expression of emotion (see pp. 34–5). The lateral dorsal thalamic nucleus may also serve a similar function because it projects to part of the limbic cortex known as the cingulate gyrus.

Some nuclei in the thalamus receive input from the cerebral cortex and project back to the cerebral cortex. The parts of the cerebral cortex involved here are not those concerned with particular senses, but are the regions involved in planning and forethought (the prefrontal cortex) or the formation of a sensory model of the world around us (the PTO association cortex). The association thalamic nuclei may control the movement of information between areas in the cortex.

Thalamic nuclei

Nuclei are clusters of nerve cells with specialist functions. The thalamus has three main types of nuclei: relay, association, and midline and intralaminar. This table shows the different thalamic nuclei, their sources of input, and the structures to which they pass information.

Type of nucleus	Name	Source of incoming information	Outgoing destination
Relay	Anterior	Hippocampus	Limbic cortex
	Lateral dorsal	Hippocampus	Limbic cortex
	Lateral geniculate	Visual	Visual cortex
	Medial geniculate	Auditory	Auditory cortex
	Ventral posterior	Touch, pain, and proprioception	Somatosensory cortex
	Ventral anterior	Basal ganglia and cerebellum	Motor cortex
	Ventral lateral		
Association	Dorsomedial	Prefrontal cortex	Prefrontal cortex
	Lateral posterior	Parietal lobe	Parietal cortex
	Pulvinar	Parietal lobe	Parietal cortex
Midline and intralaminar	Centromedian, parafascicular	Sensory, limbic, and basal ganglia	Limbic and basal ganglia

The subthalamus and epithalamus

Although medical understanding of the subthalamus (subthalamic nucleus) is far from complete, its role seems to be to regulate the level of activity in the basal ganglia circuits that control movement. Damage to the subthalamus leads to the patient developing violent flailing movements on the opposite side of the body, a disorder known as hemiballismus.

The epithalamus includes some nerve cell groups called the habenular nuclei, as well as the pineal gland. The habenular nuclei are part of a circuit that allows the emotional centers of the limbic system to change activity in the brainstem, whereas the pineal gland secretes melatonin as part of the circuit controlling the sleep–wake cycle.

The hypothalamus

The hypothalamus is a small part of the diencephalon situated just below the thalamus, but it plays a critically important role in controlling the automatic functions of

The body's master clock

The suprachiasmatic nucleus is the name given to a tiny group of nerve cells within the hypothalamus immediately above the crossing of the visual pathways in the midline. This is the master clock for our daily (circadian) rhythms and receives direct information from the retina about light levels. The suprachiasmatic nucleus is part of a complex circuit that regulates the secretion of melatonin by the pineal gland. The cells in the suprachiasmatic nucleus have a natural cycle of about 25 hours, but this is reset daily by light levels at the retina unless we cross time zones during international flights. Disruption of the circadian rhythm leads to the feeling of jetlag, which is best treated by exposure to strong natural light upon reaching one's destination.

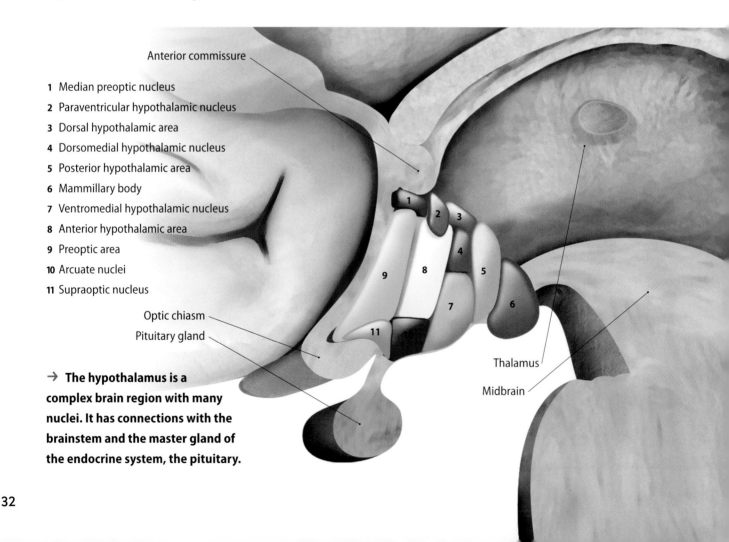

Anterior commissure

1 Median preoptic nucleus
2 Paraventricular hypothalamic nucleus
3 Dorsal hypothalamic area
4 Dorsomedial hypothalamic nucleus
5 Posterior hypothalamic area
6 Mammillary body
7 Ventromedial hypothalamic nucleus
8 Anterior hypothalamic area
9 Preoptic area
10 Arcuate nuclei
11 Supraoptic nucleus

Optic chiasm
Pituitary gland

Thalamus
Midbrain

→ **The hypothalamus is a complex brain region with many nuclei. It has connections with the brainstem and the master gland of the endocrine system, the pituitary.**

→ **Many factors influence the regulation of appetite, and the hypothalamus plays a key role. The amount of body fat influences the hypothalamus through leptin and insulin, hormones that act through the arcuate nucleus and the lateral and medial hypothalamus to tell the brainstem to stop eating or continue eating. This interacts with other signals from the liver and gut, via the nucleus of the solitary tract, to regulate how hungry we feel.**

Lateral hypothalamus
Medial (paraventricular) hypothalamus
Arcuate hypothalamus
Body fat
Leptin
Insulin
Stop eating
Keep eating
Liver
Small intestine
Stomach
Nucleus of solitary tract
Sensory nerves (transmitting stomach fullness and chemical signals)

the nervous system, the glands of the endocrine system, the blood pressure and heart rate changes that accompany emotional responses, as well as a range of complex behaviors that maintain the body and the species (feeding, drinking, and mating).

The hypothalamus is intimately connected to both the limbic system and the endocrine system, allowing it to influence the internal environment of the body in response to emotional states.

Keeping the body systems stable

Key to understanding the hypothalamus is the notion that it plays an important role in keeping the internal conditions of the body relatively stable. This is known as homeostasis. The hypothalamus can achieve this by monitoring information about the condition of the body (e.g., blood temperature) and making appropriate changes to the body to bring the condition of the body back to an appropriate set point (i.e., 98.6°F or 37°C). This could involve initiating behavioral or physiological changes (e.g., shivering, closing off skin vessels, and raising body hairs if too cold; or sweating, dilating skin vessels, and lowering body hairs if too hot).

The types of body conditions that the hypothalamus regulates include temperature, blood pressure, heart rate, and breathing, through connections with the brainstem. In this sense the hypothalamus is directing

the activities of nerve cells lower down the brain. Other types of behavior that maintain a constant internal environment involve more complexity, for example, feeding and drinking to maintain nutrients and fluids in the body. The pathways that control feeding are of particular clinical importance to clinicians because of widespread obesity in the developed world.

Sex leaves a mark on the hypothalamus

The two sexes behave differently during mating and this behavior is controlled by groups of nerve cells in the hypothalamus. It is not surprising, then, that the internal structure of the hypothalamus differs slightly between males and females. This sexual dimorphism is best studied in rodents, but it has also been reported to exist in the human hypothalamus.

The limbic system

The limbic system is a collective term for a group of interconnected structures that are broadly concerned with emotions and memory, the two being intimately linked.

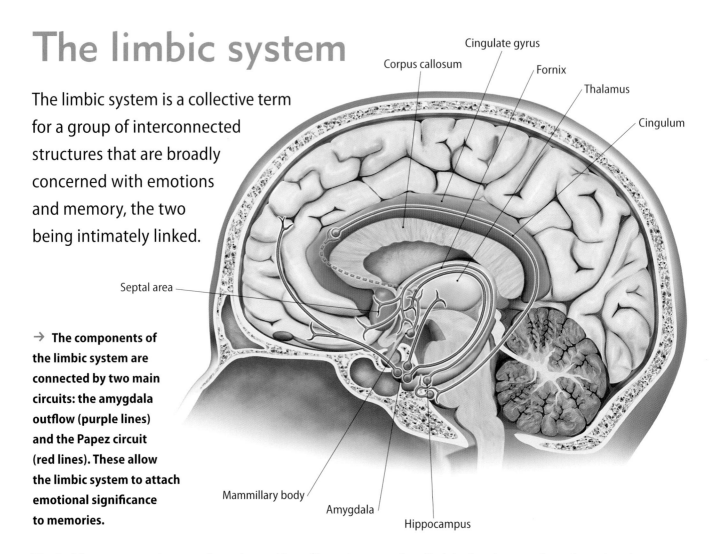

Cingulate gyrus

Corpus callosum

Fornix

Thalamus

Cingulum

Septal area

Mammillary body

Amygdala

Hippocampus

→ **The components of the limbic system are connected by two main circuits: the amygdala outflow (purple lines) and the Papez circuit (red lines). These allow the limbic system to attach emotional significance to memories.**

The limbic system gets its name from the position of its parts around the edge or border (*limbus* in Latin) of the forebrain. Ideas about this region put forward by the neuroanatomist James Papez in the 1930s emphasized that it consisted of a group of structures connected by a circuit (later called the Papez circuit), and that the system controlled drive-related and emotional behavior. We now know that the limbic system can be divided into two subsystems: one centered around a group of nerve cells called the amygdala in the temporal lobe; the other centered around a region of cortical tissue in the temporal lobe called the hippocampus.

Emotions and the amygdala
The amygdala (from the Latin for "almond," a reference to its shape) is involved in emotional responses, and processes information from a wide range of conscious senses (smell, sight, hearing, touch, and taste) and unconscious senses (from the internal organs), along with information from the cerebral cortex about the general level of physical and emotional comfort. The amygdala exerts its effects on the rest of the nervous system, and hence behavior, by pathways to the cerebral cortex and hypothalamus. The pathway to the cerebral cortex probably allows the amygdala to influence decisions about movement that serve the satisfaction of basic drives, and to create links between the perception of objects (e.g., a snake) and appropriate emotional responses (e.g., fear). In other words, it is important in emotion-related learning. The pathway to the hypothalamus allows the amygdala to initiate the physical changes in emotional responses. For example, if you are angry or afraid, your blood pressure and heart rate will increase.

When the limbic system is damaged

Damage to the temporal lobes on both sides causes a variety of problems that reflect the importance of this region in emotions and memory. Animals that have had their temporal lobes removed become fearless and show no emotional reactions, even when threatened by other animals. They show increased attention to objects, even if these have been in their environment for a long time, and will incessantly examine them. People who have undergone surgery to the temporal lobe to relieve epileptic seizures have severe anterograde amnesia and will often put inedible material such as paper into their mouths. Degeneration of the hippocampus is a feature of Alzheimer's disease and accounts for many of the memory problems in that disease.

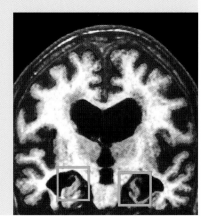

→ **This MRI scan of the brain of a man suffering from Alzheimer's disease shows the severe shrinkage of the hippocampus (lower center left and right) that is typical of the disease.**

Memory and the hippocampus

The hippocampus is a complex layered structure in the temporal lobe. It gets its name because its folded layers looked like the curled shape of a seahorse (*hippocampus* in Latin) to the early neuroanatomists.

The hippocampus and nearby entorhinal cortex are essential for memory. If the region is removed on both sides, the patient will have severe anterograde amnesia. In other words, he or she will be unable to form new memories about events or the meaning of new words from that point in time onward, although new motor skills and procedures may still be acquired. The patient may also have some retrograde amnesia (poor memory of events in the past), although this does not affect early memories from childhood. The hippocampus sends information to other parts of the brain through a large fiber bundle known as the fornix that makes up a central part of the Papez circuit.

↓ **Nerve cells in the hippocampus, such as these, are responsible for laying down new long-term memories. They do this through connections with other parts of the cerebral cortex where the memories will be stored.**

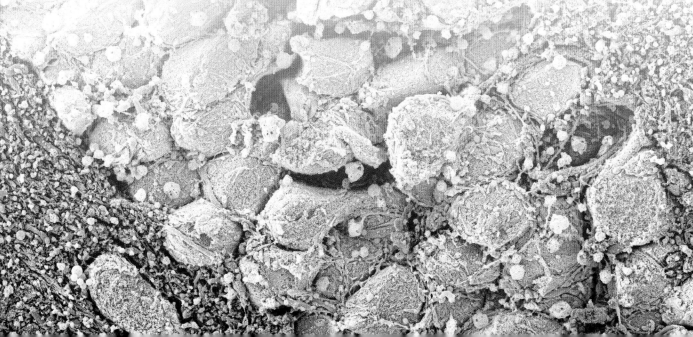

The pituitary

The pituitary is only about the size of a pea, yet it acts as the master gland of the endocrine system, producing hormones that have a powerful influence on reproduction, growth, and the internal body environment.

The pituitary sits in a bony depression below the hypothalamus. The two act together. The hypothalamus is concerned with producing appropriate behavior to maintain a constant internal environment (e.g., water and food intake) and to reproduce the species. The pituitary is concerned with directing chemical changes in the internal environment that serve similar purposes, such as reabsorbing water from the kidney to conserve water, and regulating reproductive cycles and the production of sex cells. It is not surprising, then, that these two structures lie close together at the base of the brain, or that the hypothalamus directs the activities of the pituitary by secreted chemical messengers called hormones passed down the stalk between the two. This close association of the hypothalamus and pituitary leads to the hypothalamo-pituitary axis being called the main component of the neuroendocrine system; the other being the pineal gland.

The anterior pituitary

The pituitary gland has two parts, the anterior and the posterior. Chemicals called releasing factors pass from the hypothalamus down a system of capillaries and veins (the hypothalamo-hypophyseal portal system) to the anterior pituitary, where they stimulate the cells there to release their hormones into the bloodstream. Nerve cells in two neuron clusters of the hypothalamus have axons that run down the stalk of the pituitary to end in the posterior pituitary.

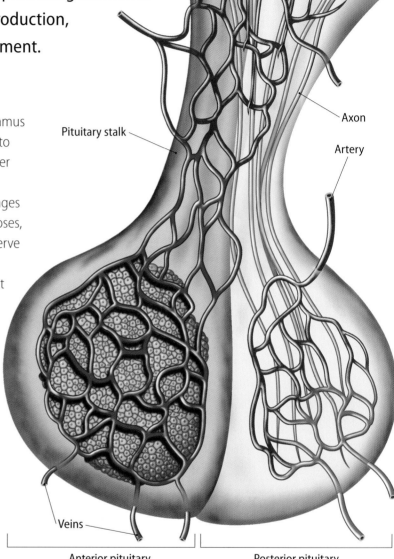

Neurosecretory cells in the hypothalamus

Axon

Artery

Pituitary stalk

Veins

Anterior pituitary

Posterior pituitary

←↑ **The pituitary lies at the base of the brain, and is connected to the hypothalamus by a stalk. The anterior pituitary is controlled by chemicals released into vessels in the stalk by neurosecretory cells (purple) in the hypothalamus. Other neurosecretory cells (green) in the hypothalamus penetrate the posterior pituitary.**

The anterior pituitary contains special cells that secrete hormones. One cell type, the acidophils, produces growth hormone, which indirectly regulates growth of bones and muscle; and prolactin, which stimulates the initiation and maintenance of milk production (lactation) after birth. Other cells, basophils, produce follicle-stimulating hormone, which stimulates development of the egg; luteinizing hormone, which stimulates the production of steroid hormones in the ovaries or testes; thyroid-stimulating hormone, which stimulates production of thyroid hormone; and adreno-corticotrophic hormone (ACTH), which stimulates the adrenal gland to produce corticosteroids.

The posterior pituitary

The posterior pituitary produces two hormones, but by a very different mechanism from the anterior pituitary. Axons from the nerve cells of the supraoptic and paraventricular nuclei of the hypothalamus run down the pituitary stalk to the tissue of the posterior pituitary, where they release two hormones into the bloodstream. In other words, unlike the anterior pituitary, there are no hormone-secreting cells in the posterior pituitary.

Nerve cells of the supraoptic nucleus primarily make antidiuretic hormone (ADH), which regulates water excretion by the kidney and, in high concentrations, is a strong constrictor of blood vessels. High levels of ADH promote water reabsorption from the urine as that fluid is being formed by the kidneys, thus making the urine more concentrated.

Nerve cells of the paraventricular nucleus primarily make oxytocin, a hormone that stimulates contraction of smooth muscle of the uterus during labor and contraction of myoepithelial cells around mammary glands of the breast to produce the milk let-down response during breast-feeding.

→ **In this micrograph of a growth hormone–producing cell (acidophil) in the anterior pituitary, the hormone is in the brown granules within the yellow cell cytoplasm. The cell nucleus is purple.**

Diseases of the pituitary

Benign tumors of the anterior pituitary may result in overproduction of hormones. Excess growth hormone results in overgrowth of the body's bones, muscles, and other tissues (gigantism in children and acromegaly in adults). If adrenocorticotrophic hormone is made in excess, the result is Cushing's disease, in which the adrenal cortex makes too much corticosteroid; resulting symptoms include fatty swellings of the face and trunk, and general weakness. Damage to the posterior pituitary leads to an inability to concentrate urine and conserve water.

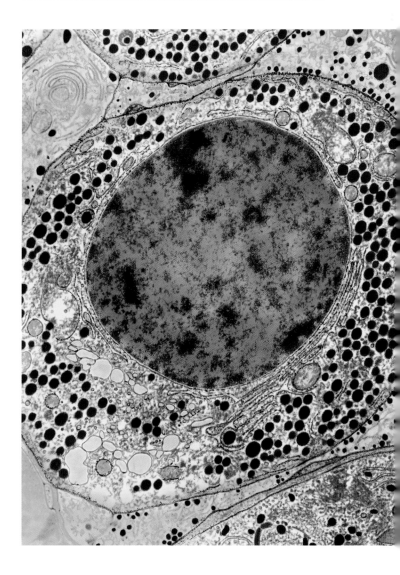

The brainstem

The brainstem contains groups of nerve cells that control vitally important functions such as breathing and heartbeat. It also controls the muscles and glands that allow us to eat, drink, and communicate.

Early anatomists divided the brainstem into three parts—midbrain, pons, and medulla oblongata—on the basis of external appearance. But these divisions do not accurately reflect the underlying internal organization of this region. Neuroscientists who study the developing brain have found that the brainstem develops from a series of as many as ten segments, arranged like body segments in a centipede down the length of the brainstem. Each segment gives rise to a characteristic group of motor and/or sensory nerve cells and is associated with a particular cranial nerve. Within each segment there is an additional level of functional subdivision, in that the brainstem is arranged like wedges in a pie: nerve cells with motor function (i.e., controlling muscles and glands) are produced close to the midline; whereas nerve cells with sensory function are made toward the side of the brainstem.

The functions of the brainstem

The brainstem has three main functions. First, it provides a highway for nerve pathways going up and down the central nervous system (the conduit function of the brainstem). The brainstem either receives, or has passing through it, pathways carrying sensory information from a wide variety of sources. These include information from the spinal cord about touch, pain, temperature, vibration, and the position of joints in the lower parts of the body. The brainstem also receives information from the inner ear about sound, the pull of gravity, and the acceleration or deceleration of the body in space. This information must be carried up to the forebrain for us to be consciously aware of these sensations, and the brainstem contains great axon bundles for conveying this information. Conversely, there are huge bundles of

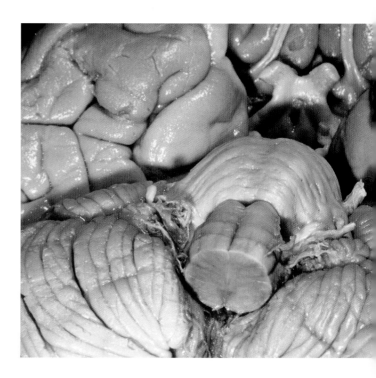

↑ **The brainstem comprises the medulla oblongata (bluish structure), the pons (just above the medulla), and the midbrain (hidden behind the pons).**

axons running from the forebrain to the brainstem and spinal cord to control the body's movements. Some of these will end in the brainstem, activating the nerve cell groups that control rhythmic movements of the head and neck or postural muscles; others will pass through without stopping, on their way to the spinal cord.

It also acts as an integrative center, processing sensory information and making commands to internal organs to control vital body functions, often without us being consciously aware of the activity. The brainstem has a core of nerve cell groups, known as the reticular

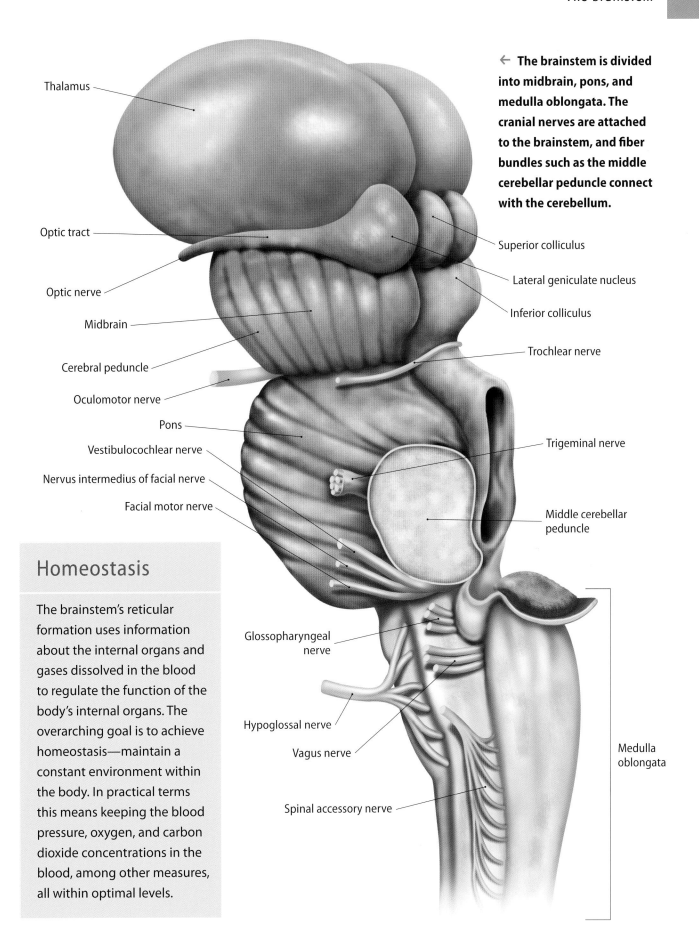

Thalamus

← **The brainstem is divided into midbrain, pons, and medulla oblongata. The cranial nerves are attached to the brainstem, and fiber bundles such as the middle cerebellar peduncle connect with the cerebellum.**

Optic tract

Superior colliculus

Lateral geniculate nucleus

Optic nerve

Inferior colliculus

Midbrain

Trochlear nerve

Cerebral peduncle

Oculomotor nerve

Pons

Trigeminal nerve

Vestibulocochlear nerve

Nervus intermedius of facial nerve

Facial motor nerve

Middle cerebellar peduncle

Homeostasis

The brainstem's reticular formation uses information about the internal organs and gases dissolved in the blood to regulate the function of the body's internal organs. The overarching goal is to achieve homeostasis—maintain a constant environment within the body. In practical terms this means keeping the blood pressure, oxygen, and carbon dioxide concentrations in the blood, among other measures, all within optimal levels.

Glossopharyngeal nerve

Hypoglossal nerve

Vagus nerve

Medulla oblongata

Spinal accessory nerve

→ **These "slices" are horizontal cross sections of points on the brainstem, from top to bottom. They show the descending motor and ascending sensory nerve pathways, as well as groups of nerve cells (nuclei) such as the substantia nigra, red nucleus, locus coeruleus, and nucleus ambiguus.**

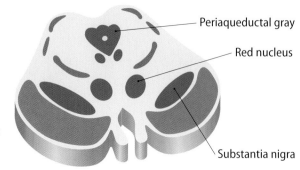

Periaqueductal gray

Red nucleus

Substantia nigra

■ Nerve pathways down the brainstem
■ Nerve pathways up the brainstem
■ Nerve cell groups

The primitive brain

Unlike many other parts of the brain, such as the cerebral cortex, the brainstem has changed very little during the evolution of back-boned animals. In fact, many of the nerve cell groups that can be found in the brainstem of a lungfish are also recognizable in the human brainstem, and there are very few differences between the brainstems of humans and chimpanzees.

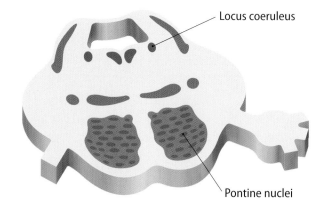

Locus coeruleus

Pontine nuclei

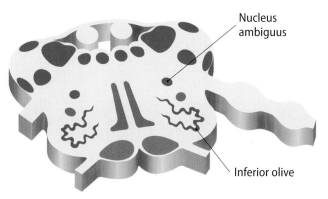

Nucleus ambiguus

Inferior olive

formation (see pp. 48–51), that use sensory information about the body's internal organs and blood gases to regulate the function of internal organs (heart, blood vessels, lungs, gut, bladder). The reticular formation also contains nerve cell groups that regulate some of the head and neck reflexes and automatic movements, e.g., the jaw and blink reflexes, the gagging reflex when an object is forced into the throat, and coordinating the movements of the eyes with head rotation.

Finally, the brainstem allows us to process sensory information from the cranial nerves, and to control the muscles and glands of the head and neck to consume and digest food, and communicate by speech and facial expressions. Most of the cranial nerves attach to the brainstem. These either receive sensory information from the head and neck, or control the muscles and glands in those regions. The brainstem contains many groups of sensory nerve cells (sensory nuclei) to process the information carried in from several cranial nerves, or motor nerve cells (motor nuclei) to control the head and neck muscles and glands through other cranial nerves.

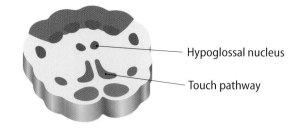

Hypoglossal nucleus

Touch pathway

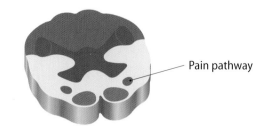

Pain pathway

Brainstem sensory nuclei

One group of sensory nuclei processes information entering the brainstem by the large trigeminal nerve, which carries information about touch, pain, and temperature from the surface of the face and from some parts of the mouth, palate, and tongue. This information can either be passed up toward the cerebral cortex for conscious awareness or be used locally in the brainstem to regulate reflexes (e.g., the corneal, or blink, reflex—an involuntary blinking of the eye in response to a foreign body touching the cornea).

A second group, associated with the vestibulo-cochlear nerve, processes sensory information from the inner ear about sound (in the cochlear nuclei) or the balance and acceleration of the head in space (in the vestibular nuclei). Like information from the trigeminal nerve, this data may be used locally in the brainstem to focus attention on important sounds or coordinate postural muscles, or be passed up the brain for conscious awareness and interpretation.

A third group of sensory nuclei in the brainstem is associated with either chemical senses (e.g., taste on the tongue or palate, and oxygen concentration in the blood) or internal organ senses (e.g., blood pressure or stretching of the stomach). This information enters the brainstem through the facial, glossopharyngeal, and vagal nerves. Some aspects of this sensation (e.g., taste) come to our conscious awareness by means of pathways to upper parts of the brain, but most will be used locally by the reticular formation to regulate functions that keep the internal environment of the body stable.

Brainstem motor nuclei

Some nuclei in the brainstem control muscles and glands. Several of these groups are much like the motor nerve cells of the spinal cord in that they control striped (skeletal) muscle and are under voluntary control. These include the nerve cells that control the muscles around the eye, the chewing muscles, the muscles of facial expression, the tongue, and two muscles of the neck (sternomastoid and the upper parts of the trapezius muscle). Other groups of nerve cells control muscles that can be controlled by will, but usually function

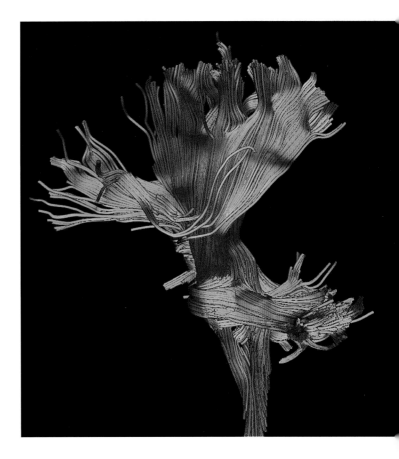

↑ **A 3-D scan highlights the bundles of white-matter nerve fibers in the brainstem. The purple fibers are ascending or descending pathways. The green fibers connect the brainstem to the cerebellum (lower right).**

as part of motor routines that are involuntary. These include nerve cells that control the muscles of the throat and soft palate that are usually activated during stereotyped or reflexive activities such as swallowing or the gag reflex. Even nerve cells that are usually voluntary in function may take part in involuntary reflexes, such as the blink reflex.

Other nerve cells in the brainstem, which are part of the parasympathetic nervous system, control the smooth muscle and glands of the head, neck, or trunk. These include nerve cells that control the smooth muscle inside the eye to close the pupil or change the shape of the lens. Other groups of nerve cells in the midbrain and pons drive the tear and salivary glands to produce secretions.

Cranial nerves

The 12 pairs of cranial nerves connect directly to the brain and serve various parts of the head and body. They control movements of the face, tongue, eyes, and throat, and receive sensory input from the organs of hearing, sight, smell, and taste.

Twelve pairs of nerves attach to the brain, rather than the spinal cord, and so are said to be cranial. Some of them convey information from the sense organs to the brain; others control muscles; and some have both sensory and motor functions. Two cranial nerves are attached to the forebrain and are concerned with exclusively forebrain senses (smell and vision), but the other ten are attached to the brainstem.

Serving the head and neck

The two nerves attached to the forebrain are very different in nature from the other ten. Both the olfactory and optic nerves are really part of the central nervous system. In fact, the entire sensory part of the eye develops as an outgrowth of the embryonic brain. By contrast, the other ten cranial nerves are part of the peripheral nervous system.

Many of the cranial nerves are critically important in some of the reflexes of the head and neck. For example, the blink reflex depends on both the sense of touch on the cornea of the eye being carried to the brainstem by the trigeminal nerve, and impulses to activate the blink muscles being carried out from the brainstem along the facial nerve.

The roaming vagus nerve

Even though the cranial nerves are all attached to the brain, one of them has a remarkably long course. This nerve is called the vagus (from the Latin *vagor* meaning "to roam"), because it wanders through the neck, chest, and upper abdomen controlling many glands and muscles in the organs of these regions, and receiving sensory information from the same organs. The vagus nerve is a key part of the para-sympathetic nervous system.

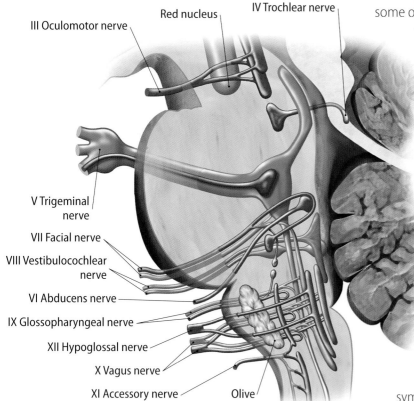

III Oculomotor nerve
Red nucleus
IV Trochlear nerve
V Trigeminal nerve
VII Facial nerve
VIII Vestibulocochlear nerve
VI Abducens nerve
IX Glossopharyngeal nerve
XII Hypoglossal nerve
X Vagus nerve
XI Accessory nerve
Olive

↑ **The cranial nerves may be sensory (blue), motor (red), or a mixture of both. Each is named for the body part it serves and also given a Roman numeral.**

→ **The 12 cranial nerves are connected with the brain and leave the cavity of the skull to reach their target organs through many fine holes.**

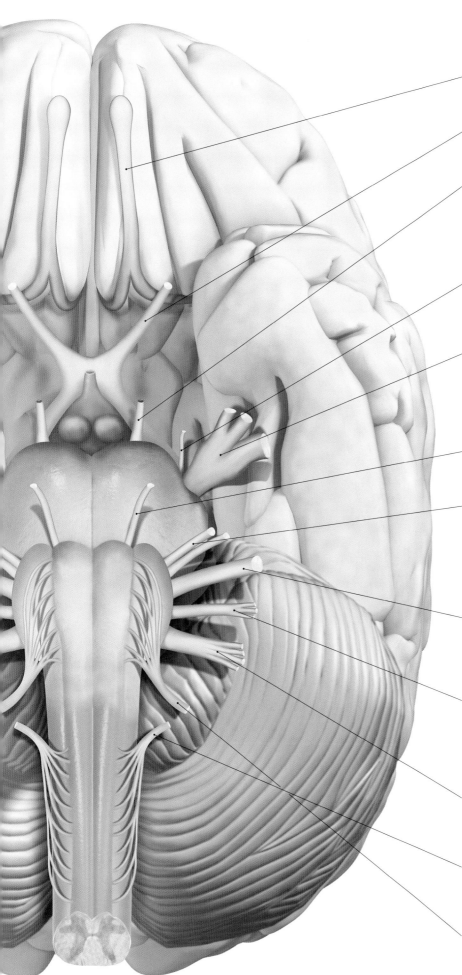

I Olfactory (sensory)

Carries impulses for the sense of smell

II Optic (sensory)

Carries impulses for vision

III Oculomotor (motor)

Controls most of the muscles that move the eyeball and elevate the eyelid; also controls the smooth muscle that adjusts the shape of the lens and the size of the pupil

IV Trochlear (motor)

Supplies a muscle that turns the eye down and to the midline

V Trigeminal (sensory and motor)

Carries sensation from the face and part of the scalp; controls the chewing muscles, muscles on the floor of the mouth, and a muscle in the middle ear that protects against loud noise

VI Abducens (motor)

Supplies a muscle that turns the eye to the side

VII Facial (sensory and motor)

Sensory: carries taste from the front two thirds of the tongue; motor: controls the muscles of facial expression, a muscle in the middle ear that protects against loud noise, the tear glands, and two types of salivary glands

VIII Vestibulocochlear (sensory)

Vestibular: carries information from the inner ear about gravity and acceleration; cochlear: transmits impulses for the sense of hearing

IX Glossopharyngeal (sensory and motor)

Sensory: carries information from the pharynx and taste buds on the back third of the tongue; motor: controls the parotid salivary glands and a muscle in the throat

X Vagus (sensory and motor)

Sensory and motor supply to the throat; supply of internal organs of chest and abdomen

XI Accessory (motor)

Controls muscles in the neck and upper shoulder

XII Hypoglossal (motor)

Controls the muscles of the tongue

The cerebellum

At the back of the brainstem sits the cerebellum, the "little brain" that coordinates muscle activity and maintains the balance and equilibrium of the body. It may even play a role in thought and emotion.

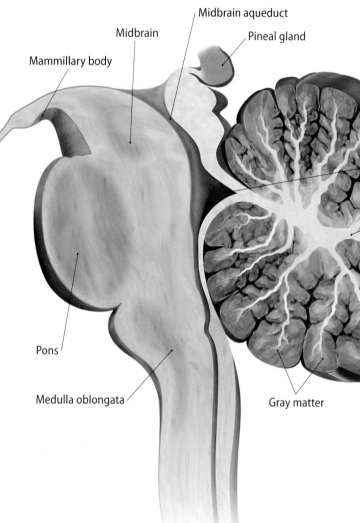

Mammillary body

Midbrain

Midbrain aqueduct

Pineal gland

Fourth ventricle

White matter

Folia

Pons

Medulla oblongata

Gray matter

← **The cerebellum is attached to the back of the brainstem. It has a cortex of gray matter, thrown into folds, or folia, around a core of white matter.**

The word cerebellum literally means "little brain," because the earliest anatomists noted its resemblance to the cerebral hemispheres. This superficial similarity is due to the folding of the cortex, or outer surface, of the cerebellum, a feature that increases the surface area of the organ and hence its information-processing capacity. Anatomically, the cerebellum's main parts include a narrow medial zone called the vermis (Latin for "worm"), and two cerebellar hemispheres, one on either side of the vermis.

The cerebellum is attached to the brainstem by three large bundles of axons called the cerebellar peduncles that carry the rich flow of information into and out of the cerebellum. It sits in the hindmost cavity of the skull interior (posterior cranial fossa) and receives blood supply from the vertebro-basilar group of arteries.

Inside the cerebellum

When examined under a microscope, the cortex of the cerebellum can be seen to have three layers: an outer molecular layer of axons and dendrites (projections

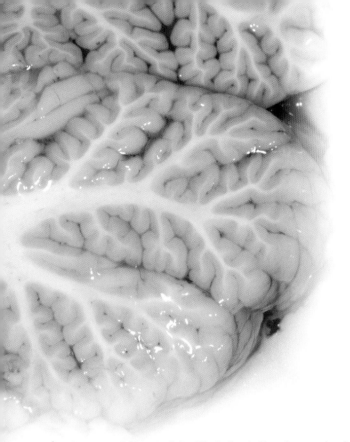

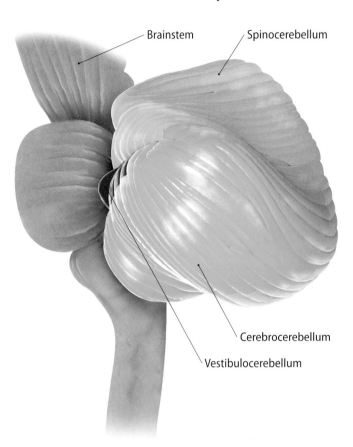

↓ **Neuroscientists divide the cerebellum in three: the vestibulocerebellum, the spinocerebellum, and the cerebrocerebellum. Each has a specific function.**

Brainstem

Spinocerebellum

Cerebrocerebellum

Vestibulocerebellum

↑ **The resemblance of the "little brain" to the cerebral hemispheres is clear in this dissected cerebellum.**

from nerve cells) with very few cells; a single layer of the cell bodies of large nerve cells called Purkinje cells; and an inner layer of the densely packed bodies of small nerve cells called granule cells. Below this is a region of white matter containing all the incoming and outgoing axons of the cortex. Inputs to the cerebellar cortex come from sensory fibers and groups of nerve cells in the brainstem, called the precerebellar nuclei, that are functionally linked with the cerebellum.

Deep inside the white matter of the cerebellum are groups of nerve cells called the deep cerebellar nuclei. These are in three groups: the fastigial near the midline; the globose and emboliform nuclei further to the side; and the large dentate nucleus at the edge of the group. The deep cerebellar nuclei are under the influence of the cerebellar cortex and are the only nerve cells to provide the output from most of the cerebellum.

Functional parts of the cerebellum

The cerebellum needs several types of information to perform its role of coordinating motor functions and maintaining balance. These include information about

Other roles for the cerebellum

Neuroscientists postulate that the cerebellum plays a role not just in movement, but also in non-motor functions such as thought, emotional processing, and language. Studies of human subjects using PET and functional MRI scanning techniques have shown increased blood flow in the cerebellum when purely cognitive tasks are being performed. The cerebellum also receives, indirectly, information from the limbic and prefrontal cortex, areas of the cerebral cortex that are concerned with emotions and planning. This is still a controversial idea, however, and not all neuroscientists support the proposition of a cognitive or emotional role for the cerebellum.

the balance and acceleration of the head and body in space, the position of the joints of the limbs, and the state of tension of the muscles. It also needs information from the motor cortex of the cerebrum about the types of movements that need to be coordinated.

Neuroscientists divide the cerebellum into three functional divisions that reflect its broad functions and sources of information: the vestibulocerebellum, the spinocerebellum, and the cerebrocerebellum (also called the pontocerebellum or neocerebellum).

The vestibulocerebellum uses information from the inner ear about the orientation of the head and its rotation in space to influence the muscles that move the eyes.

The spinocerebellum receives information from the spinal cord about the position of limbs and the state of tension or activity in muscles. This information is used to adjust the posture of the body by pathways that run, firstly to the vestibular nuclei and reticular formation of the brainstem, and from there by long pathways to the spinal cord. These pathways control the muscles that maintain the posture of the body, keeping us upright, but may also control the sorts of stereotyped movements that we perform without thinking (e.g., walking).

Some parts of the spinocerebellum receive information from the spinal cord but also get an overlapping input from the cerebral cortex. This intermediate region of the cerebellum is able to compare motor commands from the cerebral cortex with the actual position of the body part to be moved. It can issue commands that correct the position of the part of the body, even while the action is taking place.

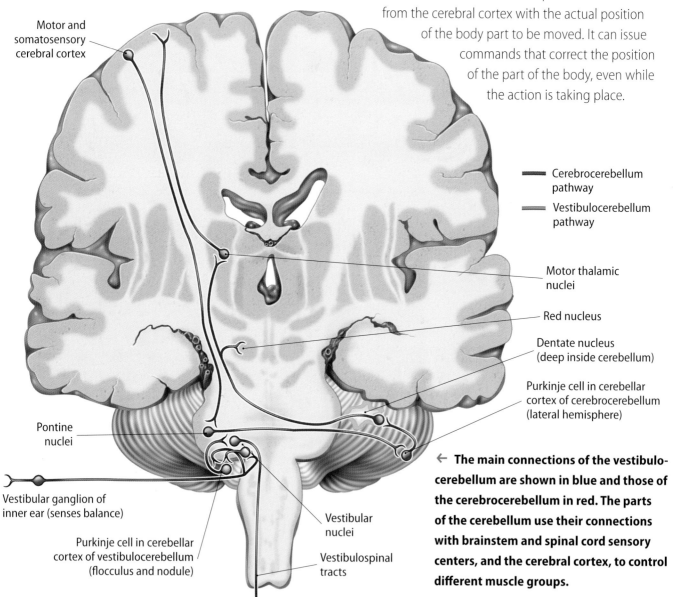

Motor and somatosensory cerebral cortex

Cerebrocerebellum pathway

Vestibulocerebellum pathway

Motor thalamic nuclei

Red nucleus

Dentate nucleus (deep inside cerebellum)

Purkinje cell in cerebellar cortex of cerebrocerebellum (lateral hemisphere)

Pontine nuclei

Vestibular ganglion of inner ear (senses balance)

Purkinje cell in cerebellar cortex of vestibulocerebellum (flocculus and nodule)

Vestibular nuclei

Vestibulospinal tracts

← **The main connections of the vestibulo-cerebellum are shown in blue and those of the cerebrocerebellum in red. The parts of the cerebellum use their connections with brainstem and spinal cord sensory centers, and the cerebral cortex, to control different muscle groups.**

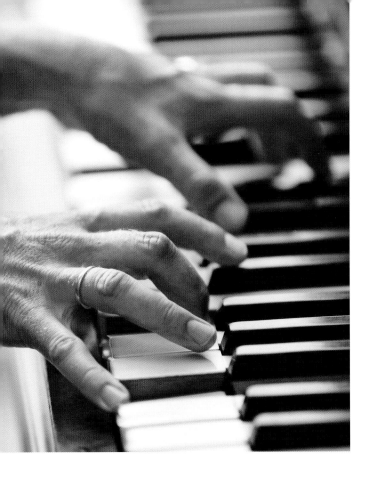

↑ **Part of the cerebellum, the cerebrocerebellum, plays a vital role in planning fine, skillful movements such as playing the piano.**

Learning and coordinating skilled movements

The lateral parts of the cerebellum (cerebrocerebellum) are very large in humans and are essential in planning the fine, skillful movements that humans perform with their upper limbs (e.g., knitting or performing surgery), particularly when those movements become more rapid, precise, and automatic with practice. It is still not entirely clear how exactly this planning is achieved, but it does depend on a great looped circuit that runs from the cerebral cortex to the pons, then up to the cortex of the cerebellum, down through cerebellar white matter to the dentate nucleus, out of the cerebellum to the thalamus, and then back to the motor and premotor cortex of the cerebral cortex. This circuit is actually active before movement commences, suggesting that some sort of plan of action for the movement is being retrieved from the cerebellum. Not surprisingly, if any part of this loop circuit is damaged, then learned skillful movements are permanently lost.

Damage to the cerebellum

The cerebellum may be damaged by tumors, strokes, or degenerative disease. Damage to one side of the cerebellum causes problems with balance and coordination on the same side of the body. Alcohol abuse is a common cause of cerebellar degeneration in the developed world. Damage to the midline of the cerebellum in chronic alcoholism causes an unstable, broad-based, staggering walk with a general lack of coordination of the limbs. If a tumor grows in the roof of the fourth ventricle, the parts of the cerebellum that control eye movement may be affected, and the patient will have difficulty following moving objects with their eyes. Damage to the lateral parts of the cerebellum causes problems with fine motor coordination of the upper limbs, leading to a tremor that gets worse on movement (intention tremor) and a type of speech where the words are broken up into individual syllables (scanning speech).

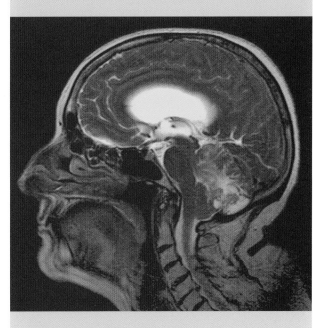

↑ **A scan reveals a tumor in the left lobe of the cerebellum. This would cause loss of coordination of the limbs on the left side.**

The reticular formation

Buried at the core of the brainstem, the reticular formation plays an important role in a wide variety of functions, including movement, the sleep–wake cycle, emotion, breathing, heart rate, and blood pressure.

The reticular formation gets its name because it has the superficial appearance of a diffuse nerve cell network (the Latin for "a small net" is *reticulum*), all located in the core of the brainstem. These groups of nerve cells have poorly defined boundaries and have been difficult to study, but some have characteristic chemical signatures because of the neurotransmitters they use.

The reticular formation has three zones, arranged in sequence from the midline to the side of the brainstem. The zone closest to the midline contains the raphe nuclei (from the Greek word *rhaphe*, meaning "seam"). Alongside the raphe nuclei is a medial (magnocellular) zone that contains a mixture of large and small nerve cells. The larger nerve cells of the medial zone give rise to most of the long ascending and descending pathways that influence other parts of the central nervous system. Further to the side is a lateral (parvicellular) zone of smaller nerve cells that is concerned with cranial nerve reflexes and control of internal organs.

↓ **A cross section reveals the three main components of the reticular formation inside the brainstem: the parvicellular and magnocellular parts, and the raphe nuclei.**

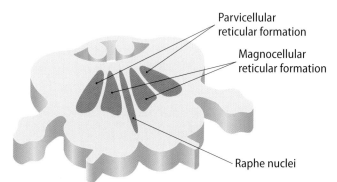

Parvicellular reticular formation

Magnocellular reticular formation

Raphe nuclei

Chemical signatures

Chemicals that pass on signals at synapses are called neurotransmitters. Some nerve cell groups in the reticular formation have characteristic chemistry because of their neurotransmitters.

Many nerve cells of the raphe nuclei use the neurotransmitter serotonin and project axons to both upper parts of the nervous system (e.g., cortex and thalamus) as well as lower parts (e.g., cerebellum, spinal cord). Serotonergic (serotonin-using) pathways are important in the regulation of the sleep–wake cycle (see pp. 234–7). The activity of dorsal raphe nerve cells is highest during waking, low during slow-wave sleep, and almost completely lost during rapid eye movement (REM) sleep. Drugs that influence the breakdown or reuptake of serotonin and make more of the neuro-transmitter available at cortical synapses are used to treat mood disorders.

The locus coeruleus and Alzheimer's disease

The cells in one part of the reticular formation, the locus coeruleus, are profoundly affected in old age, with 30 to 50 percent lost from early adulthood to old age. Patients with Alzheimer's disease have a particularly profound loss of cells in the locus coeruleus that contain noradrenaline (norepinephrine). This loss may account for much of the lost function that characterizes the disease.

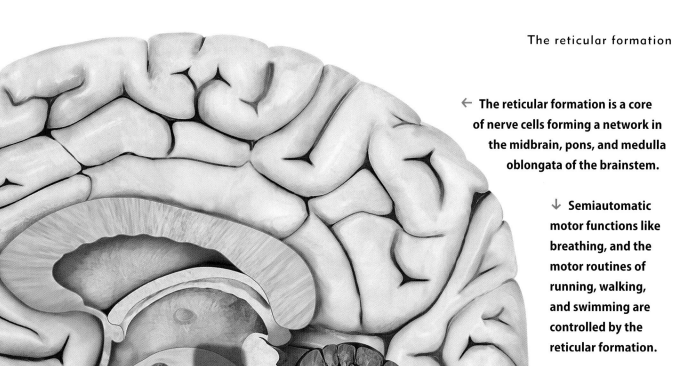

↓ **Semiautomatic motor functions like breathing, and the motor routines of running, walking, and swimming are controlled by the reticular formation.**

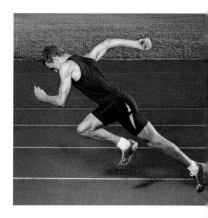

Midbrain reticular formation

Pontine reticular formation

Medullary reticular formation

Nerve cells in the locus coeruleus—a tiny part of the reticular formation—comprise most of the noradrenergic (noradrenaline-containing) nerve cells in the brain. The locus coeruleus is blue in fresh brains because a byproduct of the production of noradrenaline is a blue-black pigment called neuromelanin. Noradrenergic nerve cells in the locus coeruleus innervate almost the entire brain and are important for arousal, attention, and memory function. These pathways are most active in situations that are startling or call for watchfulness.

Many nerve cells in the part of the midbrain called the ventral tegmental area contain dopamine and use this neurotransmitter in their projections. These dopaminergic pathways reach the limbic system and medial cortex and are involved in motivation and cognition. One of these pathways, the mesolimbic dopaminergic pathway, is vital in rewarding behavior and plays a central role in addiction.

Controlling movement

The medial zone of the reticular formation plays a key role in the control of movement. The reticulospinal tracts are two pathways that come from large nerve cells in the medial zone of the upper medulla and pons. These pathways act directly on motor nerve cells in the ventral horn of the spinal cord and modify the activity of spinal cord reflexes. The reticular formation contains the neural machinery for complex patterns of movement, so nerve cell networks in the reticular formation probably control the actions of running, walking, and swimming.

The reticular formation is also closely involved in the role of the cerebellum in controlling motor functions. One large group of nerve cells, the lateral reticular nucleus, relays information about touch to the cerebellum for use in coordinating muscles. Other reticular formation nuclei in the medulla and pons relay information from the cerebral cortex to the cerebellum.

Pain modulation

The experience of pain may be profoundly influenced by a person's circumstances. Depression can make the experience of pain much more unpleasant, whereas fighting for one's life may allow people involved in combat or natural disasters to ignore pain temporarily. Pathways from the raphe nuclei of the reticular formation are crucial in modifying the experience of pain. Nerve cells of the nucleus raphe magnus of the upper medulla (part of the brainstem) have axons that run down to the spinal cord (raphespinal tract), where they terminate on nerve cells in the dorsal horn. This is the region where pain information is transmitted from spinal nerves to the pathways that will carry pain information up to the thalamus, so these descending pathways can block or modify the ascending sensation of pain. The raphespinal tract uses the neurotransmitter serotonin.

Nerve cells love to gossip

Nerve cells in the reticular formation may receive input from a variety of sources and even different types of senses (e.g., both hearing and touch) and may be influenced by stimuli on many parts of the body. Although the individual clusters of nerve cells within the reticular formation have separate functions, there is a lot of anatomical overlap between the clusters. Many reticular formation nerve cells possess long axons that extend to many levels of the spinal cord and send branches to many parts of the brainstem and diencephalon. You might even say that reticular nerve cells love gossip and like to spread it.

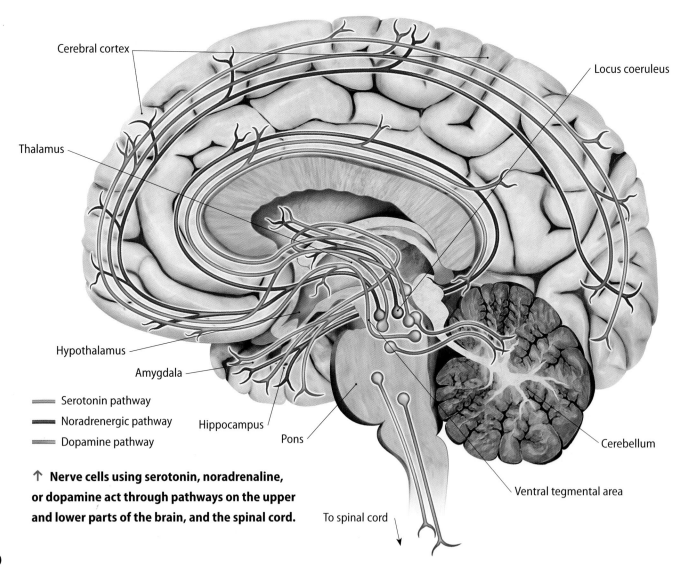

Cerebral cortex

Locus coeruleus

Thalamus

Hypothalamus

Amygdala

Hippocampus

Pons

Cerebellum

Ventral tegmental area

To spinal cord

— Serotonin pathway
— Noradrenergic pathway
— Dopamine pathway

↑ **Nerve cells using serotonin, noradrenaline, or dopamine act through pathways on the upper and lower parts of the brain, and the spinal cord.**

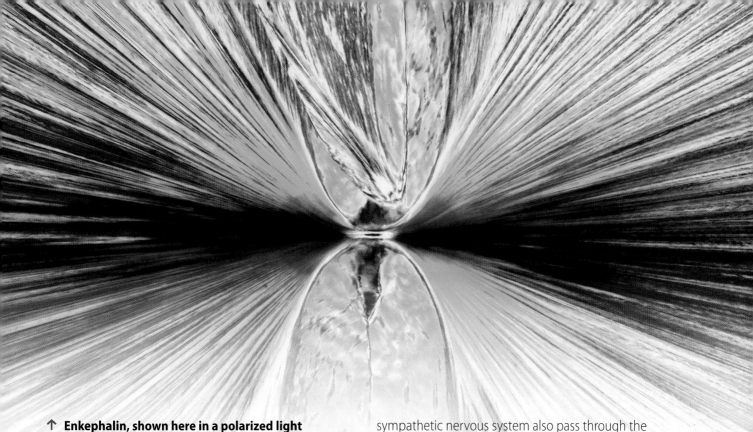

↑ **Enkephalin, shown here in a polarized light micrograph, is one of the body's naturally occurring opioid neurotransmitters. It has painkilling effects resembling those of the drugs morphine and codeine.**

Nerve cells in several parts of the pain modification pathway have receptors on their membranes for opiates (drugs, such as morphine, derived from or related to opium). The body uses naturally occurring chemicals called opioid peptides such as enkephalin and dynorphin, which have a similar molecular shape to morphine, to influence activity in the pain pathways. Therapeutic use of plant opiates, including morphine, produces a pain-relief effect when the plant opiate binds to the body's natural opiate receptors.

Controlling automatic functions

The reticular formation receives information from a wide variety of visceral organs and uses this information to control the internal organs through visceral autonomic reflexes. The reticular formation of the medulla and pons contains groups of nerve cells concerned with the control of aspects of breathing (e.g., the drive to breathe in or out, or the rhythm of the whole cycle). Other regions are concerned with the control of heart rate and blood pressure. Descending pathways for control of the sympathetic nervous system also pass through the reticular formation in the side of the brainstem.

Arousal and consciousness

The reticular formation receives input from many different senses, so it would not be surprising that it plays a role in directing sensory attention. At any time our central nervous system is bombarded with a torrent of sensory information, but not all that information is relevant to our behavior at any given moment. The pathways from the reticular formation to the thalamus and cortex are important for controlling the activity of the cerebral cortex and directing sensory attention to those senses that are of particular behavioral importance in the moment. For example, we may be sitting quietly reading a book when a child's scream outside catches our attention; suddenly we lose interest in the book and get up to investigate.

These pathways also maintain consciousness: damage to the reticular formation on both sides of the brainstem and the pathways passing through them will send the patient into a coma. Even a small hemorrhage in the pons of the brainstem may render a person unconscious despite a healthy cerebral cortex. The part of the reticular formation responsible for maintaining activity of the cerebral cortex and sustaining consciousness is the ascending reticular activating system.

The spinal cord

The spinal cord serves a host of functions, including the control of voluntary muscles, involuntary muscles, and glands, as well as the initial processing of sensory information (touch, pain, temperature, vibration, and joint position) from the body surface and interior. It also conveys sensory information up to the brain and descending pathways that allow the brain to control spinal cord function.

The spinal cord is only about 17 inches (42–3 cm) long in most men and women, somewhat less than the length of the vertebral column, and extends from the base of the skull to the middle of the back, just below the end of the rib cage. It is attached to the brain at the foramen magnum (from the Latin for "great hole") of the skull base. Since the spinal cord ends at the level of the second vertebral bone of the lumbar (lower back) region, a lumbar puncture (sampling of the cerebrospinal fluid around the nerve roots; also called a spinal tap) can be safely performed below this level, with no risk of puncturing the spinal cord.

External features
Attached to the spinal cord are dorsal and ventral nerve roots. Dorsal roots are concerned with carrying sensory information into the spinal cord, while ventral roots mainly carry motor control information out to skeletal muscles or the glands and involuntary muscle. Each dorsal root has an enlargement called the dorsal root ganglion, which contains the bodies of sensory nerve cells. The dorsal and ventral roots come together to form spinal nerves that exit between the vertebral bones. The spinal cord is enlarged in the lower neck and lower back regions where those spinal nerves that innervate the upper and lower limbs, respectively, exit.

The spinal cord is divided into a series of segments with attached spinal nerves that are named according to the region of the vertebral column through which the nerves exit. There are eight cervical (neck) segments,

twelve thoracic (chest) segments, five lumbar (lower back), five sacral (back of the pelvis), plus three to five coccygeal (tail) segments. Because the spinal cord is much shorter than the vertebral column, the segments of the lower cord are progressively higher than the vertebral bones below which the corresponding spinal nerves emerge.

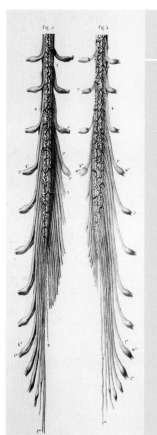

The horse's tail

Because the spinal cord does not reach the end of the vertebral column, the nerve roots leaving the lower end of the spinal cord must travel through the vertebral canal for some distance before exiting at the appropriate level. This bundle of nerves is known as the cauda equina, from the Latin for "horse's tail."

← **The "horse's tail": illustrations from an anatomical text of 1844.**

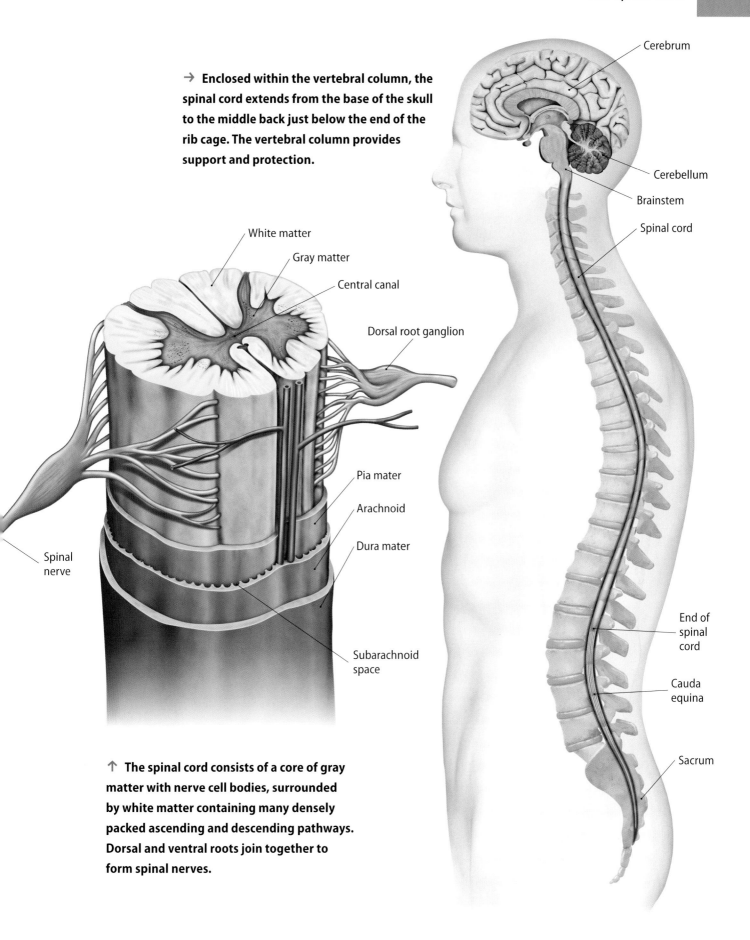

→ **Enclosed within the vertebral column, the spinal cord extends from the base of the skull to the middle back just below the end of the rib cage. The vertebral column provides support and protection.**

Cerebrum

Cerebellum

Brainstem

Spinal cord

White matter

Gray matter

Central canal

Dorsal root ganglion

Pia mater

Arachnoid

Dura mater

Spinal nerve

Subarachnoid space

End of spinal cord

Cauda equina

Sacrum

↑ **The spinal cord consists of a core of gray matter with nerve cell bodies, surrounded by white matter containing many densely packed ascending and descending pathways. Dorsal and ventral roots join together to form spinal nerves.**

53

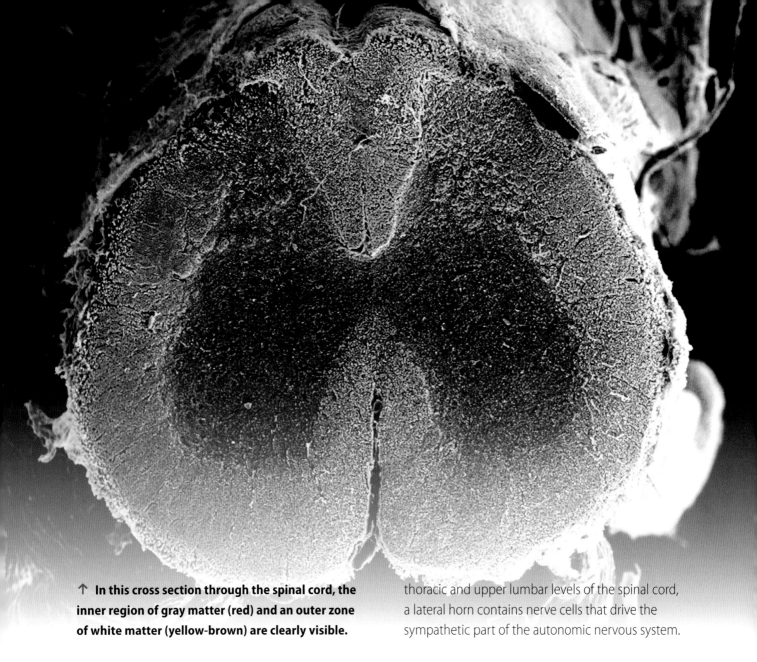

↑ **In this cross section through the spinal cord, the inner region of gray matter (red) and an outer zone of white matter (yellow-brown) are clearly visible.**

Gray and white matter

The core of the spinal cord is an "H"-shaped region of gray matter that contains the nerve cell bodies and their shorter processes. Surrounding this core is a shell of white matter containing all the axon bundles that carry information up and down the cord.

The gray matter has areas called dorsal and ventral horns throughout the length of the spinal cord (these are also sometimes known as posterior and anterior horns). Nerve cells in the dorsal horns are concerned with processing incoming sensory information, using it in local reflexes, or directing it to the appropriate ascending pathway to the brain. Nerve cells in the ventral horns control the voluntary muscles. In the

thoracic and upper lumbar levels of the spinal cord, a lateral horn contains nerve cells that drive the sympathetic part of the autonomic nervous system.

Reflexes

A reflex is an involuntary immediate response to a stimulus. The spinal cord is an important site for reflexes because its proximity to the lower parts of the body allows protective actions to be initiated quickly. All reflex circuits involve at least a sensory nerve cell and a motor nerve cell, but some reflex circuits require intervening interneurons between sensory and motor nerve cells.

The simplest type of reflex is the stretch, or myotatic, reflex. This is a reflex that is constantly active—both during movement and when standing still—to correct muscle tension and maintain posture. It consists of only a single, myelinated large-axon sensory nerve cell that carries information from stretch receptors inside the muscle belly to the spinal cord. The ends of these nerve fibers pass through the gray matter to contact the large motor nerve cells that drive the same muscle. The reflex can be elicited by tapping the tendon of a muscle (e.g., the patellar ligament at the front of the knee) with a rubber hammer. This causes a quick stretching of the quadriceps femoris muscle of the front of the thigh and the stretch receptors inside it. The impulse runs back to the spinal cord along the sensory nerves, stimulates activation of the motor nerve cells, and the resulting impulse runs back through the ventral roots to cause a jerky contraction of the quadriceps femoris muscle—the knee-jerk. Clinicians use this reflex to assess the nerve connections between muscle and spinal cord. Damage to descending motor pathways from the brain causes an increased activity in the stretch reflex circuit.

Ascending and descending pathways

The spinal cord contains sensory pathways that carry information about the body to the brain. In the white matter at the back of the cord are dorsal columns, which carry information about fine, precise touch, vibration, and joint position to the medulla of the brainstem. In the white matter to the front and side of the spinal cord are the spinothalamic tracts that carry information about simple touch, pain, and temperature from the spinal cord to the thalamus. Information in both these pathways eventually reaches the cerebral cortex and consciousness. Other ascending pathways called spinocerebellar tracts carry information about joint position and muscle tension to the cerebellum so it can use the information to coordinate muscle activity.

Pathways from the cerebral cortex and brainstem control motor activity in the spinal cord. The cortico-spinal tract allows the cortex to directly influence the activity of muscle nerve cells at levels of the spinal cord all the way to its lower end, but particularly for skillful movements of the upper limb. Other pathways from the brainstem (reticulospinal tracts) control motor behavior such as walking, running, and swimming, and regulate the activity of the autonomic nervous system.

Other descending pathways from the brainstem influence the perception of sensation and may have a profound effect on the experience of pain.

The flexion-withdrawal reflex

Step on a sharp object, such as a nail, in bare feet and you will experience the flexion-withdrawal reflex firsthand. This spinal reflex starts with the stimulation of skin receptors by painful or hot stimuli. The sensory information is carried back to the dorsal horn, where one or more interneurons carry the information to several levels of the spinal cord and activate motor nerve cells that produce contraction, not just of the nearest muscle to the stimulus, but other muscles elsewhere in the same limb, and even muscles on the other side of the body. The end result is that a potentially damaging stimulus induces a bending (flexion) and withdrawal of the entire limb on that side by contraction of many muscles acting at several joints, while causing the opposite limb to straighten to support the body weight.

↓ **Doctors test the knee-jerk reflex by tapping the ligament just below the kneecap. An abnormal response may indicate a defect in nerve conduction.**

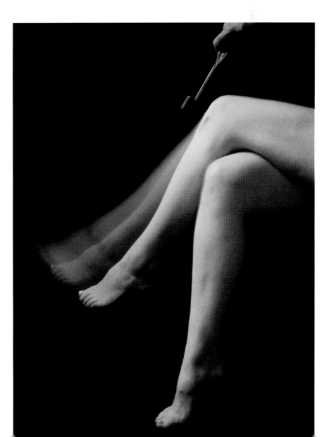

Spinal nerves

The spinal nerves carry sensory information about touch, pain, temperature, muscle tension, and joint position to the spinal cord, and motor commands out to the muscles and glands of the body.

Spinal nerves are formed when the dorsal (or sensory) roots and ventral (or motor) roots, both attached to each side of the spinal cord, come together in the space between the bones of the vertebral column. Each of the segments of the spinal cord gives rise to a pair of spinal nerves, which branch into and service particular areas of the body. Each spinal nerve contains both sensory and motor axons.

← The spinal nerves are numbered and divided into cervical, thoracic, lumbar, sacral, and coccygeal nerves.

↓ A spinal nerve is formed by the junction of the dorsal root (sensory in function) and the ventral root (motor in function). The dorsal root is thickened by a dorsal root ganglion that contains the cell bodies of sensory nerves.

The functions of peripheral nerves

Spinal nerves from the chest level have a simple course and run in the spaces between the ribs as intercostal nerves. However, the spinal nerves from most levels of the spinal cord join with each other to form nerve plexuses. The peripheral nerves emerge from these plexuses, their axons either passing to the skin, joints, muscles, and tendon sense organs if they are sensory in nature; or to muscle fibers if they have a motor function.

Peripheral nerves have layers of connective tissue to protect them, as well as accompanying blood vessels to provide them with nutrients. They contain different types of axons with different functions. The thicker the axon and its myelin coat are, the faster nerve impulses travel. Some axons have thick myelin coats (for the senses essential to muscle coordination, and high-speed conduction of motor commands), some have thin myelin coats (for simple touch and pinprick), whereas some have no myelin coats at all (for the control of glands or the sensation of heat, itch, or pain). Special cells called Schwann cells wrap themselves around individual axons to make the myelin sheath.

C1
C2
C3
C4
C5
C6
C7
C8
T1
T2
T3
T4
T5
T6
T7
T8
T9
T10
T11
T12
L1
L2
L3
L4
L5
S1
S2
S3
S4
S5
Coccygeal nerve (Co1)

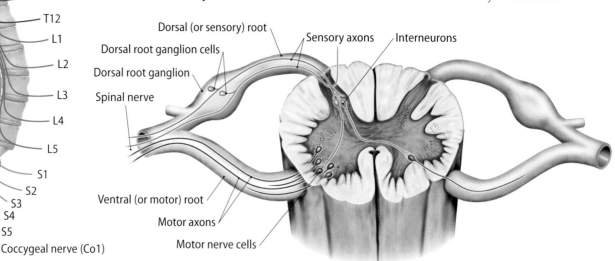

Dorsal (or sensory) root
Dorsal root ganglion cells
Dorsal root ganglion
Spinal nerve
Sensory axons
Interneurons
Ventral (or motor) root
Motor axons
Motor nerve cells

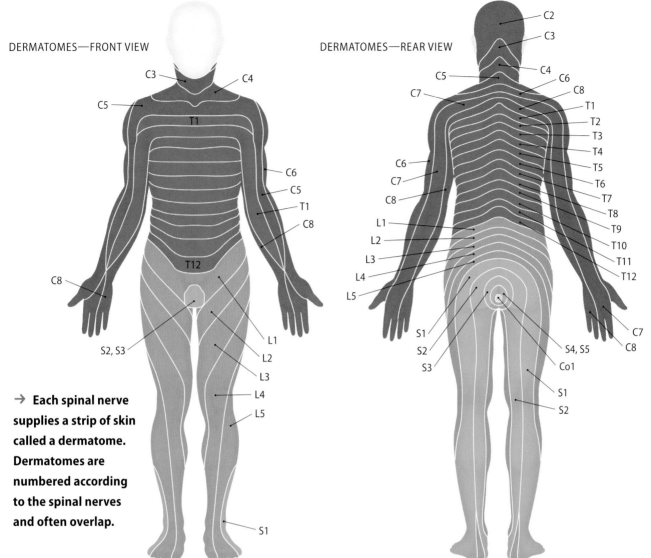

DERMATOMES—FRONT VIEW

DERMATOMES—REAR VIEW

→ **Each spinal nerve supplies a strip of skin called a dermatome. Dermatomes are numbered according to the spinal nerves and often overlap.**

Dermatomes and myotomes

The spinal cord is organized into a series of segments with spinal nerves attached to each. There are eight segments in the neck (cervical) region, twelve in the chest (thoracic) region, five in the lower back (lumbar region), five in the pelvic (sacral) region, plus a few in the tail (coccygeal) region. Each spinal nerve arising from these segments supplies a defined strip of skin called a dermatome, although there is considerable overlap between adjacent dermatomes.

This dermatomal arrangement is particularly obvious in the trunk of the body, where each nerve between the ribs (intercostal nerve) supplies a strip of skin between the ribs. Dermatomes also extend onto the limbs during embryonic development, but the growth of the limbs makes the dermatomes of the adult limb quite complex in arrangement.

Spinal cord segments also contain motor nerve cells that control the muscles of the limbs and trunk. This segmental organization of muscle control (myotomes) is relatively simple in the trunk, where intercostal nerves in the chest supply strips of intercostal muscle between the ribs. Some of these intercostal nerves extend into the abdominal wall as thoraco-abdominal nerves to supply strips of the muscle sheets that protect the abdomen. Much like the dermatomes, the myotome organization of motor control of the limbs is more complex than for the trunk, because migration of embryonic muscle cells during development stretches and distorts the segmental nature of spinal nerves to the limbs. Additionally, the spinal nerves supplying the limbs join and separate to form complex plexuses of nerves at the limb bases (brachial for the upper limb and lumbosacral for the lower limb).

Autonomic nervous system

Part of the nervous system is concerned with maintaining the body's internal environment and harnessing energy reserves during emergency situations. Because it acts automatically and is not under direct conscious control, this system is called the autonomic nervous system.

The autonomic nervous system (ANS) controls automatic functions in the internal organs of the chest, abdominal, and pelvic organs, as well as regulating sweat glands and the smooth muscle of blood vessel walls. There are three subdivisions of the ANS: the sympathetic, parasympathetic, and enteric systems. The sympathetic and parasympathetic divisions, discussed here, were traditionally described on the basis of the effects they produced on internal organs, but we now know that the simple division between the two is not an accurate reflection of reality. The enteric system is discussed on pp. 62–3.

The ANS contains clusters of nerve cells called ganglia, arranged in chains or clumps in the internal body cavities. The sympathetic and parasympathetic divisions both have chains of nerve cells in the pathways to the organs. Nerve cells with their bodies inside the central nervous system are called preganglionic. Their axons pass through the peripheral nervous system to contact postganglionic nerve cells in the many ganglia that make up both systems.

→ **Organs in the chest, abdomen, and pelvis are influenced by both the parasympathetic and sympathetic divisions of the autonomic nervous system. Autonomic innervation extends beyond these organs to include the muscles of the eyes, blood vessels, lacrimal and salivary glands, and muscles in the skin.**

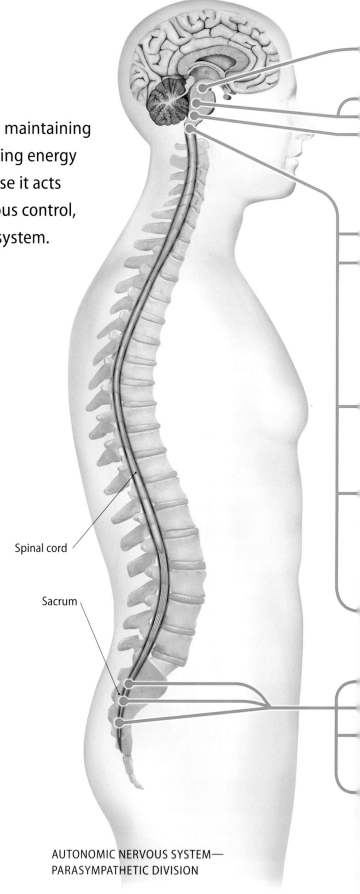

Spinal cord

Sacrum

AUTONOMIC NERVOUS SYSTEM—
PARASYMPATHETIC DIVISION

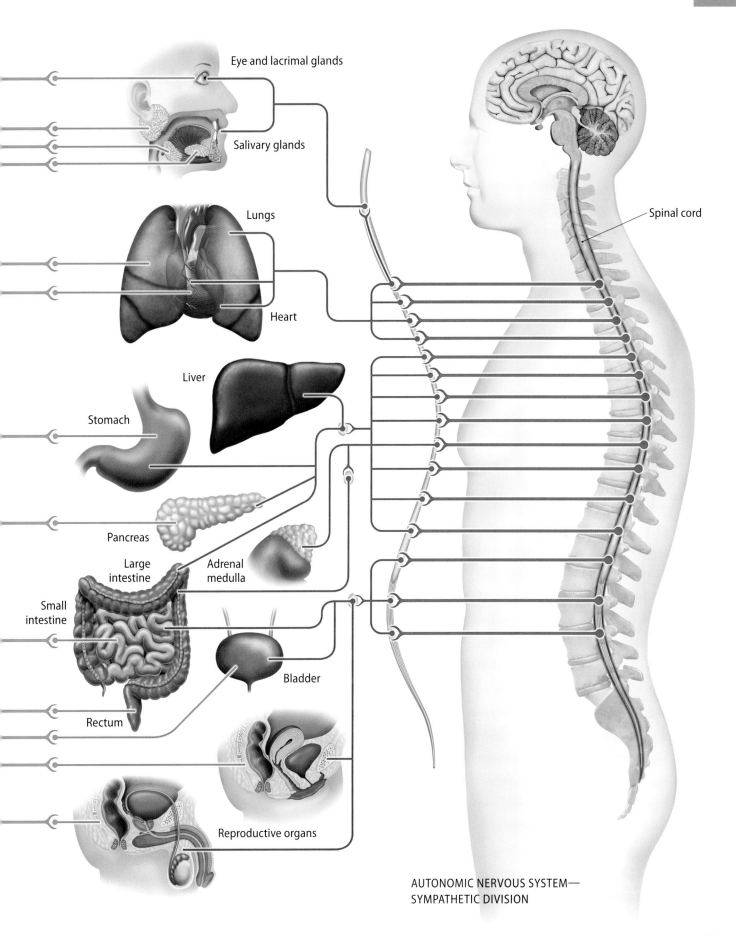

Eye and lacrimal glands

Salivary glands

Lungs

Heart

Liver

Stomach

Pancreas

Large intestine

Adrenal medulla

Small intestine

Bladder

Rectum

Reproductive organs

Spinal cord

AUTONOMIC NERVOUS SYSTEM—
SYMPATHETIC DIVISION

Regulating body temperature

Functions of the sympathetic nervous system are essential for controlling body temperature. The sympathetic nervous system controls blood flow to the skin: increasing flow to the skin when heat needs to be lost in hot weather; reducing blood flow when heat needs to be retained in cold weather. It also raises the fine hairs of the skin during cold weather (goose bumps) to reduce air flow at the skin and minimize loss of heat from the skin by conduction. In hot weather, the sympathetic nervous system activates the sweat glands to aid heat loss by evaporation.

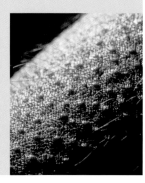

Sympathetic nervous system

The sympathetic division is mainly concerned with preparing the body for emergency action, situations where energy needs to be expended. Activation of the sympathetic nervous system increases heart rate, decreases gut movement, opens the airways, and diverts blood from the gut to the muscles.

Preganglionic nerve cells of the sympathetic nervous system are found in the lateral horn of the spinal cord in thoracic and upper lumbar levels (thoracolumbar outflow). The axons of the preganglionic nerve cells run in spinal nerves to a series of ganglia located alongside the vertebral column. This chain of ganglia is called the sympathetic trunk and extends from the base of the skull to the tip of the coccyx. The sympathetic trunk ganglia contain the postganglionic nerve cell bodies, and the axons of these cells run out to target organs in the skin (e.g., sweat glands or blood vessels). Some preganglionic axons pass through the sympathetic trunk without terminating, instead contacting postganglionic nerve cell bodies in ganglia in front of the vertebral column (the prevertebral ganglia). The postganglionic nerve cells in these ganglia then run axons out to target organs in the internal body cavities (heart, lungs, or gut). Yet other postganglionic nerve cells of the sympathetic nervous system have become modified during development to serve as endocrine glands (e.g., the adrenaline-producing cells of the center, or medulla, of the adrenal gland).

Parasympathetic nervous system

The general role of the parasympathetic division is to enhance energy storage. Activation of the parasympathetic nervous system will lower heart rate, reduce the output of blood from the heart, increase movement in the gut, and enhance absorption of nutrients from food.

Preganglionic nerve cells of the parasympathetic nervous system have their cell bodies in clusters within the brainstem and the sacral levels of the spinal cord. The axons of these nerve cells pass from the central nervous system either by the cranial nerves (facial, oculomotor, glossopharyngeal, and vagus) or by the pelvic splanchnic nerves (from sacral levels 2 to 4). The oculomotor nerve controls the muscles that constrict the pupil and change lens shape during focusing the eye on near objects. The facial and glossopharyngeal nerves carry axons that control the tear and salivary glands. The vagus is the most important parasympathetic cranial nerve, because it controls the internal organs of the entire chest cavity and most of the abdominal cavity. The pelvic splanchnic nerves from the spinal cord control the urinary bladder, rectum, and sexual organs. The preganglionic fibers in the parasympathetic nervous system are relatively long, so they contact postganglionic cell bodies located close to the target organs (e.g., the heart or urinary bladder).

Opposing and complementary roles

These two divisions of the ANS exert opposite effects for some organs (e.g., the sympathetic division increases heart rate, while the parasympathetic lowers it), but several parts of the body are predominantly controlled by one or the other. For example, the sweat glands and blood vessels of the limbs are exclusively controlled by

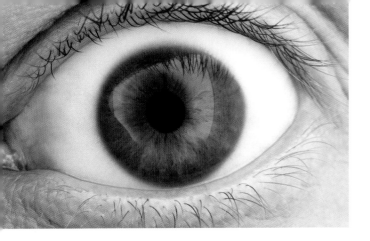

↑ **The pupil of the eye can be dilated (enlarged) by the sympathetic nervous system and constricted (narrowed) by the parasympathetic nervous system.**

the sympathetic nervous system. By contrast, the parasympathetic nervous system has the major control of the pupil and the bladder.

The sympathetic and parasympathetic divisions are traditionally treated as separate systems, but it is important to remember that the two divisions often act together to perform complex activities. For example, male sexual behavior depends on erection of the penis (produced by the parasympathetic division) that is seamlessly followed by ejaculation (controlled by the sympathetic division).

Furthermore, both of the so-called autonomic divisions are rarely activated in their entirety, so they should not be considered as functional blocks. It may be more accurate to consider each division as consisting of groups of functional pathways that act independently.

Internal organ sensation

An important part of the ANS is the visceral sensory component. This consists of sensory nerve cells whose axons accompany the parasympathetic and sympathetic motor pathways to organs. The functions of these visceral sensory nerve cells differ depending on whether they run in parasympathetic or sympathetic nerves. Sensory nerves associated with the parasympathetic nervous system carry information back to the brain or spinal cord about blood pressure, oxygen concentration of the blood, and fullness of the bladder and gut.

On the other hand, sensory nerve cells associated with the sympathetic nervous system carry information to the spinal cord about the distortion and inflammation of internal organs, which will be interpreted as pain by the person. Since this information is carried by spinal nerves to particular spinal cord segments, the pain will be interpreted as arising from the body surface or wall along particular dermatomes. This confusion of internal organ with body surface pain is known as referred pain and is an important symptom that clinicians use in the diagnosis of internal organ disease.

Neurotransmitters of the ANS

Preganglionic nerve cells of both sympathetic and parasympathetic divisions use acetylcholine as the neurotransmitter to activate postganglionic nerve cells. The situation with the postganglionic fibers is much more complex. Many axons may contain more than one type of chemical, with some chemicals acting to modify the action of the principal neurotransmitter.

For example, postganglionic nerve cells of the sympathetic division use a variety of neurotransmitters depending on where they terminate. Axons to blood vessels use adenosine triphosphate (ATP),

noradrenaline (NA), or neuropeptide Y (NPY); axons to sweat glands use acetylcholine (ACh), vasoactive intestinal peptide (VIP), peptide histidine methionine (PHM), or calcitonin gene-related peptide (CGRP); and axons to the smooth muscle that raises hairs on the skin (goose bumps) use NA.

Postganglionic nerve cells of the parasympathetic division also use different neurotransmitters depending on their target. Axons to the heart muscle use ACh; those to the smooth muscle of the gut use either ACh, ATP, nitric oxide (NO), or VIP; whereas those to the glands of the gut use ACh, NO, or VIP.

The little brain in your gut

The enteric nervous system controls the bodily processes involved in the movement and digestion of food in the gastrointestinal tract. From mouth to anus, it seems, the gut has a mind of its own.

How the enteric nervous system moves food through the gut

When a region of gut tube is dilated, sensory nerve cells known as intrinsic primary afferent nerve cells, or IPANS, are activated. These nerve cells have axons that run toward the mouth to induce activity in excitatory motor nerve cells and toward the anus to cause relaxation. Excitatory motor nerve cells may run up to 0.4 inches (11 mm) toward the mouth, whereas inhibitory motor nerve cells project up to about twice that length toward the anus. So when the gut tube is dilated by a lump of food, the gut muscle contracts above the lump to squeeze the food down, and the gut muscle relaxes below the lump to receive the food. When this process occurs in successive lengths of gut, the food is slowly but surely moved downstream.

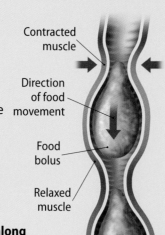

Contracted muscle

Direction of food movement

Food bolus

Relaxed muscle

→ **Food is moved along by squeezing from muscle above and relaxation of muscle below.**

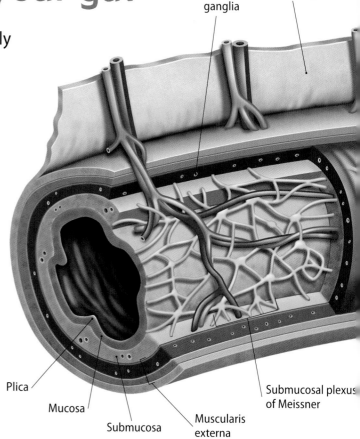

Myenteric ganglia

Mesentery

Plica

Mucosa

Submucosa

Muscularis externa

Submucosal plexus of Meissner

The wall of the gut, the gastrointestinal tube that starts at the mouth and ends at the anus, is endowed with a network of nerve cells and their processes collectively called the enteric nervous system. Many neuroscientists regard it as part of the autonomic nervous system (ANS), because it is an entirely self-regulating, automatic system that controls not only the activity of the smooth muscle and glands of the gut, but also absorption across the gut lining, and the local control of blood flow in the gut. It is surprisingly large, containing 100 million nerve cells, as many as in the spinal cord.

The enteric nervous system is made up of two networks (plexuses) of nerve cells and their axons in the wall of the gut: the submucosal plexus of Meissner is located just below the surface lining of the gut; and the myenteric plexus of Auerbach is found between the layers of smooth muscle, deeper in the gut wall. The submucosal plexus is principally concerned with

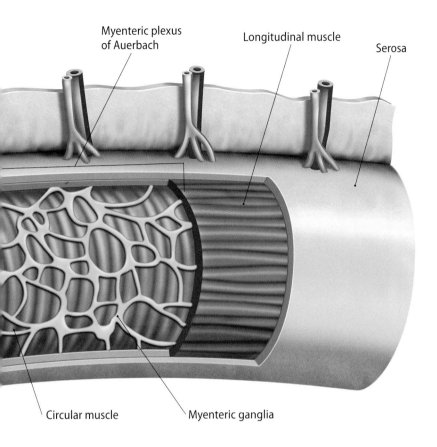

Myenteric plexus of Auerbach

Longitudinal muscle

Serosa

Circular muscle

Myenteric ganglia

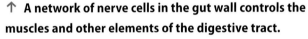

↑ **A network of nerve cells in the gut wall controls the muscles and other elements of the digestive tract.**

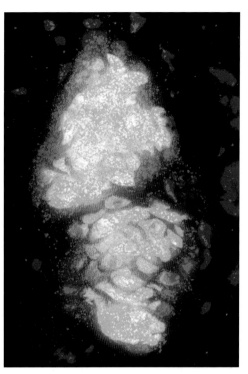

↑ **Nerve cells of the enteric nervous system (above) regulate the secretions of glands, and the contraction or relaxation of smooth muscle in the gut wall.**

the control of secretion from gut glands, while the myenteric plexus deals mainly with the regulation of gut movement.

The enteric nervous system at work

Like other parts of the nervous system, the enteric nervous system has sensory nerve cells that detect changes in the internal environment (e.g., stretching of the gut wall), interneurons that process that sensory information, and visceral motor nerve cells that produce changes in the smooth muscle and glands. This efficient network is able to produce coordinated movements by sequential contraction of smooth muscle in the gut wall to break up the gut contents into smaller chunks (segmentation) and to move those contents toward the anus (peristalsis). These movements can proceed even if the enteric nervous system is completely separated from the rest of the nervous system.

The enteric nervous system uses an array of neuro-transmitters, including nitric oxide, acetylcholine, adenosine triphosphate, and many neuropeptides. Working out how all this chemical variety translates to function is a goal for ongoing research in this area.

The little brain gets a little help

The enteric nervous system can act in isolation from the rest of the nervous system, but its activities can be modified by nerve impulses in the parasympathetic and sympathetic nervous systems. The parasympathetic nervous system tends to increase the activity of the smooth muscle and glands of the gut to improve the absorption of nutrients. By contrast, the sympathetic nervous system reduces the activity of gut glands through connections with the submucosal plexus; and reduces gut movement by lowering the activity of the excitatory motor nerve cells in the myenteric plexus.

Protecting the brain

The brain is soft, gelatinous, and vulnerable, so some form of protection is necessary to prevent injury to its delicate structure.

The brain is protected by bone, membrane, and fluid: an external rigid bony framework (the skull), a series of membranes to hold the brain in place (the meninges), and a fluid space to cushion brain movement (the cerebrospinal fluid in the subarachnoid space).

In the natural world, the brain is usually exposed to only the gentle acceleration of minor head-knocks, so the protective mechanisms evolved in the distant past are often inadequate for our modern high-speed world. For example, an automobile crash at high speed can cause sudden deceleration of the head from a velocity of 100 feet per second (nearly 70 miles per hour or 110 km per hour) to zero in less than 3 feet (1 m). This is equivalent to 30 to 40 times the force due to gravity and will overwhelm the mechanisms that have evolved to minimize brain injury.

The skull

The braincase is made up of a skull base including the occipital, sphenoid, petrous temporal, and frontal bones, which together form three bowl-shaped depressions into which the lower parts of the brain fit snugly. The upper parts of the brain are protected by a skullcap of flattened sheets of bone that are either extensions of

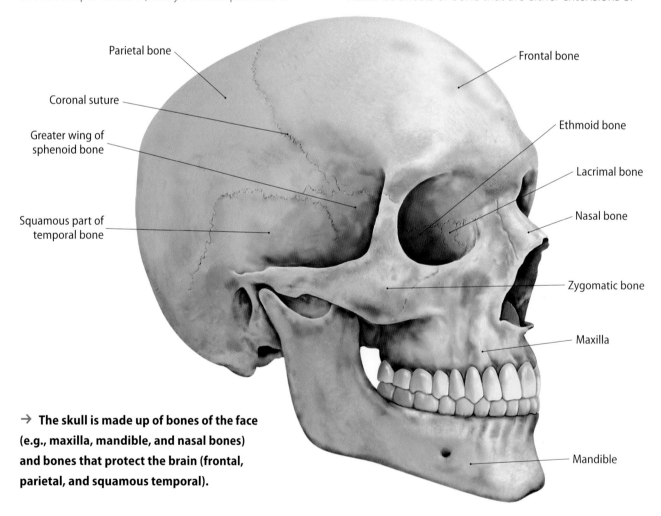

Parietal bone

Coronal suture

Greater wing of
sphenoid bone

Squamous part of
temporal bone

Frontal bone

Ethmoid bone

Lacrimal bone

Nasal bone

Zygomatic bone

Maxilla

Mandible

→ **The skull is made up of bones of the face
(e.g., maxilla, mandible, and nasal bones)
and bones that protect the brain (frontal,
parietal, and squamous temporal).**

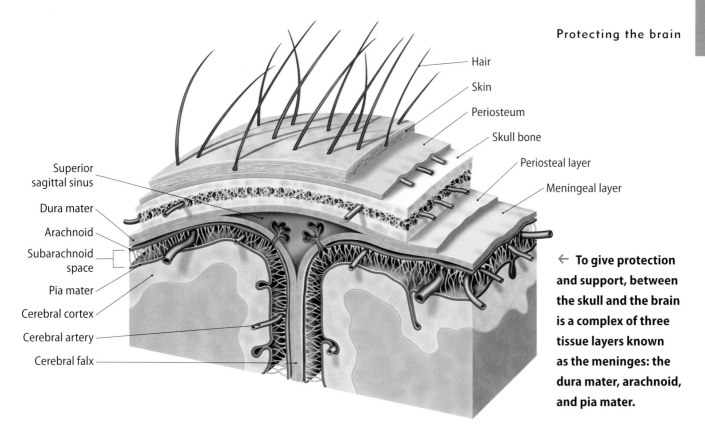

Hair
Skin
Periosteum
Skull bone
Periosteal layer
Meningeal layer

Superior sagittal sinus
Dura mater
Arachnoid
Subarachnoid space
Pia mater
Cerebral cortex
Cerebral artery
Cerebral falx

← **To give protection and support, between the skull and the brain is a complex of three tissue layers known as the meninges: the dura mater, arachnoid, and pia mater.**

the skull base bones (frontal, squamous temporal, and occipital bones) or confined to the skullcap region itself (parietal bone). In adults, these bones are joined together by tight fibrous joints with an interlocking joint-line like the edges of a jigsaw puzzle piece, but during fetal and early postnatal life the bones are only lightly attached to each other by fibrous tissue. This has some benefits during childbirth in that overlapping of the bones allows molding of the skull to squeeze through the narrow human birth canal.

The meninges and cerebrospinal fluid

For protection and cushioning, the brain and spinal cord are enclosed within three membranes called meninges: the dura mater, arachnoid, and pia mater. The dura mater forms a thick, strong membrane attached to the inside of the skull and reinforces the veins of the skull interior (dural venous sinuses). The folds of dura also form supporting walls between the two hemispheres in the midline and between the cerebral hemispheres and the cerebellum. When movements of the brain occur slowly in the skull (e.g., when a tumor grows), brain tissue may be injured by compression against these dural folds. Sudden movements during motor vehicle accidents may also throw the brain against these ridges and folds, tearing the delicate brain tissue.

The arachnoid is a delicate weblike tissue attached to the inner surface of the dura mater. It is separated from the pia mater by the subarachnoid space, containing cerebrospinal fluid (CSF) that provides a fluid space to cushion sudden brain movements during deceleration of the head. The CSF is discussed further on pp. 66–7.

The innermost layer of the meninges is the pia mater, which contains many blood vessels and follows every contour of the brain, so that it dips into all the grooves of the brain surface, carrying blood vessels with it.

The skull's weak spots

Although the rigid skull allows protection against most forces in the natural world, sudden application of extreme forces in our modern world can fracture the skull at its weak points. One of these is in the temple region, 1½–2 inches (4–5 cm) to the side and behind each eye, where thin sheets of bone from the frontal, temporal, sphenoid, and parietal bones come together. A blow here from a baseball, golf ball, or malicious boot will fracture the bones, cut the underlying artery, and cause serious bleeding inside the head.

Ventricles and cerebrospinal fluid

The deep interior of the brain contains fluid-filled spaces called the ventricles. These are the remnants of the embryonic tubular brain, but they are far more than developmental leftovers, because they play a critical role in the circulation of tissue fluid from the brain.

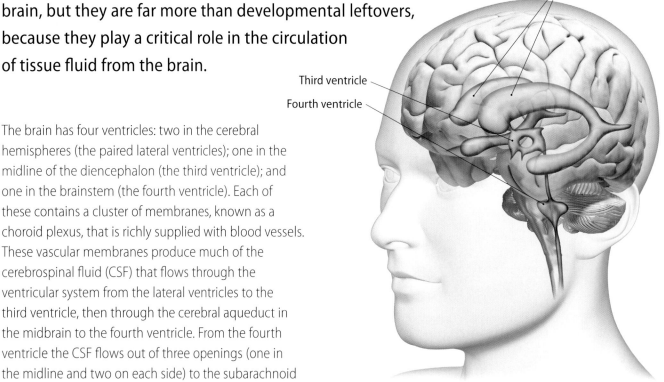

Lateral ventricles

Third ventricle

Fourth ventricle

↑ **Four fluid-filled spaces, the ventricles, lie deep inside the brain. The cerebrospinal fluid they contain bathes the surfaces of the central nervous system.**

The brain has four ventricles: two in the cerebral hemispheres (the paired lateral ventricles); one in the midline of the diencephalon (the third ventricle); and one in the brainstem (the fourth ventricle). Each of these contains a cluster of membranes, known as a choroid plexus, that is richly supplied with blood vessels. These vascular membranes produce much of the cerebrospinal fluid (CSF) that flows through the ventricular system from the lateral ventricles to the third ventricle, then through the cerebral aqueduct in the midbrain to the fourth ventricle. From the fourth ventricle the CSF flows out of three openings (one in the midline and two on each side) to the subarachnoid space around the brainstem. From here the fluid flows over the top of the brain to be absorbed into the venous blood at the reinforced venous channels, called the dural venous sinuses.

What is cerebrospinal fluid?

The CSF is essentially a clear fluid with dissolved ions (electrically charged atoms). The choroid plexus makes most CSF, but about 25–30 percent may come from brain tissue itself. The rate of production of the fluid is about 1 US pint (500 ml) per day, and this rate is relatively constant regardless of changes in blood pressure. The total volume of the CSF is about 12 cubic inches (200 ml), so the entire CSF is replaced two to three times each day. The CSF is similar in composition to the plasma of the blood (the fluid part without the red blood cells), but is richer in magnesium and chloride and poorer in potassium and calcium than you would expect if it were simply filtered blood. The cerebrospinal fluid has very few cells and proteins, unless micro-organisms reach the meninges and induce an immune response (meningitis). The watery cushion of the CSF fills the subarachnoid space, protecting the central nervous system from blows and trauma, and providing buoyancy. The CSF also contributes to control of the composition of the tissue around nerve cells, because tissue fluid from the brain continually drains to the CSF spaces. The CSF buffers changes in the volume of the intracranial space: if a tumor grows inside the brain, the volume of CSF may be reduced to accommodate the increased brain volume. The CSF also provides a route for neuroactive hormones secreted in the brain to move through the nervous system.

Blockage of CSF pathways

The CSF is replaced a few times each day, so obstruction of the CSF pathways will cause accumulation of the fluid in those parts of the ventricle system that are "upstream." In fetuses or infants with unfused skulls, this will cause enlargement of the ventricles, like expanding balloons, and swelling of the entire head, a condition called hydrocephaly. The resulting stretching of the young brain tissue tears axons and kills nerve cells. In adults, who have a fused skull, the accumulation of CSF will cause severe headaches and vomiting without enlargement of the skull.

Tapping the spine's fluid

The cerebrospinal fluid may be sampled by a lumbar puncture. In this procedure, also called a spinal tap, a needle is inserted into the lower back and through to the subarachnoid space surrounding the nerve fibers below the end of the spinal cord. The sample can be examined by microscope for the presence of blood (indicating hemorrhage into the subarachnoid space), bacteria, yeast, or parasites; analyzed for inflammatory molecules like antibodies (indicating inflammatory processes); or cultured for the presence of microorganisms (indicating bacterial meningitis).

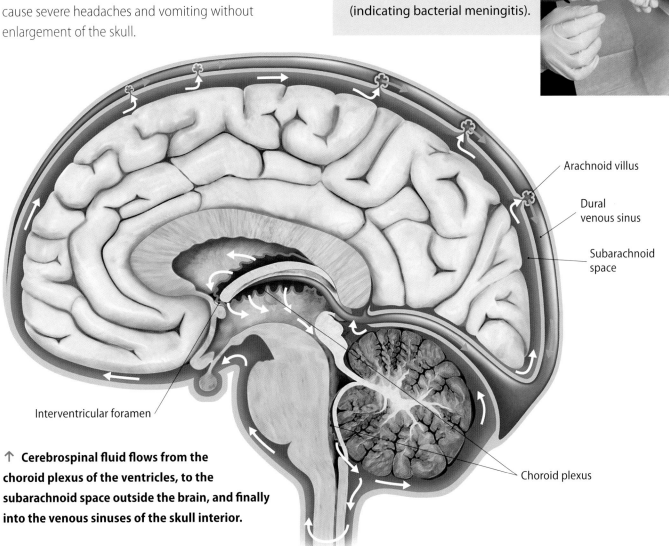

Arachnoid villus

Dural venous sinus

Subarachnoid space

Interventricular foramen

Choroid plexus

↑ **Cerebrospinal fluid flows from the choroid plexus of the ventricles, to the subarachnoid space outside the brain, and finally into the venous sinuses of the skull interior.**

Blood supply to the brain

Like other organs, the brain has an arterial supply to bring nutrients and oxygen from the heart; a capillary bed for exchange of oxygen, nutrients, and waste products with the brain tissue; and veins to drain blood back to the heart. But there are some special features of the brain that make its blood supply a little different.

The brain is very expensive metabolically, with a huge demand for oxygen and nutrients: the human brain makes up only 2 percent of the body weight but consumes 16–20 percent of the body's oxygen and nutrients. Interruption of the arterial supply for just a few seconds can cause the death of large volumes of brain tissue. And, because we walk upright, our brains are up to 18 inches (45 cm) above the heart, so arterial blood must be pumped uphill and the pressure inside cerebral veins may fall below that of the atmosphere. The biggest veins inside the skull are reinforced with a tough layer of dura mater (dural venous sinuses) to prevent collapse.

Arteries to the brain

Oxygenated and nutrient-rich blood from the left ventricle of the heart passes through one of four arteries to reach the brain. At the front of the neck are the paired internal carotid arteries that supply blood to most of the forebrain, including the bulk of the cerebral cortex. Two other (vertebral) arteries ascend through the vertebrae of the neck and enter the interior of the skull through the large hole in the occipital bone called the foramen magnum. The vertebral arteries supply the brainstem, cerebellum, and the back (occipital) parts of the cerebral cortex in a group of arteries known as the vertebro-basilar system.

The blood–brain barrier

The lining cells of the cerebral capillaries have very tight junctions between them. This blood–brain barrier maintains the special environment of the brain and protects its tissue from potentially damaging proteins in the blood, but it can be a problem when clinicians want to get therapeutic drugs into the brain. Other barriers are found at the interface between the brain tissue and the subarachnoid space, and between brain tissue and the ventricular system.

← **An MRI scan reveals some of the cerebral arteries. In the center is the circle of Willis, where the vertebral and carotid arteries from the neck are interconnected.**

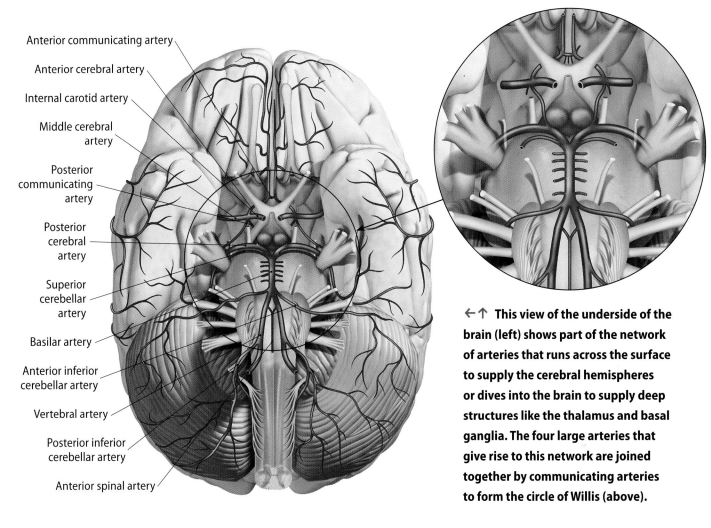

Anterior communicating artery

Anterior cerebral artery

Internal carotid artery

Middle cerebral artery

Posterior communicating artery

Posterior cerebral artery

Superior cerebellar artery

Basilar artery

Anterior inferior cerebellar artery

Vertebral artery

Posterior inferior cerebellar artery

Anterior spinal artery

←↑ **This view of the underside of the brain (left) shows part of the network of arteries that runs across the surface to supply the cerebral hemispheres or dives into the brain to supply deep structures like the thalamus and basal ganglia. The four large arteries that give rise to this network are joined together by communicating arteries to form the circle of Willis (above).**

Smaller branches of these four arteries run in the subarachnoid space across the surface of the brain and follow the pia mater membrane as it dips into the grooves and fissures of the brain surface. Many important penetrating arteries supply the deep groups of nerve cells in the basal ganglia and the large axon bundles that connect the cerebral cortex with lower parts of the brain.

The circle of Willis

Ongoing supply of blood to the brain is so critical that there is a circle of arteries around the base of the brain that connects all four of the arteries. This allows arterial supply to be maintained even if one vessel is obstructed. The communicating arteries that join the four big ones are usually quite small, but can enlarge progressively if the obstruction to flow develops slowly. Although all human brains have some form of the circle of Willis,

there is much variation in the size of both the main and communicating arteries that make up the circle.

Regulation of arterial flow to the brain

Although the brain is very metabolically active, it has no way to store either oxygen or glucose (its main energy source). It is therefore vital that the flow of blood to the brain is kept at a constant rate regardless of changes in blood pressure. The cerebral blood vessels themselves are one of the sites at which this auto-regulation takes place. The smooth muscle in the walls of cerebral arteries contracts when blood pressure is high, raising resistance to flow, and relaxes when blood pressure is low, lowering resistance to flow. There are also local regulatory mechanisms in the brain tissue itself. When nerve cells are more active they release the neuro-transmitter glutamate, which causes the release of chemicals to open cerebral vessels.

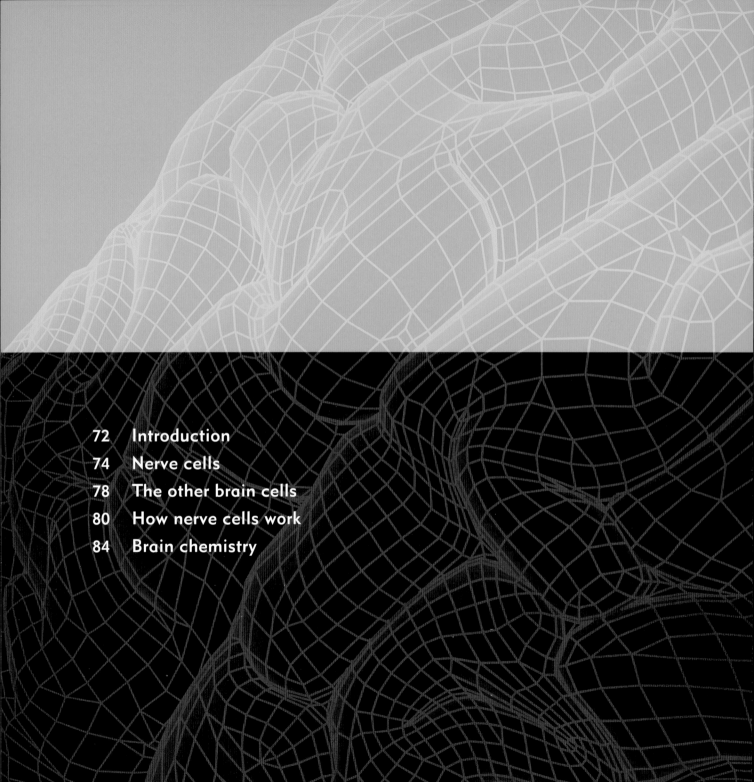

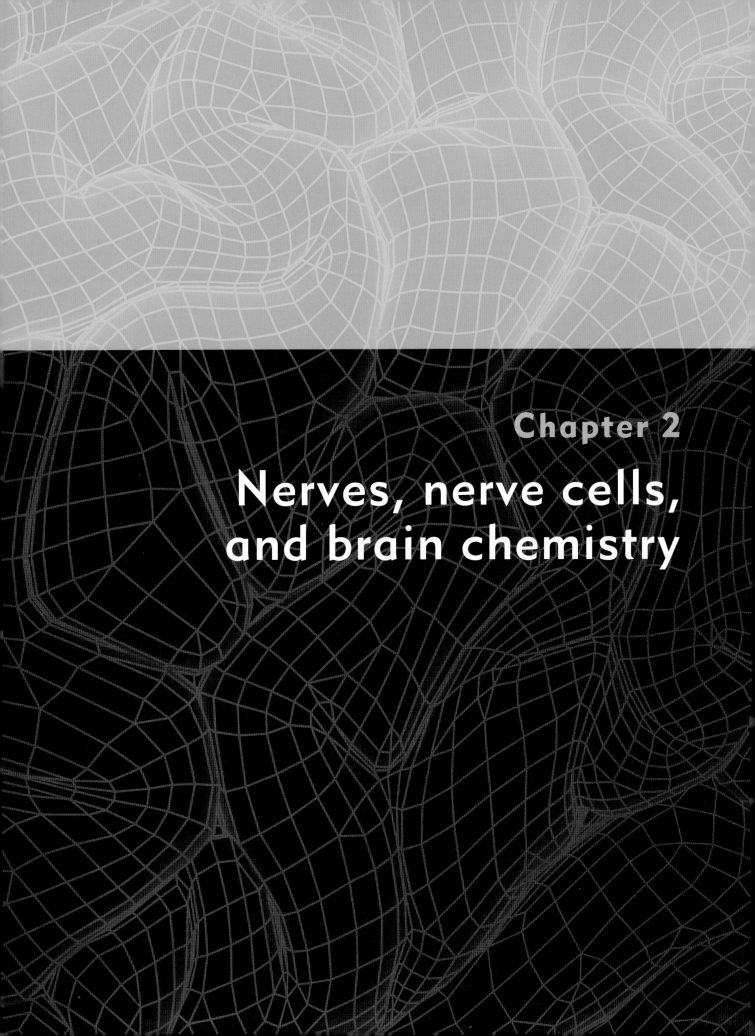

Chapter 2

Nerves, nerve cells, and brain chemistry

Introduction

To better understand how the brain and spinal cord control our sensations, thoughts, voluntary actions, and much more, we need to know about the fundamental unit of the nervous system—the nerve cell—as well as its supporting cells and chemical and electrical networks.

Nerve cells, also called neurons, are concerned with processing information and transferring that information to other nerve cells in the complex networks that make up the brain. It is tempting to compare nerve cells to components in electronic circuits, but although there are some similarities, there are also significant differences.

Electrical and chemical signaling

Nerve cells must be able to transfer information over large distances (more than 3 feet/1 m in some cases) with no, or minimal, loss of signal. They achieve this by a mechanism known as the action potential. The action potential is a moving wave of change in the electrical state of the membrane of the axon, the nerve cell's elongated projection. It has the important feature of being "all-or-none." In other words, once an action potential is started it runs to completion, spreading down the axon to the end. Trains, or sequences, of action potentials running down an axon provide the highly reliable transmission of data. Most nerve cells convey information down their axon by the number of action potentials per second.

Once an action potential reaches the end of the axon, information must be signaled to other nerve cells. At this point, nerve cells can use either a chemical or electrical mechanism, but the chemical method is more usual. Chemical transmission depends on the release of chemical messenger molecules called neurotransmitters onto the surface of another nerve cell. Neurotransmitters, in turn, induce electrical changes in the membranes of the nerve cells they contact, leading to changes in the electrical behavior of those cells and in the passage of information further down the chain of nerve cells.

Support from other cells

Nerve cells are so specialized for their task of processing information that they need several groups of other cells to support them and keep their local environment in an optimal state. These cells make the fatty sheath around the axons to assist electrical conduction, or keep the balance of charged atoms and chemicals in the tissue space outside the nerve cells at the most suitable level for nerve cell function. Other cells act as sentinels, monitoring brain tissue for invaders and signaling the body's immune system when defense is necessary.

The tissue of the brain has so many delicate processes packed tightly together that special barriers must be put in place to stop large molecules, bacteria, and even the body's own red blood cells from entering it. These barriers are found between the brain tissue and the fluid spaces around it (the blood and cerebrospinal fluid) and depend on special tight junctions between the lining cells of cerebral blood vessels. Many of the support cells also have processes that contact blood vessels and assist with the transfer of nutrients to nerve cells.

→ **Central nervous tissue is made up of nerve cells and supporting cells (astrocytes, oligodendrocytes, and microglia), as well as blood vessels, and cells that line the ventricles (ependymal cells).**

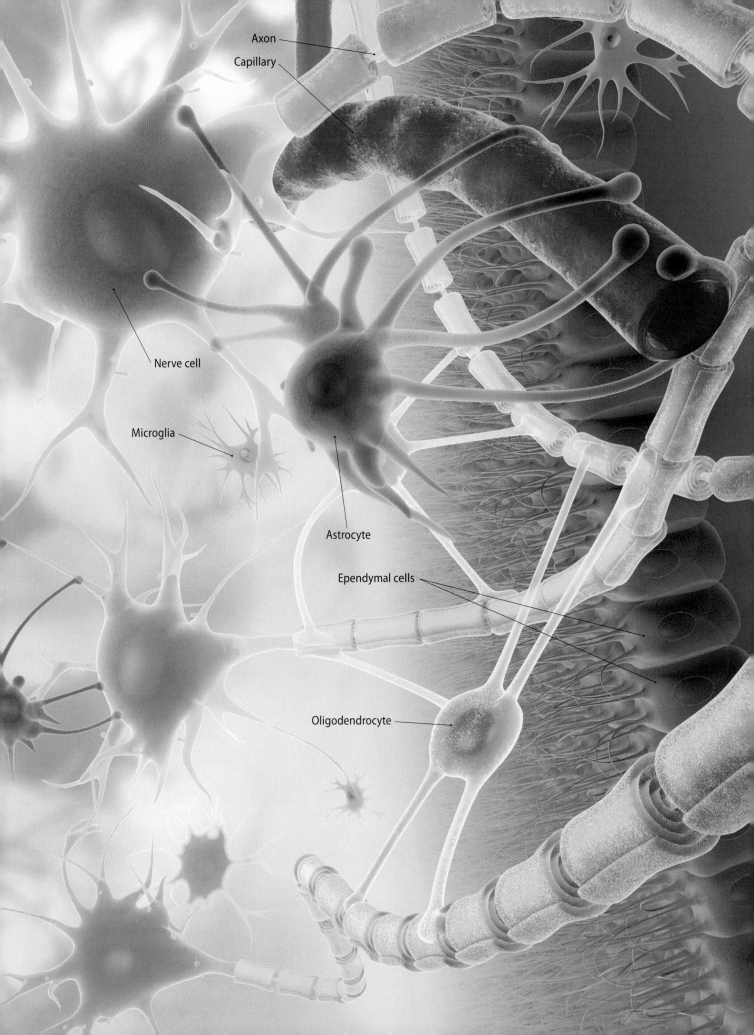

Axon

Capillary

Nerve cell

Microglia

Astrocyte

Ependymal cells

Oligodendrocyte

Nerve cells

Nerve cells are specialized cells found in the nervous system that conduct nerve impulses. They are like cells elsewhere in the body in that they have a nucleus and surrounding cytoplasm, but they also have special features that serve their information-processing function.

A typical nerve cell has a body that, like other cells, contains a nucleus and the surrounding cytoplasm. The nucleus contains the genetic information (in the form of the genetic code of DNA) responsible for directing the chemical activity of the nerve cell. Nerve cells often have a well-developed nucleolus inside the nucleus. The nucleolus directs the manufacture of chains of nucleic acids called messenger RNA, which then move from the nucleus to the rest of the cell body to instruct the manufacture of protein.

The cytoplasm around the nucleus contains all the chemical machinery to produce usable energy for the nerve cells, manufacture proteins and chemical messengers (neurotransmitters), and package these substances ready for transport to distant parts of the cell. Energy is produced in structures called mitochondria; small protein factory units called ribosomes make the proteins and some neurotransmitters; and the manufactured materials are packaged for transport in the Golgi apparatus.

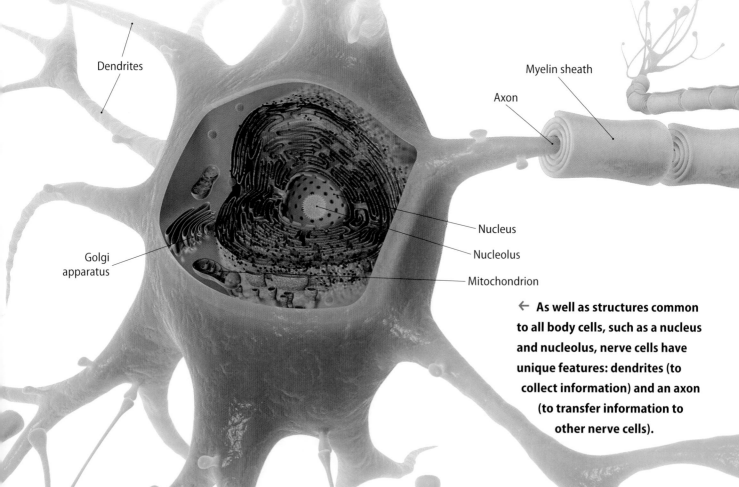

Dendrites

Myelin sheath

Axon

Golgi apparatus

Nucleus

Nucleolus

Mitochondrion

← **As well as structures common to all body cells, such as a nucleus and nucleolus, nerve cells have unique features: dendrites (to collect information) and an axon (to transfer information to other nerve cells).**

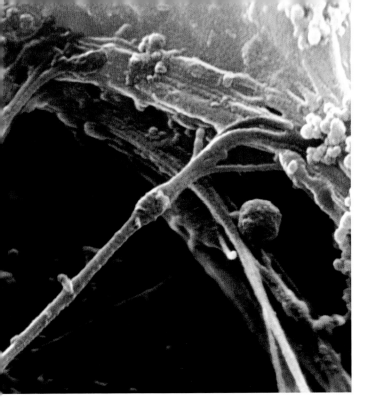

Multiple sclerosis and the vanishing myelin sheath

The proteins contained in myelin are powerful inducers of immune responses. If the body mounts an immune response against its own central nervous system myelin, the resulting disease is called multiple sclerosis. This is a serious disease characterized by recurring bouts of loss of myelin (plaques) in the brain, optic nerves, and spinal cord. Loss of the myelin sheath causes disordered conduction of nerve impulses along the affected axons.

↑ **At the top of this micrograph is the surface of a nerve cell (yellow) on which the nerve axons (pink) have formed synapses.**

What sets a nerve cell apart

The structures discussed above are present in all body cells, but the nerve cell possesses two distinctive features associated with its information-processing role. These are the fine branching projections called dendrites, and a single elongated projection, the axon.

A typical nerve cell has a widely branching dendritic tree, which consists of dendrites extending for up to 0.2 inches (several millimeters) in some cases. The dendritic tree receives information from other nerve cells, usually by chemical synapses, sites where neuro-transmitters are released onto discrete areas of the surface of the dendrite. The dendritic tree carries electrical impulses toward the body of the nerve cell.

Axons may extend for distances from 0.01 inches (a few tenths of a millimeter) to almost 3 feet (1 m) in the case of some nerve cells with axons that run down the spinal cord. Long axons are usually seen in the main nerve pathways that control motor function or carry sensory information up from the spinal cord. The end of the axon may be widely branched, so that one nerve cell can make contact with many other nerve cells.

Axons carry impulses away from the body of the nerve cell. The electrical transmission of impulses down the axon is made both faster and more reliable by a special fatty substance called myelin that surrounds the axon (the myelin sheath). The very end of each axon (axon terminal) may terminate in fine, buttonlike processes, called terminal boutons, which are the sites of direct contact with the dendritic trees, nerve cell bodies, or even the axons of other nerve cells.

Through their dendrites and axons, nerve cells connect together to form nerve circuits, in much the same way that a computer is made up of many electrical components joined together to form electrical circuits.

Nerve cells' skeleton and transport system

Within the axon, and some parts of the nerve cell body, there is a network of strands known as neurofilaments, which provide the skeleton of the nerve cell. They give strength to the nerve cell body and maintain its shape.

Neurotubules are tiny tubular structures that provide a transport system through the cell body, the dendrites, and along the length of the axon. There are two types of transport along the axon: fast and slow. Fast transport (4–16 inches, or 10–40 cm per day) is designed to move neurotransmitters, the enzymes that make neurotrans-mitters, and membrane components to the end of the axon. Slow transport (0.004–0.08 inches, or 0.1–2 mm per day) moves the components of the cell skeleton down to the end of the axon to rebuild the internal structure of the nerve cell. Transport back from the axon end to the cell body is important for sampling of the local environment at the axon terminal. This "backward transport" is particularly important during development, when axons must sample the region through which they are growing in order to choose the correct path. It is also used to remove debris, but this can be dangerous if the debris being removed to the cell body is infectious, e.g., the viruses that cause rabies or poliomyelitis.

Gray and white matter

When the first neuroanatomists began to study brains recently removed from the skull, they noticed that some parts of the brain had a grayish color, whereas other parts were whiter in appearance. We now know that the gray matter contains the nerve cell bodies and dendrites with some axon ends, while the white matter is devoid of nerve cell bodies and consists of tightly massed axons with myelin sheaths—the white coloration is due to the high content of fat from the myelin wrappings of the axons. In some parts of the brain the gray matter is on the outside and the white matter contained within (e.g.,

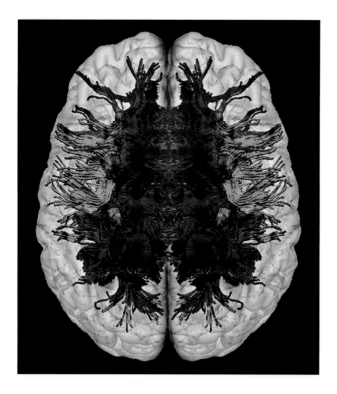

the cerebral cortex), whereas other parts of the central nervous system (e.g., the spinal cord) have the gray matter in a central core, surrounded by white matter. Other parts of the brain (e.g., the brainstem) have gray and white matter mixed together, but the white matter is usually formed into columns, ribbons, or tracts.

Types of nerve cells

Nerve cells come in an astonishing variety of shapes and sizes that reflect their function. The variety largely hinges on the shape of the dendritic tree, but some nerve cells also have remarkably complex axons.

The simplest type of nerve cell has a cell body and just one or two processes. These include the sensory ganglion cells that carry information from sense organs in the skin, muscles, joints, or gut wall into the central nervous system. The nerve cell bodies are located in clusters outside the central nervous system (in the sensory ganglia on cranial or spinal nerves). One process of the cell runs out to the skin or joint; the other runs into the spinal cord or brainstem. In the case of sensory ganglion cells carrying information about fine touch or vibration from the foot, the process from the foot to the cell body may be as long as 3 feet (about 1 m), and the process entering the spinal cord may run for up to about 2 feet (60 cm) to the brainstem before making a contact on another nerve cell.

Deeper inside the nervous system are nerve cells with extraordinarily complex shapes. The most striking example is the Purkinje cell, found in the cerebellum. Purkinje cells consist of a cell body with a complex dendritic tree that spreads in a fanlike shape oriented at right angles to the folds of the surface of the cerebellum. The fan-shaped dendritic tree is designed to provide a large surface area for contacts from the axons of other nerve cells.

← **White matter consists of masses of axons. This 3-D scan allows us to see the normal orientation of white matter fibers in a top view of the brain. Descending and ascending fibers are in green, corpus callosum in red, and local connections in purple.**

Turning stimuli in the physical world into nerve signals

Some types of sensory cells are highly specialized for their function. For example, photoreceptors in the retina are highly specialized to respond to the impact of light packets (photons). They turn this impact into electrical signals (a process called photonic transduction) that will eventually be interpreted in the brain as visual information. Other sensory cells in the inner ear are specialized for mechanical transduction, which is the process of converting the mechanical distortion of fine hairs on the tip of the cell—such as occurs when a pressure wave in the inner ear moves across the cell—into electrical signals that can be sent to the brain to be interpreted as sound.

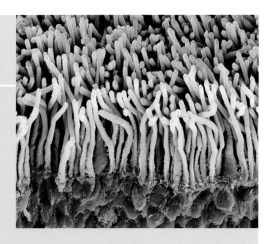

↑ **Photoreceptors in the retina of the eye turn information in photons of light into electrical signals.**

↓ **These two Purkinje nerve cells are growing in a lab in tissue culture. Their cell bodies extend dendrites across the surface of the culture dish.**

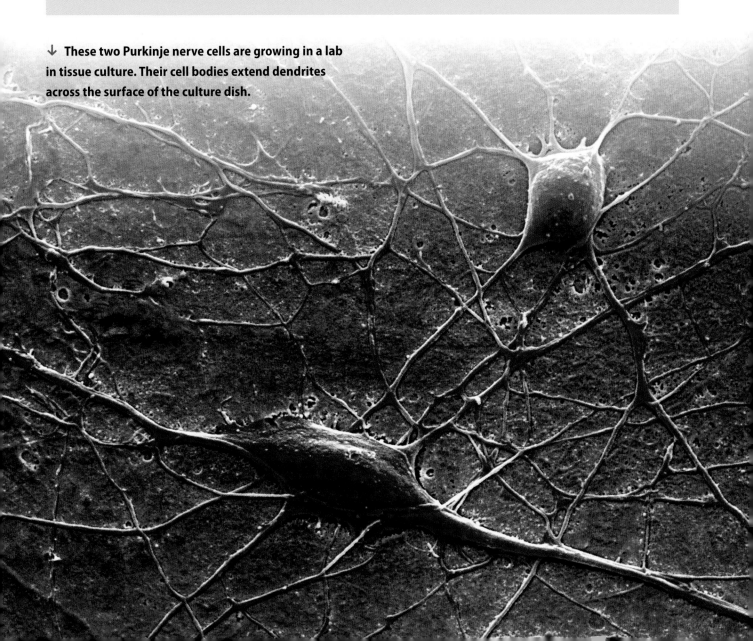

The other brain cells

Apart from nerve cells, the other large group of cells in the brain is the glia. Glial cells make up the brain's connective tissue and carry out such tasks as transporting nutrients, helping nerve cells to grow and function properly, fending off pathogens, and repairing damage.

Glial cells are named after the Greek for "glue," because early neuroscientists imagined that they formed a glue to hold the nerve cells together. Glia do make an important contribution to holding central nervous tissue together and serve the same function as connective tissue elsewhere in the body, although they have many other functions too.

Glia are about as numerous as nerve cells. The three main glial cell types are astrocytes, oligodendrocytes, and microglia.

↓ **Glial cells like these make up about half the volume of the brain and spinal cord.**

Astrocytes
These star-shaped cells come in two different types: fibrous astrocytes, found in white matter, and protoplasmic astrocytes, in gray matter. Both have cell processes that end in expansions called end-feet. These surround the capillaries of the brain and the pia mater of the meninges to control the concentrations of ions in the tissue fluid and the transfer of chemicals through the tissue spaces. Other end-feet cover the dendrites and cell bodies of nerve cells and those surfaces of axons that are not covered by myelin. These latter contacts allow the astrocytes to control the concentration of ions (sodium and chloride) around the parts of the axons where nerve impulses (action potentials)

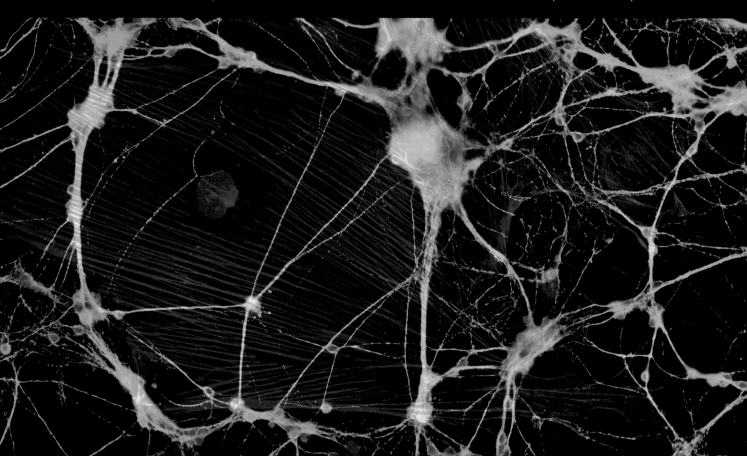

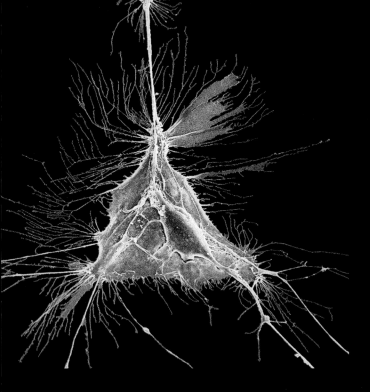

← **Oligodendrocytes, such as the one shown here, form the myelin sheaths around nerve fibers in the central nervous system.**

many different axons by wrapping its process repeatedly around each axon. Those parts of the axon not covered by oligodendrocyte processes are contacted by the end-feet of astrocytes.

Microglia

Microglia are smaller than the other glia and serve an immune protective function in the brain and spinal cord. Their primary role is to engulf debris (a process called phagocytosis) and present the foreign molecules to other immune system cells to induce an immune response. When nerve cells die during development or after injury or disease, microglia clean up the cellular debris. Microglia also produce molecules that attract other immune cells, such as white blood cells, from the blood to enter the brain and start an immune response.

The activity of microglia is increased in the brains of patients infected with Human Immunodeficiency Virus Type 1 (HIV-1). This virus does not directly affect nerve cells, but causes microglia to produce toxic molecules called cytokines, which are damaging to nerve cells. The resulting damage causes loss of nerve cells and a type of AIDS-related dementia.

are elicited. Astrocytes also transfer the chemical products of metabolism to and from nerve cells and are able to form dense scars in brain tissue after injury.

Oligodendrocytes

Oligodendrocytes (from the Greek for "cell with a few branches") serve the vital function of forming the myelin sheath around axons in the central nervous system (in the peripheral nervous system, Schwann cells do this). The myelin sheath insulates the axon and makes the transmission of electrical impulses down the axon both faster and more reliable. A single oligodendrocyte may form myelin sheaths around

The trouble with glia

Glial cells retain the ability to divide into daughter cells well into adult life, unlike nerve cells. This has its dangers, because glia and their precursors can give rise to certain highly aggressive brain tumors. Another problem with glia concerns brain repair. When the brain or spinal cord is injured, glial cells mobilize to clean up the debris. They leave behind a glial scar, which seals off the wound, but it can also interfere with the regrowth of axons.

→ **A very malignant glial cell tumor, or glioblastoma, shows as an orange patch in these CT scans of the brain.**

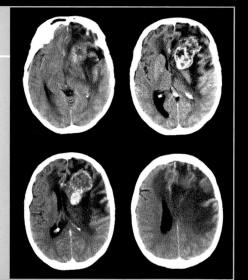

How nerve cells work

Nerve cells have a fundamental role of processing and communicating information. Some of the information processing is achieved at the level of the individual nerve cell, but most information processing requires networks of nerve cells acting together.

Nerve cells perform their information-processing functions in part by the spread of electrical impulses through their appendages. These impulses may be spread in two ways: passively, i.e., without any active changes of the channels in the nerve cell membrane that allow the movement of charged particles (positively charged sodium or potassium atoms) across the membrane; or actively, by the activation of an "all-or-none" change in the electrical properties of the membrane that must run to completion.

Active or passive?

Passive, or electrotonic, spread of electrical signal is best seen in the dendrites of nerve cells. The dendrites of a nerve cell may be contacted by thousands of synapses (nerve junctions). Each synapse is a site where the nerve cell membrane is bombarded with neurotransmitter chemicals that cause changes in the electrical properties of the dendritic

membrane by opening channels in the nerve cell membrane and allowing charged particles to move across the membrane. The activation of each of these sites creates a spreading electrical field down the dendritic tree toward the cell body. The sum of all these spreading electrical fields from thousands of synaptic sites will influence the total electrical activity of the nerve cell at the cell body. Both the shape of the dendritic tree and the relative positions of different types of synapses (whether excitatory—increasing activity; or inhibitory—decreasing activity) profoundly influences the sum activity in the nerve cell as a whole. This is one mechanism by which decision-making occurs in nerve networks.

Active spread of an electrical signal is called an action potential, or nerve impulse. This is a spreading wave of electrical activity that flows down an axon to its end. Action potentials are initiated at the axon hillock, the region where the axon is attached to the nerve cell

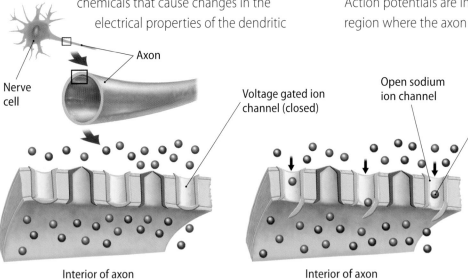

Axon

Nerve cell

Voltage gated ion channel (closed)

Open sodium ion channel

Sodium ion moving through open ion channel

Interior of axon
Sodium ion channels closed before or after action potential

Interior of axon
Sodium ion channels open during action potential

← **The membranes of nerve cell axons have tiny channels that can be opened to permit the movement of ions across the membrane. These movements change the voltage across the membrane and underlie the action potential.**

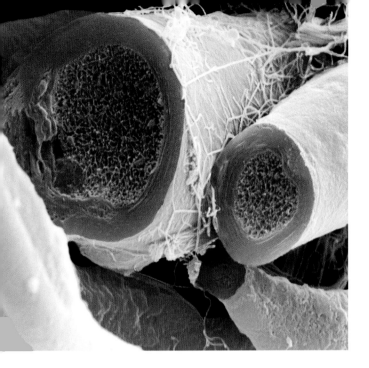

The fastest axons in the body

Some of the largest and most thickly myelinated nerve fibers in the human body are those that either carry information about muscle stretch (proprioception), or control the voluntary muscles themselves. This is because the precise control of voluntary movement (e.g., in running, jumping, or dancing) needs rapid information flow, more than any other system in the body. Pain fibers conduct more slowly.

↑ **A nerve axon's myelin sheath (colored pink in this micrograph) is an insulating layer that allows the rapid and efficient conduction of nerve impulses.**

body. Some nerve cells generate action potentials continuously (tonically active), whereas others generate action potentials only when stimulated (phasically active). Regardless of which type it is, the chance that a given nerve cell will produce an action potential is strongly influenced by the strengths of the passively spreading electrical fields generated in the dendritic tree by synaptic inputs from other cells.

How an action potential is generated
The initiation of an action potential depends on the opening of tiny channels in the nerve cell membrane that allow sodium atoms to enter. This changes the voltage across the membrane (a process known as depolarization) and is followed a few thousandths of a second later by the opening of tiny channels that allow potassium atoms to flow out of the cell to return the voltage across the membrane to normal (a process called afterhyperpolarization).

The important point is that depolarization in one part of the axon (usually the axon hillock) will induce currents around the axon that activate sodium channels in the next segment of axon, thereby spreading the wave of depolarization down the axon as an action

potential. Axons may perform this process hundreds to thousands of times per second, and information is usually conveyed by the number of times per second that an action potential is activated. So a strongly painful stimulus elicits many more action potentials per second in a pain fiber than a faintly painful stimulus.

Moving impulses faster with myelin
Given that information is conveyed by nerve impulses, you would expect that faster impulse conduction would allow the nervous system to do its work more quickly. The speed of an action potential depends on the diameter of the axon (the fatter the axon, the faster the conduction) and whether it is wrapped in a fatty substance called myelin. An axon without a myelin sheath (e.g., some pain fibers) can carry nerve impulses at only 19 inches (50 cm) per second. If the axon is coated with myelin, the speed of the nerve impulse may reach as high as 330 feet (100 m) per second.

The myelin sheath can be thought of as the insulation that surrounds an electrical wire, but the analogy is incomplete: the myelin sheath is not a continuous coat along the entire length of the axon, but a series of little coats down the axon with intervening spaces (the nodes of Ranvier). The nerve impulse runs down a myelinated axon by causing depolarization *only* at the nodes of Ranvier. This jumping activation is called saltatory conduction (from *saltare*, Latin for "to jump") and is much faster than activating every part of the axon.

Chemical synapses

We have seen how signals arise in and travel along the axons of individual nerve cells. But how do nerve cells communicate with each other? Most nerve cells do so by means of chemical synapses. These use special chemicals called neurotransmitters, which are stored within tiny synaptic vesicles in the buttonlike end of the axon of one nerve cell and released on demand to act on the membranes of another nerve cell. They are usually released into a minute space called the synaptic cleft, a region that lies between the membrane of the axon terminal of one nerve cell (presynaptic membrane) and the membranes of the dendrites, cell body, or even the axon of another nerve cell (postsynaptic membrane). This synaptic cleft is minuscule (perhaps less than a thousandth the diameter of a human hair) and

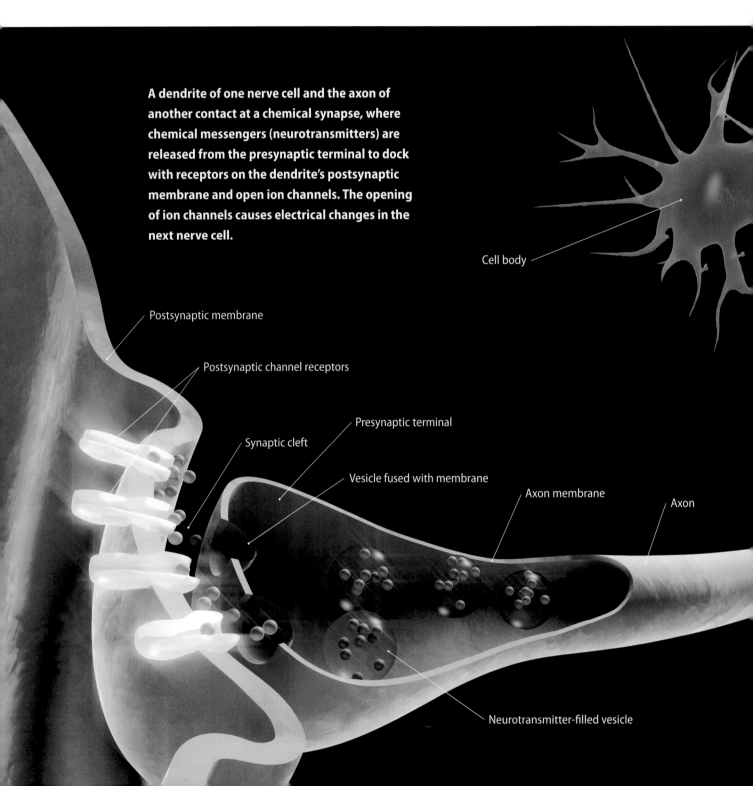

A dendrite of one nerve cell and the axon of another contact at a chemical synapse, where chemical messengers (neurotransmitters) are released from the presynaptic terminal to dock with receptors on the dendrite's postsynaptic membrane and open ion channels. The opening of ion channels causes electrical changes in the next nerve cell.

Cell body

Postsynaptic membrane

Postsynaptic channel receptors

Synaptic cleft

Presynaptic terminal

Vesicle fused with membrane

Axon membrane

Axon

Neurotransmitter-filled vesicle

chemicals released into this space will bind with complex structures in the nerve cell membrane called receptors. When a neurotransmitter binds to a receptor it will initiate changes in the conductance of the membrane to different ions (e.g. sodium, potassium, or chloride ions). These changes in conductance of the membrane will in turn cause changes to the electrical properties of the nerve cell.

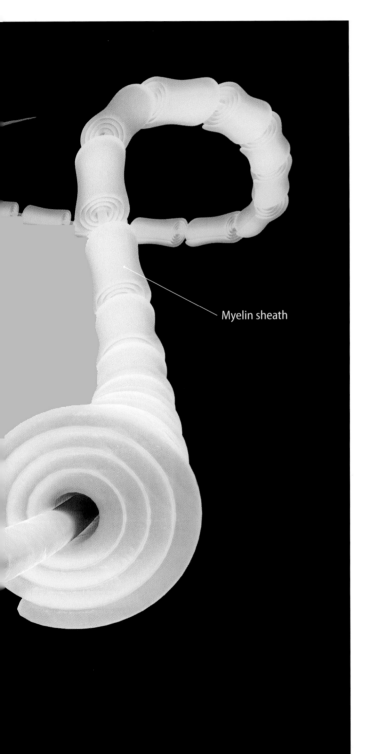

Myelin sheath

Cleaning up synapses

A neurotransmitter that has been released into the synaptic cleft must be removed to avoid an ongoing activation of receptors. If the neuro-transmitter is never removed, the chemical will stay bound to the receptors, keeping the ion channels constantly open and exhausting the stimulated nerve cell. Removal is achieved by either reuptake of the neurotransmitter into the axon that produced it, diffusion out of the cleft, or breakdown of the neurotransmitter into inactive components. Some drugs act on this process. One group of anti-depressants, the SSRIs, increases the availability of serotonin in the cerebral cortex by slowing the reuptake of serotonin at synapses. Increasing available serotonin in the synaptic cleft improves mood.

Electrical synapses

Some nerve cells communicate with other nerve cells by electrical synapses—sites where the cell membrane of one cell is in close contact with the cell membrane of another with no intervening gap. Special protein molecules called connexins bind the membranes together, so that electrical activity in one cell can be directly transferred to the other. This type of synapse is seen in a group of nerve cells in the eye's retina (the horizontal cells), and during development when cells need to share information to regulate growth processes.

Electrical synapses have the advantage that they allow direct transfer of a signal from one cell to another with no delay, but their use in the human nervous system is relatively rare. This is because coupling nerve cells by electrical synapses turns them all into a single electrical unit. In mammals, nervous systems prefer to keep nerve cells as separate electrical units that com-municate by chemical synapses. Chemical transmission between nerve cells allows them to act as discrete units, with each one able to perform a different task.

Brain chemistry

The special ability of the nervous system to process information and control behavior depends on the amazing features of the chemistry of nerve cells. These mainly concern the special structure of the membranes of nerve cells, which allows them to generate waves of electrical activity down their own axons and to reliably transmit information to nearby nerve cells.

All cells in the body have a cell membrane that separates the cytoplasm of the cell from the surrounding extracellular fluid. The electrical properties of this membrane are extremely important for the signaling and information-processing abilities of nerve cells.

The cell membrane is a complex double layer of fat molecules known as phospholipids. On its own, this double layer (called the lipid bi-layer) would be impervious to water molecules and charged chemical particles (sodium, potassium, and chloride ions). Floating in the lipid bi-layer are protein molecules

that can permit the movement of water and ions under special circumstances. Some of these proteins are only exposed at the outer or inner surface of the membrane, but many of the proteins span the entire thickness of the membrane. The most important of the membrane-spanning proteins are those that control the movement of ions into or out of the cell, because it is the flow of these ions that underlies the electrical activity of the nerve cell membranes. These ion channel proteins have a central pore that can either be opened, to allow movement of ions, or closed, as required.

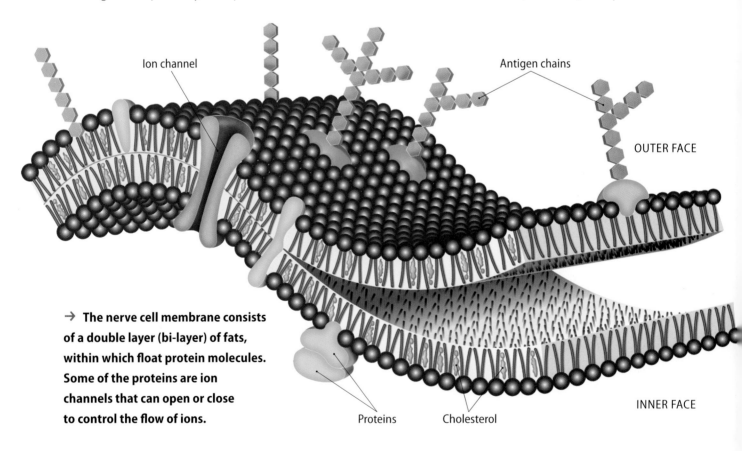

Ion channel

Antigen chains

OUTER FACE

INNER FACE

Proteins   Cholesterol

→ **The nerve cell membrane consists of a double layer (bi-layer) of fats, within which float protein molecules. Some of the proteins are ion channels that can open or close to control the flow of ions.**

→ **An ion channel opens in response to changes in voltage across the membrane or when neurotransmitters dock with receptors on the binding sites on the channel. Movement of ions through the channels changes the electrical properties of the nerve cell membrane.**

Ion (charged atom)

Receptor part of channel protein

Neurotransmitter

Ion channel closed

Ion channel open

Ion passing through channel with surrounding water molecules

Neural gateways: ion channels

Some ion channels open in response to changes in the distribution of charge across the membrane and are known as voltage-gated channels. They are vital for the production of the "all-or-none" response that is the action potential. In other words, once a change in voltage across the nerve cell membrane of one part of an axon is started, it induces the opening of voltage-gated sodium channels that perpetuate the voltage change and spread it to the next length of axon. By successive opening of these channels down the axon, the nerve impulse or action potential is reliably carried down the axon to its end.

Other ion channels open when chemicals bind to them. These ligand-gated channels (from the Latin *ligare* meaning "to bind") are found on the dendrites and other parts of nerve cells, wherever there is a synaptic contact from another nerve cell. When the neurotransmitter chemical is released onto the membrane, the binding of the neurotransmitter to the ligand-gated channels causes them to open and allow ions to move through the membrane, with consequent changes in the electrical properties of the nerve cell.

Yet further ion channels open in response to mechanical stimulation. A good example of these is in the inner ear. These mechanically gated channels are found on the tips of the hair cells of the inner ear. When the pressure wave of sound moves through the inner ear, it distorts the hair processes on the tips of these cells and opens the mechanically gated channels, leading to electrical changes in the hair cells that are transmitted to the brain and perceived as sound.

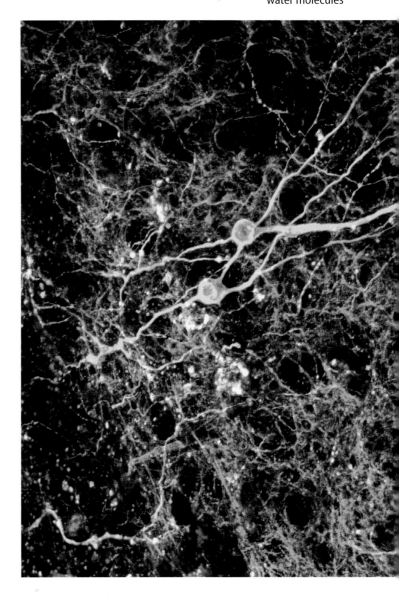

↑ **The gold areas in this micrograph of brain tissue are ion channels, which allow the exchange of ions across cell membranes. Green areas are nerve cells.**

Sex on the brain

Some nerve cells in the brain that control sexual behavior have receptors on their membranes that bind with sex hormones and move the hormone into and through the cell cytoplasm to the cell nucleus where the manufacture of protein and other chemicals is altered. In fact, sex hormones may act on a variety of nerve cells, even those not directly involved in sexual function. For example, many nerve cells in the cerebral cortex can be influenced by estrogen, accounting for the changes in mood and cognitive function when estrogen levels drop after menopause.

Finally, some ion channels open in response to changes in temperature and are useful as biological thermometers. These channels are found in the skin, where changes in skin temperature cause opening of the channels and changes in the electrical properties of the sensory nerve axons. Those changes are converted to nerve impulses that are perceived in the brain as hot or cold.

Membranes in different parts of a nerve cell have different types of ion channel. The dendrites that receive most of the synaptic contacts have a high proportion of ligand-gated channels. Conversely, the axons that carry the action potential have a high proportion of voltage-gated sodium and potassium channels.

Chemical messenger systems inside nerve cells

Although most chemical and electrical interaction between nerve cells occurs at the cell membranes, there are some chemicals that alter the function of nerve cells by entering the cell and changing the internal metabolic machinery. These may bind to proteins in the nucleus and have long-term effects on nerve cell function. A good example of these involves sex hormones that adjust the function of nerve cells.

Making and transporting neurotransmitters

Neurotransmitters used in the central and peripheral nervous systems include acetylcholine, noradrenaline (norepinephrine), serotonin, dopamine, glutamate, and gamma aminobutyric acid (GABA). Some of these have excitatory effects, in that they stimulate the postsynaptic membrane to become more conductive (i.e., open particular ion channels) and make the nerve cell more electrically active. On the other hand, others are inhibitory, in that they electrically stabilize the postsynaptic membrane and make the nerve cell less electrically active.

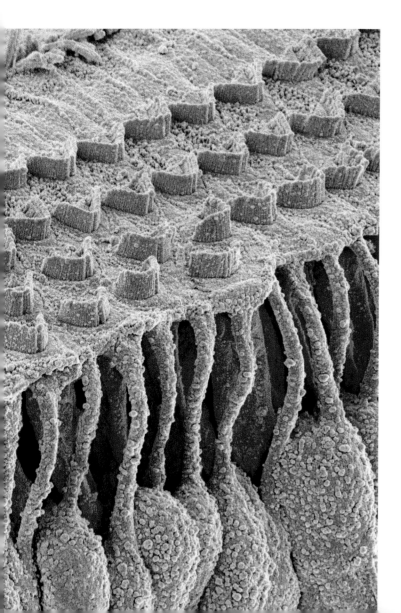

← **Some ion channels can be activated by mechanical force, such as those in the hair cells of the inner ear (pictured). Sound waves bend the hairlike processes on the cells and trigger a nerve impulse to the brain.**

Neurotransmitters

Neurotransmitters are chemicals made by one nerve cell to act on other nerve cells, usually at a chemical synapse. They must be produced continuously by nerve cells, transported to the end of the axon and stored before release. Most neurotransmitters are small molecules: either modified from the amino acids that make up proteins, or consisting of short chains of amino acids called peptides. The small size of neurotransmitters is important because they are simple to make and can diffuse quickly when released.

→ **Neurotransmitters (in synaptic vesicles) are transported to the end of the axon and released into the synaptic cleft between the axon and the next nerve cell.**

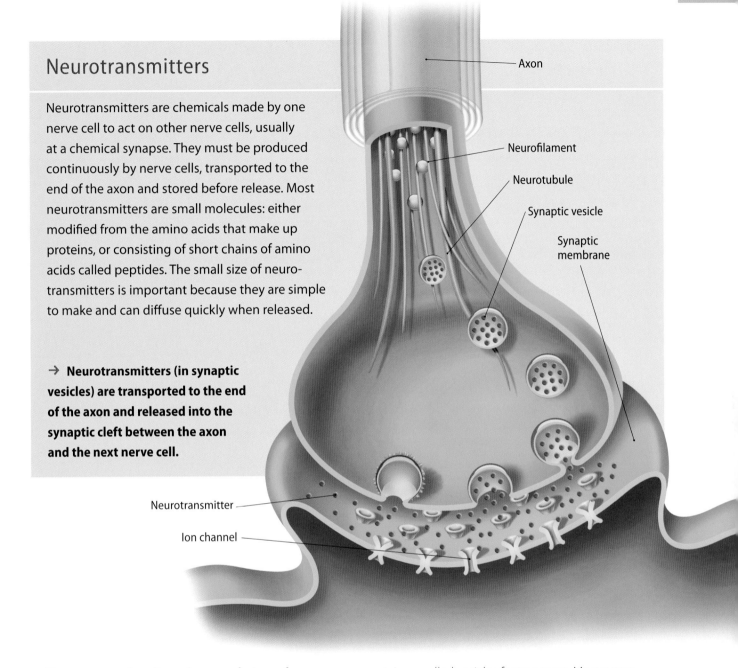

Axon

Neurofilament

Neurotubule

Synaptic vesicle

Synaptic membrane

Neurotransmitter

Ion channel

The programs that direct the manufacture of neurotransmitters are stored in the DNA (deoxyribonucleic acid) of the nerve cell. This information is carried out of the cell nucleus by a type of molecule called messenger RNA (ribonucleic acid). The ribosomes in the cytoplasm of the nerve cell use the information coded into the messenger RNA to either manufacture the enzymes that in turn make the neurotransmitters, or to manufacture the small amino acid chains that are themselves the peptide neurotransmitters.

Once the neurotransmitters have been made, the Golgi apparatus packs them into membrane-covered containers called vesicles for transport. Most neurotransmitters will be released at a distance of 0.2 inches to 3 feet (many millimeters to a meter) away from the cell body, so the neurotransmitters must be carried for long distances down the axon. The fast axonal transport system moves these vesicles down the neurotubules of the axon at a speed of 4–16 inches (10–40 cm) per day. A few neurotransmitters (e.g., acetylcholine) that are made locally in the axon end from available molecules do not need to be transported down the axon, but the enzymes used to make them do come from the cell body.

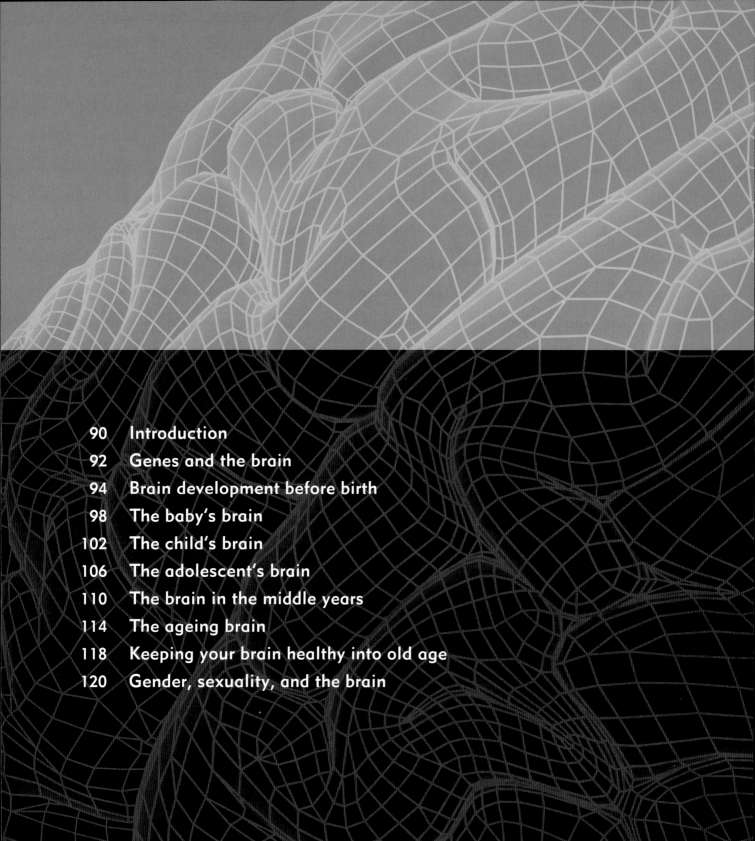

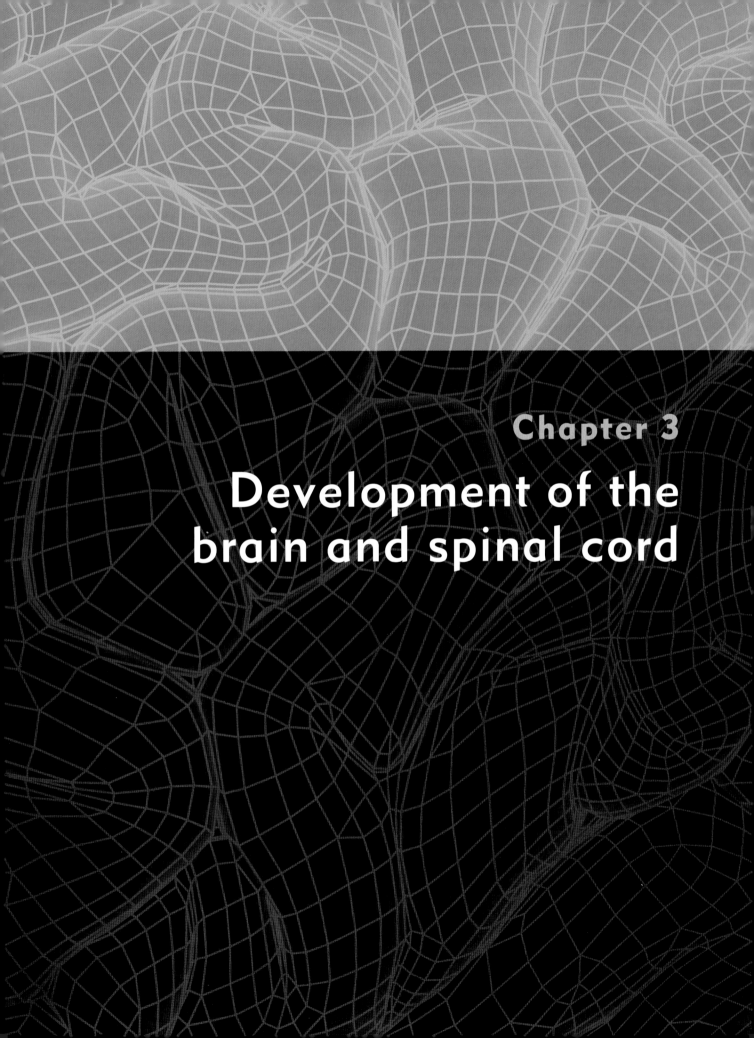

Chapter 3

Development of the brain and spinal cord

Introduction

Our brains grow from a single cell, the fertilized egg that carries genetic information from our parents. How is that genetic code used to build the brain and how do genes and the environment interact during brain growth? At the other end of life there are other questions to consider. How do we avoid brain disease and keep our brains in optimal health?

The structure of the nervous system is far too complex for the genetic code to specify the position and connections of every single nerve cell. Genes that control the development of the brain act as regulators, switching on or off key developmental processes (e.g., the cell division that generates the nerve and glia cells) and setting general rules for the interactions between nerve cells. Much of the complex structure of the adult nervous system is actually the result of competition between nerve cells in the brain as it develops. Many different types of nerve cells are produced in greater numbers than will survive to adulthood. Nerve cells must compete through their axons for growth factors from target structures, and those cells that obtain too little support will die. The connections between brain regions are also formed through a competitive process which ensures that the most effective connections are those that are maintained into adult life.

Maturity and the ageing brain

There are inevitable changes in the brain as we age. These mainly involve the gradual loss of connections between nerve cells, rather than the loss of nerve cell bodies themselves. Some of these lost connections may have been redundant anyway, and do not necessarily cause a reduction in functional ability. The greater experience of mature brains can also counterbalance some of the effects of lost processing speed, particularly in the fifth and sixth decades of life. On the other hand, the loss of connections accelerates as we reach our 70s and 80s and we gradually lose speed of action in both our intellectual and motor functions. The gradual and relentless loss of sensory receptors may deprive us of the taste and aroma of food, and erode the ability to balance our body and avoid falls. These effects can compound and accelerate the mental ageing process so that loss of function in one area makes it difficult to retain functions in other areas.

Maintaining brain health

Many of the degenerative processes that erode our brain function as we age can be held at bay by maintaining an active lifestyle. By training the remaining circuits and stimulating the production of growth factors, physical and mental activity help to stave off the loss of sensory, motor, and cognitive function. Physical activity also slows down the process of atherosclerosis that narrows the arteries to the brain.

→ **The human brain undergoes profound changes in shape and size during embryonic life and childhood, to reach a maximum size in early adulthood before slowly shrinking in old age.**

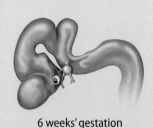

6 weeks' gestation

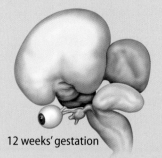

12 weeks' gestation

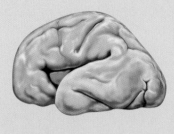

37 weeks' gestation

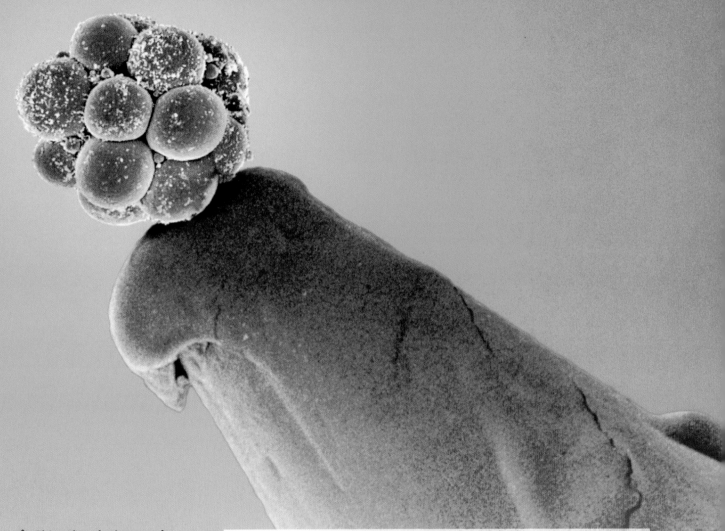

↑ **This colored micrograph shows a human embryo at the 16-cell stage (about three days old) sitting on the tip of a pin. The nucleus of each cell contains the genetic information that will give rise to the embryonic nervous system and other parts of the body.**

Environmental factors in brain development

The developing brain is exquisitely sensitive to environmental factors at all stages of development. These could be in the environment of the womb, when the embryo and fetus can be exposed to fluctuations in maternal nutrition or temperature, or toxic agents like alcohol, viruses, or methyl mercury; or a complex array of factors that are important during life after birth (nutrition, emotional support, social experience, and intellectual stimulation).

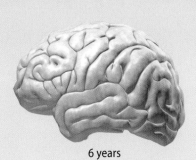

6 years

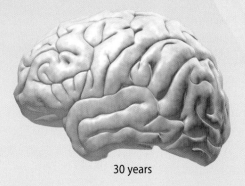

30 years

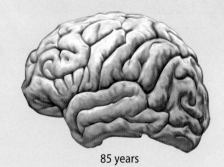

85 years

Genes and the brain

Our genomes differ by only about 1 percent from that of our nearest relatives, the chimpanzees, but our brains are three times the size and many times more cognitively able. It appears that changes in a few key genes can have profound influences on the size and internal organization of the brain.

Gene expression is the conversion of information in a gene into proteins which are used either to influence other genes or perform cellular functions. Studies of gene expression in the developing brain show that almost 600 genes are up-regulated (increased in activity) in the cerebral cortex. Many of these are recently evolved genes that play vital roles in the growth of the cerebral cortex in general and the prefrontal cortex in particular. The lateral prefrontal cortex is a key region for decision-making. It is particularly well-developed in humans.

Another important set of genes is that controlling the development of language areas. As yet, not all of these genes have been identified, but it is clear that some genes like *FOXP2* play a critical role in forming the circuitry that allows us to comprehend and use grammatical rules.

New or improved genes?

The overall structure of the vertebrate brain is at least 400 million years old and yet the large human brain, with its lateralization of function and special language areas, may be only a few hundred thousand years old. This raises the question of whether the human brain developed by changes in old genes, or by the emergence of radically new or recently evolved genes. Studies comparing the genomes of vertebrates indicate that the recent expansion of the human brain is due to the emergence of new human-specific genes, particularly involving the prefrontal cortex.

Genes do not explain everything

Although genes critically influence the processes of brain development, they should be seen more as switches that set developmental processes in action and establish the main rules for interaction between growing nerve cells. Much of the complex architecture of the brain emerges as a result of competition between nerve cells and their axons for contacts and growth factors. In this sense, the development of the brain is as dependent on non-genetic factors as it is on genetic control. Some of these factors are internal to the brain, such as competitive interactions between different nerve cells for growth factor support and targets for their axons; whereas others are external to the brain but within the body, including hormonal support from the endocrine system and nutrition from the placenta. Yet more important factors that influence brain development are outside the body, including maternal nutrition during pregnancy, nutrition of the infant after birth, and the experiential environment during childhood and adolescence.

→ **Each chromosome in every cell of the body is made up of strands of chromatin, which consists of lengths of DNA that encode genes, and the accompanying protein molecules (histones). Although necessary for setting developmental processes in action, genes do not account for all the complexity of the brain. That is the product of an interaction between genes, competition between nerve cells, and the environment.**

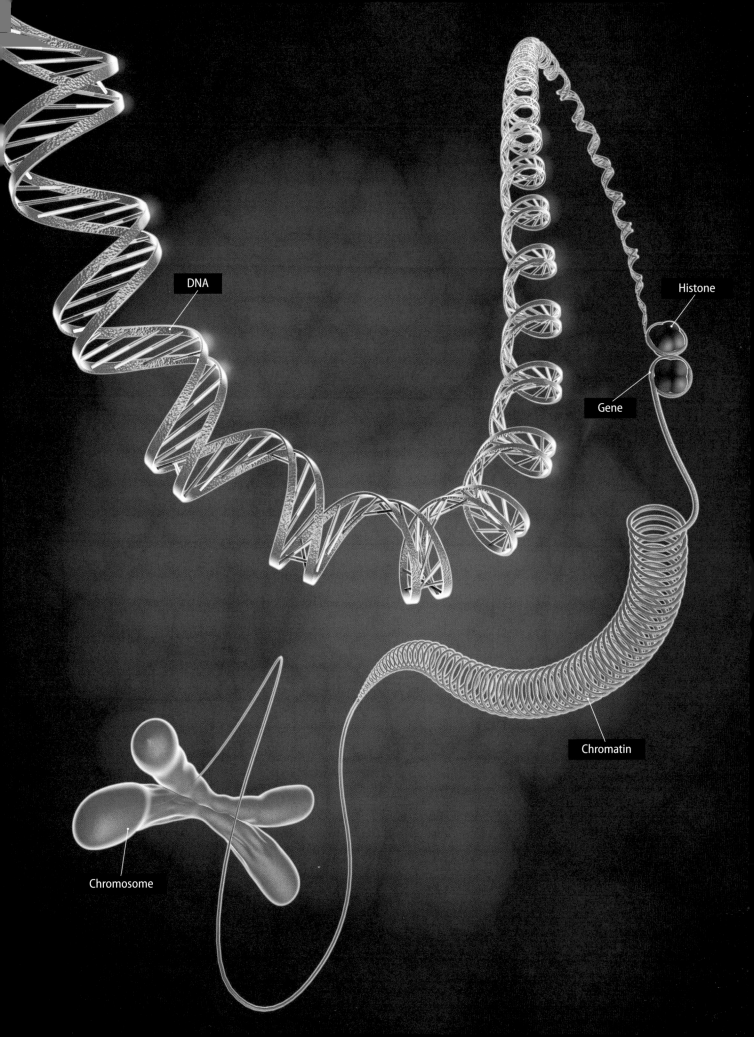

DNA

Histone

Gene

Chromatin

Chromosome

Brain development before birth

The human brain is a complex structure with hundreds of billions of nerve cells and glia. It is constructed using information stored in the genetic programs in the DNA of the fertilized egg, but is also strongly influenced by both the internal environment of the embryo and fetus as well as the environment in the womb and beyond, particularly during the later stages of pregnancy.

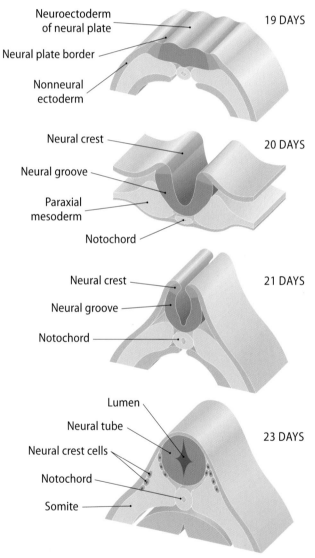

19 DAYS
- Neuroectoderm of neural plate
- Neural plate border
- Nonneural ectoderm

20 DAYS
- Neural crest
- Neural groove
- Paraxial mesoderm
- Notochord

21 DAYS
- Neural crest
- Neural groove
- Notochord

23 DAYS
- Lumen
- Neural tube
- Neural crest cells
- Notochord
- Somite

↑ **In utero, the nervous system develops from a neural plate that is induced by the notochord. The plate folds into a neural groove and eventually a neural tube. Neural crest cells at the edge of the neural plate form the peripheral nervous system.**

The brain is initially formed from a flat tadpole or tennis racket-shaped neural plate, which lies on the upper surface of the 18-day-old embryo. The neural plate is induced by the notochord—a rodlike structure that coordinates developmental events of nearby tissue. Even at this early stage, the parts of the adult brain are mapped out onto the flat surface. The very front part of the plate will give rise to the forebrain, whereas the "tail" or "handle" at the back will form the spinal cord.

The neural tube

The sides of the neural plate begin to fold upward to form a tube over the next three days. This neural tube closes first in a region that corresponds to the lower neck area

Neural tube defects

Failure of the two neuropores to close (a type of abnormality called a neural tube defect) results in incomplete development of the front and back ends of the nervous system. If the anterior neuropore does not close, the brain cannot develop and the condition is called anencephaly (from the Greek for "without a brain"). If the posterior neuropore fails to close, the spinal cord will not develop properly and the condition is called spina bifida (from the Latin for "split spine"). Extra folate in the mother's diet before becoming pregnant can reduce the chance of her child developing a neural tube defect.

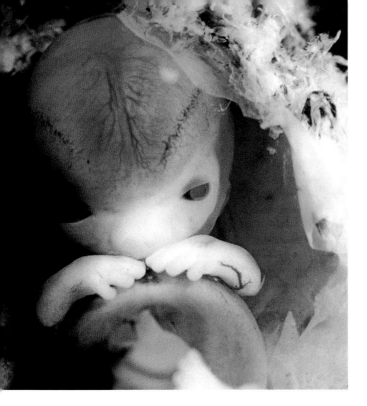

← **This embryo is about seven weeks old. The brain is developing rapidly by cell division. The eyes are developing but not yet functioning.**

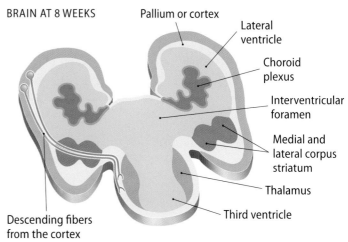

BRAIN AT 8 WEEKS

Pallium or cortex
Lateral ventricle
Choroid plexus
Interventricular foramen
Medial and lateral corpus striatum
Thalamus
Third ventricle
Descending fibers from the cortex

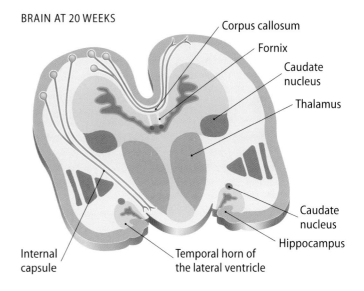

BRAIN AT 20 WEEKS

Corpus callosum
Fornix
Caudate nucleus
Thalamus
Caudate nucleus
Hippocampus
Internal capsule
Temporal horn of the lateral ventricle

of the adult, so initially the tube is open at the brain and lower spinal cord ends. These are called the anterior and posterior neuropores, respectively, and remain open to the amniotic fluid around the embryo for almost a week. The anterior neuropore eventually closes at 25 days and the posterior neuropore at 27 days.

Neural crest cells

The ridges at the side of the closing neural plate give rise to a special group of cells (neural crest cells) that migrate to diverse areas of the body. These cells give rise to all the cells of the peripheral nervous system, including the sensory dorsal root ganglion cells that lie alongside the spinal cord and autonomic ganglion cells that control the internal organs. The Schwann cells that form the myelin coat of nerves in the peripheral nervous system are also of neural crest origin, as are the cells of the adrenal medulla that make adrenaline (epinephrine).

A host of other cells with no obvious nerve cell function also originate from the neural crest. These include the melanocytes of the skin that produce the melanin pigment to protect against ultraviolet exposure, as well as parts of the heart, some parts of the skeleton in the head, and even the teeth. This means that any congenital abnormality that stops the neural crest cells migrating through the body can give rise to problems in many organs.

↑ **Nerve cells of the developing forebrain are formed by cell division in the wall of the brain vesicles (lateral and third ventricles). Once nerve cells have reached their resting place they begin to grow axons (green lines) to connect to other parts of the brain. These connections include those across the midline (corpus callosum), as well as those to the brainstem and spinal cord (internal capsule).**

The brain takes shape

During the later stages of embryonic life (28 to 50 days) the neural tube grows into a complex shape. Initially the tube develops three bulges at the brain end. These are known as the primary brain vesicles and will give rise to the fore-, mid-, and hindbrain parts of the mature brain. The cerebral hemispheres are formed when the neural tube bends at the midbrain location while the side of the forebrain section expands.

Brain cells are born

Nerve cells and glia are produced in several sites within the developing brain and in several waves of cell division. The most important site is known as the ventricular germinal zone, which is a region lying close to the cavity of the brain vesicles. This is the most active site of young nerve cell production, especially of larger nerve cells such as the pyramidal neurons of the cerebral cortex. This area is active from about 6 weeks to 26 weeks of prenatal development. Gradually the activity of the ventricular germinal zone winds down and a second significant site for neuron generation is formed a little further away from the cavity of the brain vesicles. This second site is known as the subventricular zone and is important for production of small nerve cells and some of the glia (astrocytes and oligodendrocytes). Some special areas in the brain, such as the cerebellum, have additional areas where nerve cells are produced (e.g., the external granular layer that covers the cerebellum during late fetal life and early postnatal life).

Interrupted migration

Interruption of the normal process of migration, whether by preventing the correct signaling between young nerve cells and radial glia, or by damage to the scaffolding, can result in nests of nerve cells being left stranded close to the brain ventricles. This could be the result of abnormal genes or environmental factors like viral infection. These displaced clumps of nerve cells around the brain ventricles are often unable to form correct connections, with the result that the person will have some degree of intellectual disability.

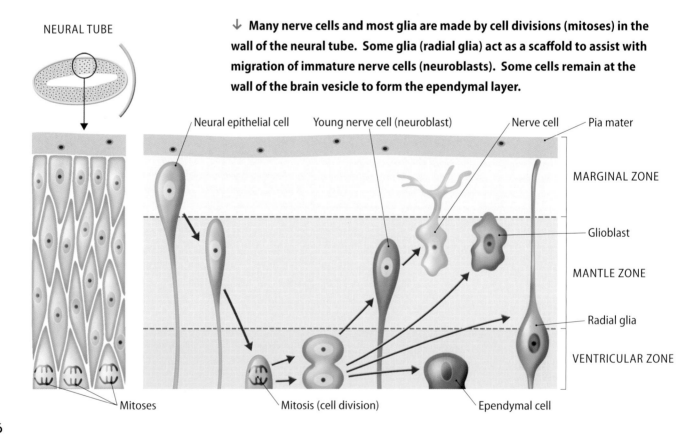

NEURAL TUBE

↓ **Many nerve cells and most glia are made by cell divisions (mitoses) in the wall of the neural tube. Some glia (radial glia) act as a scaffold to assist with migration of immature nerve cells (neuroblasts). Some cells remain at the wall of the brain vesicle to form the ependymal layer.**

Neural epithelial cell   Young nerve cell (neuroblast)   Nerve cell   Pia mater

MARGINAL ZONE

Glioblast

MANTLE ZONE

Radial glia

VENTRICULAR ZONE

Mitoses   Mitosis (cell division)   Ependymal cell

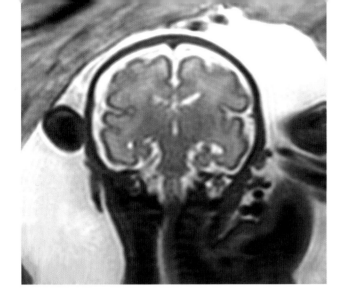

← At 25 weeks' gestation, connections within the fetal brain are developing, especially in the areas responsible for emotions, perception, and conscious thought.

↓ The shape of the brain is produced by bending of the neural tube and thickening of its walls. The eye is an outgrowth of the forebrain.

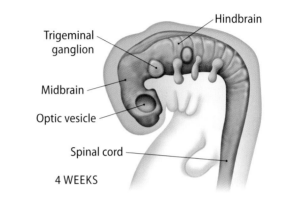

Hindbrain

Trigeminal ganglion

Midbrain

Optic vesicle

Spinal cord

4 WEEKS

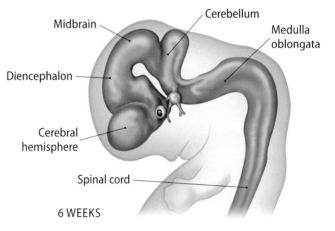

Midbrain

Cerebellum

Medulla oblongata

Diencephalon

Cerebral hemisphere

Spinal cord

6 WEEKS

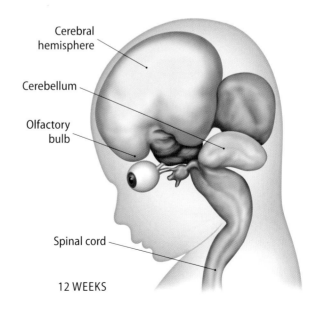

Cerebral hemisphere

Cerebellum

Olfactory bulb

Spinal cord

12 WEEKS

Nerve cell migration

Newly made nerve cells in the ventricular germinal zone need to migrate to their final locations in the cerebral cortex or other brain regions. For the large nerve cells that are made very early in development, this migration occurs along scaffolding provided by a special elongated type of glial cell known as radial glia. Some migration occurs independent of this scaffolding. Tracing studies using virus labeling of embryonic brain cells have shown that some sideways spread occurs once nerve cells enter the general area of their destination. Small nerve cells are made later in development and eventually make up the internal circuits of the cerebral cortex. These cells migrate long distances around the curvature of the brain during fetal life. Some of this migration may be along the pathways made by large nerve cells during earlier stages of development.

Development during the last half of pregnancy

During the last half of pregnancy, nerve cells complete their migration to their final locations and begin to grow axons to other parts of the brain and spinal cord. Some areas of the brain continue to actively generate young nerve cells by cell division (including the subventricular zone of the forebrain and the external granular layer of the cerebellum). This ongoing cell division means that the brain continues to be extremely sensitive to adverse environmental factors (drugs, radiation, viruses, and elevated temperature of the mother) for the entire pregnancy. Some of this cell division continues into postnatal life and the potential to produce new nerve cells may even be retained into adulthood.

The baby's brain

At birth the brain is only about 25 percent of its final adult weight. Most brain growth occurs in the first two years after birth when experience drives the growth of nerve cell processes (axons and dendrites) and myelin coats form around axons.

At the time of birth all the major grooves on the surface of the cerebral cortex have formed and the brain weighs about ¾ pounds (350 g). Brain weight more than doubles in the first year after birth, reaching more than 2 pounds (900 g) by one year and about 2.2 pounds (1,000 g) by two years. A very important area of brain growth is the cerebral cortex, where profound changes in the complexity of the dendritic trees of nerve cells occur during the first few postnatal years. This is the period when nerve cells of the cerebral cortex grow dendritic branches that extend distances many hundreds of times the diameter of the nerve cell body. As these dendrites grow, they begin to contact axons from other parts of the cerebral cortex.

↓ **Newborn infants are routinely tested for effective nervous system function. This baby is being checked for a healthy grasping reflex.**

Nerve cell production in postnatal life

Some nerve cell production continues into postnatal life (such as nerve cells for the olfactory system and cerebellum). Recent studies have revealed a stream of nerve cells migrating from the subventricular zone around the lateral ventricle of the infant brain to two main sites. The first of these is a stream toward the olfactory bulb, the second is toward the lower and midline parts of the prefrontal cortex. These cells seem to be destined to form interneurons that make up the nerve circuits within the cortex. The streams of young nerve cells are best developed during the first 18 months of life and provide a steady supply of cells to the cortex during the period of life when social development is blossoming. They may also provide new nerve cells in the event of early brain injury. Recent studies also indicate that stem cells capable of producing new nerve cells may be present into adult life in the remains of the subventricular layer.

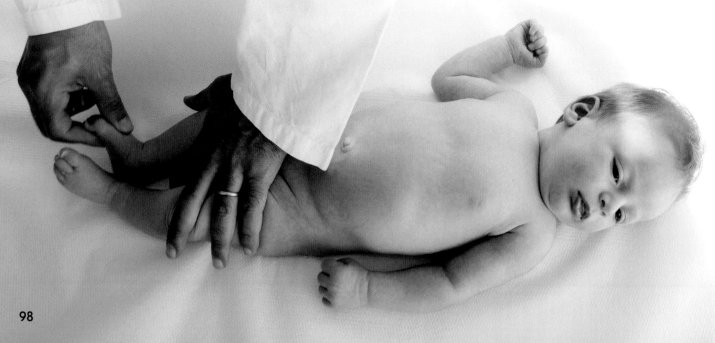

Axon competition in the postnatal brain

Nerve cells often grow several axon branches during development, some of which reach parts of the brain that are not normally contacted in adult life. These excess connections compete with each other to contact dendrites. Those connections that are functionally useful are retained, whereas those that are not useful are pruned. The interaction between sensory and motor experience and the evolving connections in the brain allows the immature brain to be shaped by experience. Enriching the environment of the infant with lots of sensory stimulation and activity during this critical period can help build cognitive function and motor skills in subsequent life. This axonal exuberance is also an important component of the plasticity of the young brain and allows the brain to recover from injury by growing new axons when others are damaged.

On the other hand, sensory deprivation and bodily confinement can permanently disable the sensory and motor centers in the cortex and limit the child's potential. This is why any medical condition (e.g., a squint, or strabismus) that interferes with the ability of the infant or child to see objects simultaneously with both eyes (binocular vision) must be treated early in life before the visual cortex loses its plasticity. If the eyes are not correctly aligned early in life, the child may preferentially use only one eye and never gain the ability to form a single fused image from the input of both eyes.

→ **An excess of embryonic nerve cells and nerve connections is eliminated by competition between nerve pathways.**

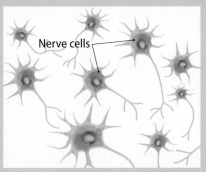

1. The embryonic brain produces extra nerve cells.

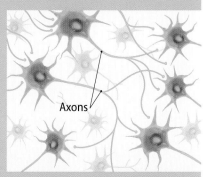

2. Surviving nerve cells produce multiple branches at the axon ends.

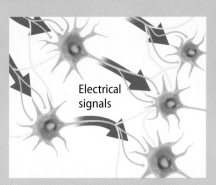

3. Electrical activity strengthens some connections while others atrophy.

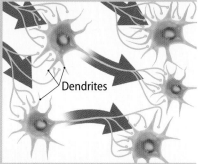

4. After birth, the brain experiences a second growth stage as axons and dendrites make new connections.

Hormones and brain development

The early postnatal brain may be strongly influenced by the hormones circulating in the blood. Sex hormones during early postnatal life alter the structure of the hypothalamus and basal forebrain nuclei to produce the nerve cell groups that control sexual function. Thyroid hormone is essential for dendritic development of cortical nerve cells. Insufficient thyroid hormone, whether from a deficient thyroid gland or poor dietary intake of iodine, results in a form of intellectual and physical disability known as neonatal hypothyroidism (formerly known as cretinism).

Key milestones from birth to 18 months

Age	Posture and movement	Vision and manipulation	Hearing and speech	Social behavior
3 months	Lifts head and chest when placed on stomach. Head bobs when held upright.	Visually alert and watches movements of adults. Follows toys held close to the face.	Stays quiet for interesting sounds. Chuckles and coos when pleased.	Shows pleasure when happy.
6 months	Lifts body up on straight arms when placed on stomach. Sits upright. Takes weight on legs when held standing.	Watches rolling ball 2 yards (2 m) away. Reaches out for toys and grasps them.	Turns to soft sounds 1½ feet (0.5 m) to the side of the head. Makes double syllable sounds.	Alert and interested in surroundings. Still friendly with strangers.
9 months	Wriggles and crawls. Sits unsupported for 10 minutes.	Looks for dropped toys. Transfers gripped objects to other hand.	Quickly locates soft sounds at the side of the ear. Babbles tunefully.	Distinguishes strangers and shows apprehension of them. Chews solid food.
12 months	Crawls on all fours. Walks with hands held. Stands alone for a second or two.	Drops toys deliberately and watches where they go. Pincer grip and use of index finger to touch tiny objects.	Understands simple commands. Babbles incessantly.	Cooperates with dressing (holding up arms). Waves "bye-bye."
18 months	Walks alone and can pick up toys from floor without falling.	Builds tower of three blocks and scribbles.	Uses several words.	Drinks from cup using two hands. Demands attention from mother.

Cerebral palsy

Cerebral palsy is a disorder of posture and movement that is caused by nonprogressive damage to the developing brain. It occurs once in every 300 births and can result from problems during late pregnancy (e.g., infections or abnormal genes), problems around the time of birth (e.g., birth injury, poor oxygen supply during delivery, low blood glucose, or severe neonatal jaundice), and illness during early infancy (e.g., infection, trauma, and problems with brain vessels).

Cerebral palsy is most often suspected around the age of six months, when the child is noticed to have delayed motor development. Children may go on to develop rigidity of the limb muscles

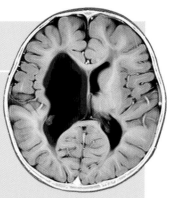

→ This MRI section through the brain of a child with cerebral palsy reveals an abnormal cavity filled with cerebrospinal fluid.

(spasticity), be unsteady and uncoordinated (ataxia), or be paralyzed in the limbs (hemiplegia or paraplegia). They may also have involuntary movements such as chorea and athetosis (see p. 179). Early physiotherapy, medication, and orthopedic surgery can help to alleviate the symptoms and signs, but a complete cure is not possible at this stage.

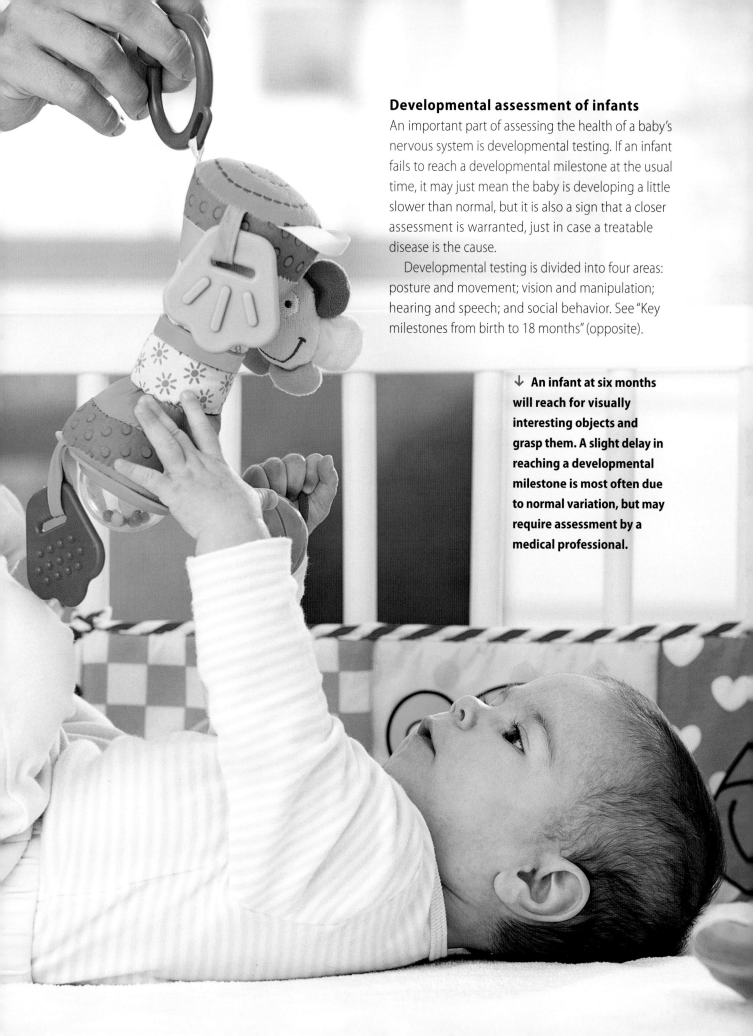

Developmental assessment of infants

An important part of assessing the health of a baby's nervous system is developmental testing. If an infant fails to reach a developmental milestone at the usual time, it may just mean the baby is developing a little slower than normal, but it is also a sign that a closer assessment is warranted, just in case a treatable disease is the cause.

Developmental testing is divided into four areas: posture and movement; vision and manipulation; hearing and speech; and social behavior. See "Key milestones from birth to 18 months" (opposite).

↓ **An infant at six months will reach for visually interesting objects and grasp them. A slight delay in reaching a developmental milestone is most often due to normal variation, but may require assessment by a medical professional.**

The child's brain

The rate of brain growth slows after the age of two years. From the age of two to eight years, the child's brain grows by only 20 percent by weight, but that modest portion of extra brain tissue contains a wealth of new connections that make possible the acquisition of vitally important cognitive and motor skills for later life.

Parents are naturally very concerned when their child appears to be slow to reach developmental milestones. In most cases this is simply a normal child who is at one end of the normal range of when a child reaches a milestone. The pediatrician will need to assess the child carefully and exclude any diseases that might be the cause.

It should be remembered that developmental skills are stepping-stones. Not all children progress at the same pace, e.g., some may go from shuffling on their bottoms to walking, without any appreciable time spent crawling. Some children appear to be stuck at a particular level for a few weeks before suddenly acquiring new skills almost overnight. Sometimes the child appears to be devoting all of his or her time to progressing in one area, while others remain static.

A common cause for concern is when a child is slow to speak. This could be due to many causes, including motor problems with the throat and soft palate, deafness, intellectual problems, autism, or an environment lacking sufficient exposure to speech. Being spoken to and mixing with talkative children will encourage speech development.

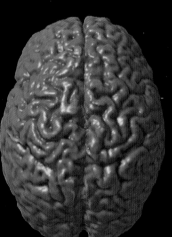

← **The brain of a child has the same overall shape as an adult brain but may still be growing as new connections are coated in myelin.**

→ **Childhood is a time when many connections are made between nerve cells (left and center). Many of these "exuberant" connections will be pruned later in adult life (right).**

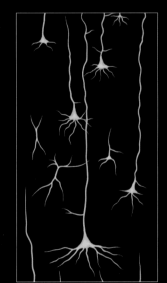
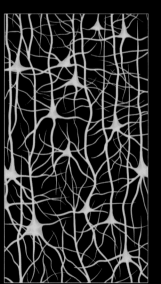
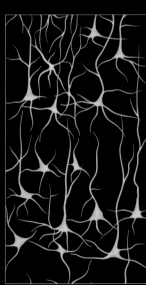

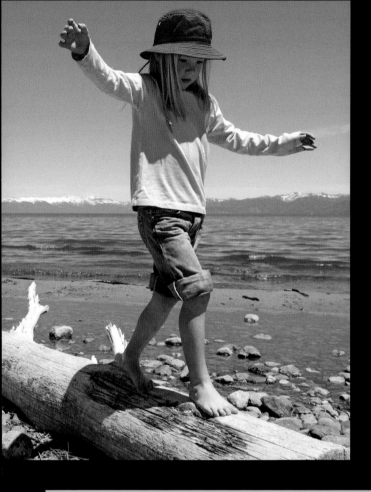

← **Exercise, good diet, and exposure to stimulating experiences are important for healthy brain development during childhood.**

The effects of stress

Experiences during early childhood—good and bad—can have long-lasting effects on behavior during later life. Many studies have shown that children who have been abused or neglected during childhood are at a much higher risk of developing anxiety and depression during adult life. Stress early in life causes a rise in the stress hormone cortisol in the blood and a reduction in the number of receptors for cortisol in the brain. These changes are believed to predispose the person to anxiety and depression when stress and misfortune occur during adult life.

Key milestones for young children

Sensory and motor development continues throughout the preschool years. Doctors recognize a number of key milestones against which a child's progress can be measured.

Age	Posture and movement	Vision and manipulation	Hearing and speech	Social behavior
2 years	Runs. Walks up and down steps two feet to a step.	Builds a tower of six blocks.	Joins words together in simple phrases.	Uses a spoon. Says when they need to use the toilet. Dry during the day.
3 years	Stands on one foot for a second or two. Walks up steps using one foot per step.	Builds a tower of nine blocks. Can copy a circle.	Speaks in sentences. Can say his/her own name in full.	Eats with spoon and fork. Can undress with assistance.
4 years	Stands on one foot for five seconds. Walks up and down steps using one foot per step.	Can build three steps from six blocks. Can copy a circle and a cross.	Talks a great deal. Speech contains many infantile substitutions of words.	Dresses and undresses with assistance.
5 years	Skips and hops. Stands on one foot with arms folded for five seconds.	Draws a human figure. Copies a circle, a cross, and a square.	Speaks fluently.	Dresses and undresses alone. Washes and dries face and hands.

Stress, food, and exercise

When the effects of early stress are studied in experimental animals, the inclusion of comfort foods in the diet and regular exercise appear to protect against the adverse effects of elevated stress hormone levels. These beneficial effects are due to effects on the cortisol receptors and neurotrophic chemical factors in the hippoc-ampus. The number of cortisol receptors and the expression of brain derived neurotrophic factor (BDNF) in the hippocampus are reduced when young rats are stressed by being separated from their mother, but providing fat-rich comfort foods and exercise brings these back to normal.

Of course, consuming a diet rich in fat has hazards of its own for future health, so it would be preferable, firstly to reduce sources of stress in the child's environment; and secondly, to encourage regular exercise as a means of dealing with unavoidable stress during childhood.

Seizures during childhood

A seizure is the result of an abnormal electrical discharge of a group of nerve cells in the cerebral cortex. About 4 percent of preschool children (six months to five years) have had a seizure, and the commonest form is a febrile convulsion. These are precipitated by any illness that causes a rise in body temperature, commonly upper respiratory tract infections. In about 20 percent of cases there is a family history. Often the EEG is normal between febrile convulsions and although half the children who have had one febrile convulsion will have another, these become much rarer after the age of five.

Febrile convulsions are treated by a combination of laying the child in the recovery position to keep the airway clear, cooling the child gently with tepid sponging, and medications to control the infection.

↓ **Most seizures during childhood are isolated events due to fever, but sometimes neurological abnormalities may be present. An EEG may detect abnormal electrical activity in the cortex.**

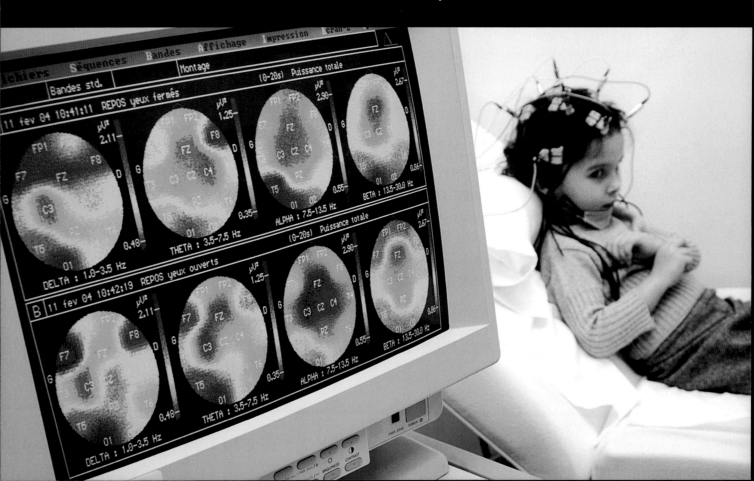

→ **Unlike spoken language, reading is not an innate skill. It requires training over many years and may be more difficult to acquire for boys than girls.**

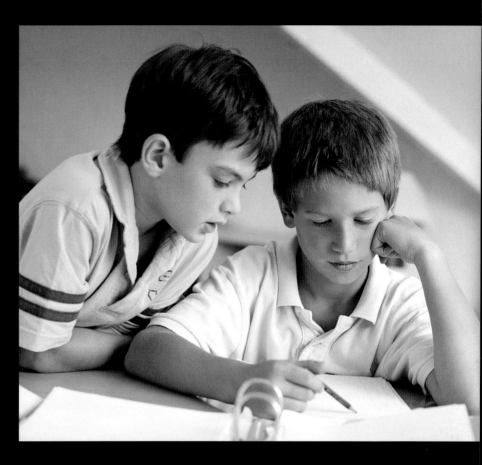

Anticonvulsant drugs may be used while the child continues to have a fever.

Epilepsy is the usual cause of seizures in the ages between 5 and 15 years. This may include seizures that seem to involve much of the brain, such as grand mal or petit mal, or seizures that appear to involve only select parts of the brain, e.g., temporal lobe epilepsy. Grand mal is a major convulsion of the entire body followed by a period of unconsciousness. It may be triggered by viewing flashing lights on television. Petit mal is a very brief period of loss of awareness (absence attack) lasting less than five seconds and accompanied by blinking. Intelligence is usually normal. Temporal lobe epilepsy often involves hallucinations and strange behavior and is associated with behavioral problems and poor intelligence.

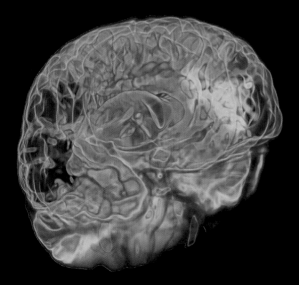

↑ **This is an MRI brain scan of a child who is looking at themselves in a mirror. The part of the frontal cortex associated with the sense of self is activated. True self-consciousness is usually achieved by age four.**

The development of reading

Reading is usually acquired by consistent training in the school environment and any unhappiness at school or home can profoundly affect its development. Usually reading ability becomes a cause for medical concern when the child's reading level is more than two years behind that of his or her peers. Reading problems are more common in boys, particularly those from lower socioeconomic backgrounds, and in larger families. All children with significant reading problems need skilled assessment and help from specialists, sometimes including clinical and educational psychologists.

Recent imaging studies of the brains of children with reading problems have shown that low volume of the cerebral cortex and a reduced asymmetry of the auditory areas (i.e., less of a difference between the left and right hemispheres) of the cerebral cortex are associated with reading delay. These anatomical features, in combination with a low processing speed of visual information, may be major contributors to reading problems.

The adolescent's brain

The teenage years are a time when most of the processes that have built the brain have slowed to a halt, but subtle maturation of the important executive areas of the cerebral cortex is still going on. It is also a time when complex cognitive abilities and demanding motor skills are acquired, as the young person prepares to take on adult responsibilities.

Imaging studies have shown that the volume of the white matter of the brain increases by about 5 percent between age 10 years and adulthood. The thickness of gray matter in the cerebral cortex rises during childhood to peak at age 11 in girls and age 12 in boys and then begins to fall during adolescence. This is probably associated with maturation of nerve cells, pruning of excess synapses, and thickening of axons in the white matter and does not necessarily imply a loss of function. Not all parts of the

cerebral cortex mature at the same pace: the motor and sensory cortex mature faster than the association cortex that is concerned with judgment and planning.

Brain growth during adolescence also appears to differ between the sexes. The amygdala tends to increase in size most in boys, whereas the hippocampus increases most in girls. Both of these regions have a high density of sex hormone receptors, suggesting that their growth is controlled in part by hormonal surges during puberty.

Not all people undergo the same degree of brain growth during adolescence. This may explain why an individual's verbal and nonverbal intelligence may rise or decline relative to that of their peers during this period of life. Changes in verbal intelligence appear to be closely correlated with changes in the part of the left

↓ **The gray matter of the cerebral cortex wanes in a back-to-front wave as the brain matures through adolescence. This is due to pruning of unnecessary connections as cognitive abilities improve.**

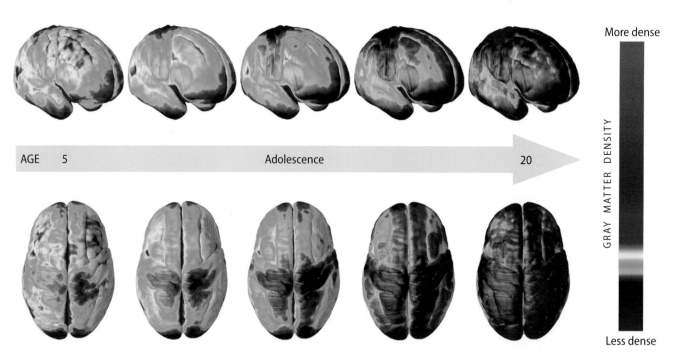

AGE   5   Adolescence   20

More dense

GRAY MATTER DENSITY

Less dense

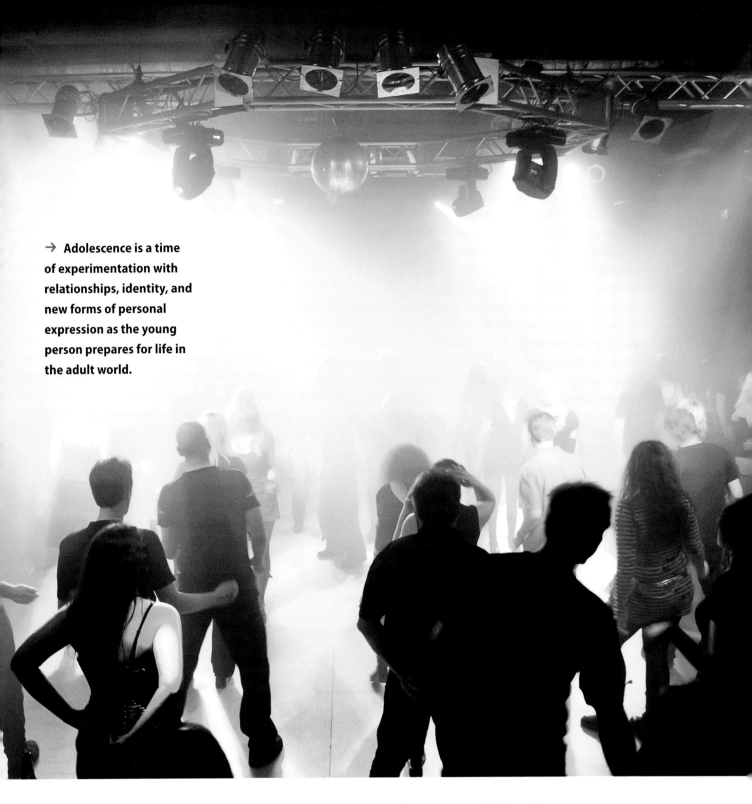

→ **Adolescence is a time of experimentation with relationships, identity, and new forms of personal expression as the young person prepares for life in the adult world.**

hemisphere that is concerned with the articulation of language (Broca's area). On the other hand, changes in nonverbal intelligence test performance are most closely correlated with changes in the front of the cerebellum. In other words, improvement in an individual's performance as they grow through adolescence may slow if they fall behind in the rate of maturation of one of these brain regions.

Adolescents and risk taking

Adolescents (12 to 18 years) and young adults (18 to 25 years) are more likely than older adults to use illicit or dangerous drugs, to drive recklessly or while intoxicated, and to engage in antisocial behavior. Risk-taking is associated with an increased tendency toward sensation-seeking and immediate reward-seeking, and a lack of inhibition. Some researchers have linked this to the pace

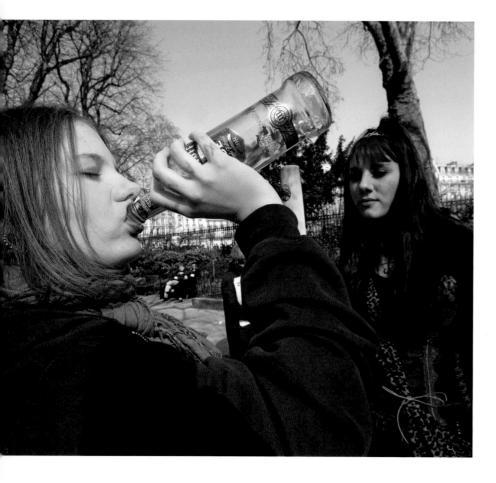

← **Adolescent experimentation with mood-altering drugs, including alcohol, carries significant risks because the adolescent brain is still structurally and functionally immature. Patterns of binge drinking are particularly damaging and may lead to risk-taking behavior.**

of structural brain changes during adolescence. The parts of the brain that are concerned with high-level executive functions, such as judgment, planning, and organization (the upper temporal lobe and the upper lateral prefrontal cortex) are the last to mature (after 16 to 17 years). At the same time, the surge in the male hormone testosterone during early puberty causes an enlargement of the amygdala, a part of the limbic system concerned with emotion-driven impulsive behavior. It has been proposed that risk-taking behavior among adolescents is due to a mismatch between the prefrontal and limbic control systems. During childhood both the limbic and prefrontal regions are still developing, but during adolescence the limbic region develops before the prefrontal cortex (particularly in males), causing impulsive behavior, while in adulthood the prefrontal cortex has fully matured and is in control of social behavior.

Adolescence and recreational drug use

Risk-taking behavior of adolescents and the need to fit in with their peer group can often lead them to experiment with recreational drugs (including alcohol). The adolescent brain is still immature, so exposure to addictive and neuroactive substances may have very different adverse effects from those on the adult brain.

The most prevalent type of alcohol consumption among teenagers is heavy episodic, or "binge," drinking, usually defined as four or more standard drinks on any

The social brain of adolescence

Adolescence is a time of profound changes in identity, self-consciousness, and relations with others. It is not surprising then that adolescent brains have slightly different patterns of activity from adult brains. When adolescents and adults are given the task of determining whether a speaker is being sincere or ironic, adolescents show more activity in the upper and medial part of the prefrontal cortex than do adults. On the other hand, adults show more activity in the upper temporal lobe. These findings suggest that adolescents and adults process information about the intent of another person differently, but further research is necessary to determine how this difference might influence adolescent behavior in day-to-day life.

occasion for females and five or more standard drinks on any occasion for males. As many as 30 percent of adolescents in their final school year have reported binge drinking during the past month. Binge drinking among adolescents is a serious public health concern because of reduced judgment and increased tendency toward risky behavior, with a range of potential adverse consequences (violence, motor vehicle accidents, pregnancy, sexually transmitted disease). Adolescents who engage in binge drinking have been shown to have poorer performance in working memory, particularly those involving visuo-spatial tasks. These abnormal test results appear to be due to abnormal function in the cerebral cortex of the frontal lobe, anterior cingulate gyrus, and upper parietal lobe. Females appear to be more susceptible than males to the adverse effects of binge drinking.

A particular social problem in developed countries in recent years is the epidemic of methamphetamine abuse among adolescents. Abuse of this powerful and dangerous drug of addiction is associated with agitation in 39 percent of users, and increased rates of depression and suicidal thoughts (31 percent of users) and suicide attempts (21 percent of users).

Adolescent depression and suicide

Adolescent depression is a worldwide problem, affecting 4 percent of adolescents in any one year, with as many as 20 percent of adolescents experiencing depression by

Bullying during adolescence

Bullying victimization is a common problem among adolescents of both sexes, affecting between 10 and 30 percent over the teenage years. Victims of bullying not only suffer distress, but can also be socially marginalized and have low status among their peers. Boys who have suffered bullying are four times more likely to engage in self-harm in later life and to suffer low self-esteem.

the end of the period. Among major risk factors for adolescent depression are a family history of depression and exposure to psychosocial stress (such as bullying, family discord, or poverty). Suicide is a significant risk and is the second or third leading cause of death in this age group. Depression is often missed in adolescents because this age group are frequently subject to irritability and mood fluctuations as part of the usual adolescent experience, and because the main symptoms may not be an obvious change in mood: eating disorders, refusal to attend school, substance abuse, and decline in school performance may all be signs of depression. Treatment of mild depression is usually by cognitive behavioral therapy and interpersonal psychotherapy in the first instance. Some controversy exists about the safety of using antidepressant medication in this age group because their brains are still immature, but these drugs may be required if the depression is severe.

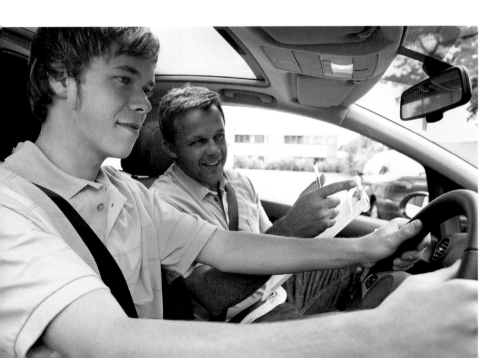

← **Adolescence is a time when new complex motor skills (like driving) are developed and new adult responsibilities are taken on. These skills may be acquired before fully adult judgment is developed.**

The brain in the middle years

Brain function may appear relatively stable between late adolescence and middle age, but there are subtle behavioral and cognitive changes that are due to slow, age-related physical changes in the brain. Most of these are beneficial, but we also gradually lose the mental flexibility and easy acquisition of skills and information that we enjoyed during our youth.

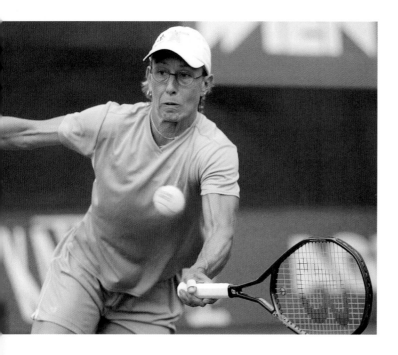

↑ **Athletic performance peaks during late adolescence and early adulthood, after which reaction times and muscle strength gradually decline. Most professional athletes have retired by their mid-30s, although some exceptional athletes like Martina Navratilova continue playing professionally into their late 40s.**

There may be as much as a 30 percent reduction in brain volume between adolescence and old age, and that process starts as early as age 25. This loss of volume appears to be due to a loss of nerve cell processes (dendrites and axons). The earliest changes probably involve the pruning of redundant connections and so make very little difference to brain function, but the acceleration of the process as people reach the end of the middle years can begin to erode behavioral flexibility and reaction time speed. These physical changes to brain structure cannot be avoided, but maintaining physical and mental activity can slow their effects.

Experience has benefits

Most routine activities during middle age are affected very little by ageing. This is because many of our brain functions, whether intellectual or motor actions, become highly automated over many years of practice and remain resistant to the gradual loss of brain volume.

Studies of bank employees have shown that although older employees had poorer performance on reasoning tests than younger ones, their job performance was just as good. This suggests that specific experience in tasks, as well as continuous training, is able to preserve performance in the face of this kind of slight age-related decline in speed and precision.

Nerve cell pathways that are continuously used are probably more resistant to age-related loss of function, perhaps because more nerve cells are recruited into task-specific circuitry. Continuous exercise of mental abilities may also stimulate the production of growth factors that help to maintain nerve connections.

A fit body for a bright brain

Physical exercise in general, and cardiovascular training in particular, may be able to protect against the effects of brain ageing. Studies suggest that having a good aerobic capacity (the ability to effectively transport and use oxygen), is linked with better preservation of cognitive

Menopause and brain function

For women, a significant event during this period of life is menopause. This is a permanent change in the function of the ovaries such that they no longer produce eggs or cyclically release female hormones. Nerve cells in the cerebral cortex are sensitive to the effects of estrogen, and the relatively sudden loss of hormonal support at menopause (around age 50) can have significant effects on mood and cognitive function. Women may complain of insomnia, fatigue, forgetfulness, increased susceptibility to stress, decreased libido, and mood changes at this time. Menopause may also coincide with many social changes in a woman's life, including children leaving home, having to care for frail or demented elderly parents or cope with their death, and a transition to grandmotherhood. Depression is an important condition that may emerge at this time and may respond to treatment with hormone replacement therapy or antidepressants.

Men are less obviously affected by changes in hormonal levels as they age, because testosterone levels in the blood usually decline gradually during the middle years.

↓ **Exercise is essential throughout adulthood for maintaining the health of body and mind into old age. Exercise slows the progression of atherosclerosis and maintains coordination.**

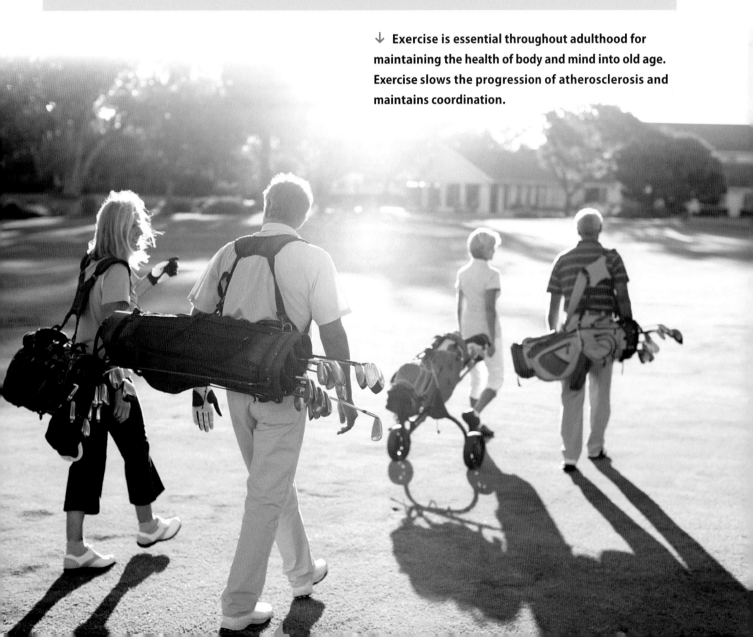

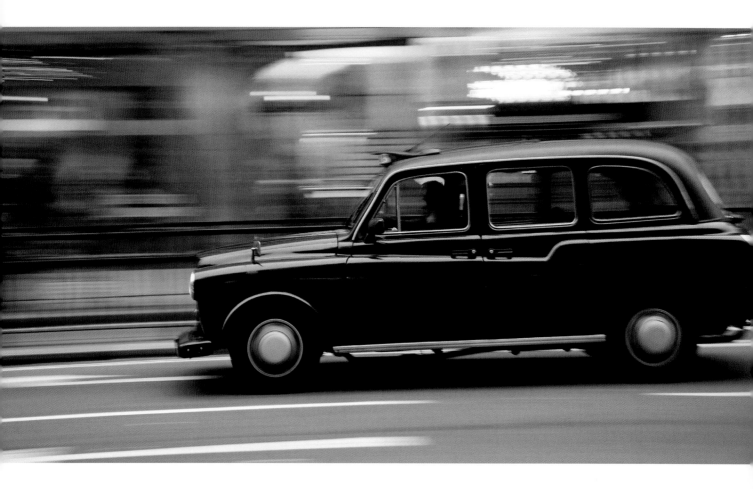

function into old age. Planning, coordination of tasks, and working memory are best preserved when subjects engage in regular aerobic exercise. Some of this effect may be due to slowing the advance of atherosclerosis, a condition that narrows the arteries supplying the brain. People living in developed countries who consume an excessively energy-rich diet and do not exercise, are susceptible to this condition.

There are also benefits from keeping the nervous system in an active state through exercise. Increased physical activity may increase the production of neuro-trophic factors that support nerve cell survival. One of these, brain-derived neurotrophic factor (BDNF), is produced in greater amounts following exercise and is known to enhance nerve cell plasticity into middle age.

The beneficial effects of exercise are likely to be greatest when aerobic exercise is practiced throughout adult life and particularly during middle age. However, even exercise taken up during later years can help to maintain a sense of balance and reduce the risk of falls.

↑ **The middle years are not necessarily a time of inexorable mental decline. Studies of London cab drivers show that the more experienced the driver, the larger the hippocampal volume thanks to the need to memorize the intricate road network of the city.**

Training of the nervous system to perform motor tasks that demand coordination and balance keeps the vestibular system pathways and the cerebellar circuits capable of peak performance well into old age.

Maintaining healthy brain vessels

Although the adverse effects of constricted and damaged arteries do not usually become apparent until old age, the middle years are important for adopting a healthy lifestyle that keeps the brain's blood vessels healthy.

The main problem is a condition called atherosclerosis. This disease involves the progressive accumulation of fatty, fibrous, and even calcified material in the walls of

Keep-fit tips for the brain

Most good health practices for a healthy brain in later life derive from the dictum, "Use it or lose it." The brain stays at its healthiest when all its functions are given gentle, extending exercise throughout life. Follow these tips to keep your brain young:

- Keep mentally active throughout life
- Maintain a regular routine of age-appropriate physical activity
- Engage emotionally and socially with family, friends, and society
- Adopt good sleep habits
- Avoid toxic substances (excess alcohol, smoking, illegal psychoactive drugs)
- Have regular health checks (blood pressure, blood fats, fasting blood glucose)

large- and medium-sized arteries. These changes constrict the vessels and weaken their walls, potentially causing either sudden or gradual obstruction of the blood supply to the brain, as well as increasing the risk of arterial wall rupture. The effects of these changes can be a catastrophic stroke or a gradual decline of intellectual function (vascular dementia).

Minimizing vessel disease

The main risk factors for atherosclerosis are well known: high blood pressure, obesity, smoking, lack of physical exercise, diabetes mellitus, elevated blood fats, and excess alcohol intake. The middle years are the best time to take control of one's health and work hard to avoid these risk factors.

Everyone in the fifth decade of their life should take time to reassess their priorities and follow some active steps to improve their future health. Regular checks of blood fats and blood pressure, as well as a program of aerobic and weight training exercise to keep one's body weight within recommended levels, are essential.

↓ **Atherosclerosis is a disease of arteries where fat, cholesterol, and fibrous and calcified material collect in the vessel wall. The accumulated material thickens the wall, reducing blood flow, and may be accompanied by thrombosis (blood coagulation) if the endothelial surface is ulcerated.**

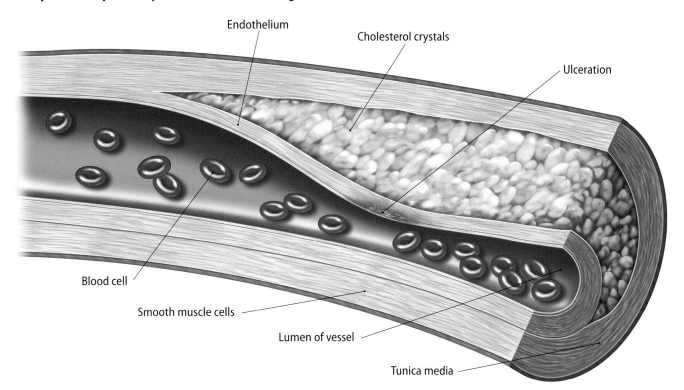

Endothelium · Cholesterol crystals · Ulceration · Blood cell · Smooth muscle cells · Lumen of vessel · Tunica media

The ageing brain

Brain ageing is accompanied by changes in brain weight, the number of nerve cells and synapses, and levels of neurotransmitters. Although we usually associate ageing with diseases such as Alzheimer's and Parkinson's, it is quite possible to reach advanced old age without developing any neurodegenerative diseases.

When we consider the changes in brain structure and function during ageing, we need to remember that not all brains age in the same way. Studies of memory for recent events among elderly people have found that, although there is a decline in this skill with old age, the abilities of about half the elderly population overlapped with the range for normal 25-year-olds!

Elderly people tend to have slower psychomotor speed (the speed of processing information and responding to commands) than the young, but often these differences do not show up unless there is a high performance demand. Elderly people who have been mentally active their entire life and have maintained an ongoing level of physical fitness, tend to preserve their brain function best into old age.

Resilient functions

There are some aspects of brain function that change very little with old age. Personality remains relatively stable from early adulthood through to old age and may only change when severe degenerative changes in the prefrontal cortex make it impossible to maintain

Changes in nervous system structure and function with age

Age-associated change	Effect on daily life
Loss of brain volume in association areas of the cortex	Overall decline in cognitive ability
Reduced blood flow to the brain	Poorer cognitive performance. Greater susceptibility to strokes and vascular dementia
Loss of synapses and reduction in the size of dendritic trees of nerve cells	Poorer cognitive performance. Slower reaction times due to reduction in psychomotor speed
Slower conduction of nerve impulses	Slower reaction times due to reduction in psychomotor speed
Loss of neurotransmitters (e.g., glutamate, acetylcholine, dopamine, and noradrenaline) and their receptors	Problems with cognitive function, poorer ability at maintaining attention and focus, higher tendency to make errors
Reduced plasticity	Poorer ability at recovering from brain injury including strokes
Shrinkage of the hippocampus	Poorer memory for recent events
Shrinkage of the prefrontal cortex	Poorer performance in the ability to hold items temporarily in memory while performing tasks
Shrinkage of the lateral cerebellum	Poor coordination of fine motor activity
Loss of sensory receptors and nerve cells (taste, smell, hearing, balance, vision)	Loss of enjoyment of food, problems with hearing speech, falls and fractures, trouble reading

Our brain shrinks as we age

Studies of brain size have found that at 25 years of age the average male and female brain weighs 3 and 2.9 pounds (1,400 and 1,300 g), respectively. By age 80 these values have dropped to 2.75 and 2.5 pounds (1,250 and 1,150 g), a loss of about 10 percent; but this may be an underestimate because it does not take into account the enlargement of the ventricles within the brain. In fact, loss of brain tissue volume may be as high as 20 to 30 percent between adolescence and old age.

→ **A typical brain at 30 years of age (left) has between 10 and 30 percent more volume than a typical brain at 90 years of age (right). This shrinkage involves loss of both surface gray matter and interior white matter.**

Not all brain regions are affected equally by this shrinkage. Most shrinkage occurs in the higher processing and executive areas of the frontal, parietal, and temporal lobes. Other affected areas include the hippocampus, lateral parts of the cerebellum, and the caudate nucleus of the basal ganglia.

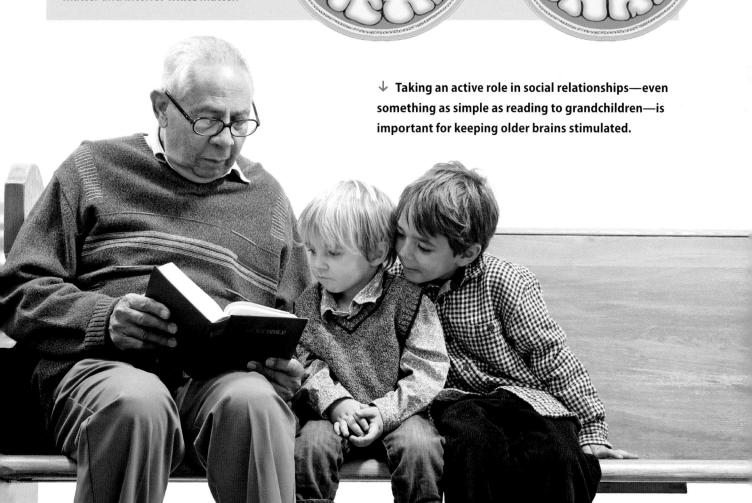

↓ **Taking an active role in social relationships—even something as simple as reading to grandchildren—is important for keeping older brains stimulated.**

long-held patterns of behavior. Long-term memory is also relatively well preserved into old age, so older people can become a valuable source of wisdom and mature insights.

Although plasticity declines in old age, some retained plasticity may help the elderly shift function from regions of the cortex where connections have been lost, to other parts of the brain.

Loss of sensory cells

Sensory cells are lost from all the body's sensory systems during ageing. Loss of taste buds and olfactory receptors rob many elderly of the ability to savor the taste and aroma of food. Loss of proprioceptive fibers from the muscles and joints of the limbs and receptor cells from the inner ear make the elderly more vulnerable to problems with balance, leading to falls and fractures of the hip and wrist.

The ageing nervous system is particularly vulnerable to loss of sensory cells because of the nature of nerve connections in the sensory pathways. In the brain, processing of information is often done by multiple channels acting in parallel, so loss of one set of connections may have little effect on the overall

How many nerve cells do we lose when we age?

Although there is a significant loss of brain volume when we age, the number of nerve cells is less affected. Some studies have found a loss of only 10 percent of cortical nerve cells between early adulthood and age 90, whereas other studies find no change at all. It is important to remember that the number of nerve cells in the cerebral cortex may vary by as much as 100 percent between individuals, so a loss of 10 percent of nerve cells may not be significant.

function; but many peripheral sensory pathways rely on nerve cells linked in series or chains, so loss of one nerve cell completely disconnects the whole pathway.

The larger myelinated nerve fibers tend to be more vulnerable to the effects of ageing than thinner nerve fibers. Larger fibers conduct nerve impulses faster so their loss slows the overall flow of information from sense organs to the brain.

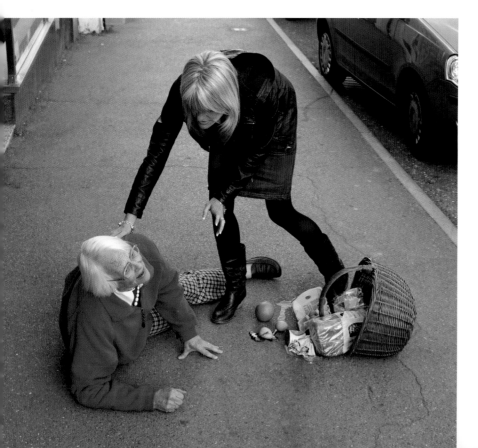

Lost connections

Very few nerve cells are lost from the brain during old age, but there is a significant loss of volume. Almost all the lost volume is due to a reduction in the number and size of the nerve cells' processes, whether the branches of the dendritic tree or the axon ends and synapses. The loss of these is far more functionally significant than any lost nerve cells, because the loss of processes

← **Falls are a common problem in the elderly because of a decline in the quality and speed of transmission of the sense of balance, and the slowing of motor reaction times.**

Neurofibrillary tangles
inside nerve cells

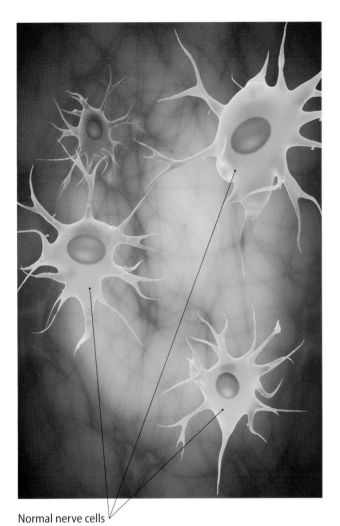

Normal nerve cells

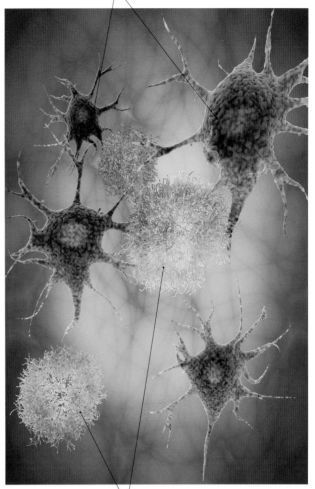

Senile (amyloid) plaques

represents a reduction in established connections that underlie already learned behavior and a diminished ability to form new connections when learning.

Most of the lost brain volume is due to the loss of thinly myelinated axons that interconnect cortical regions. The structure of myelin is also changed, causing the conduction of nerve impulses to slow. Connections between parts of the cortex, e.g., between the prefrontal and parietal or temporal association cortex, are essential for the rapid and efficient transfer of information that underlies thought and reasoning. A loss of these connections would explain why mental processes and reaction times are slower in elderly people.

Synapses are also lost during ageing. Studies in monkeys suggest that as many as 30 percent of the synaptic connections in the cerebral cortex are lost from early adulthood to old age. Most of these are lost from

↖↑ **The ageing brain undergoes changes that include the accumulation of neurofibrillary tangles within nerve cells and the formation of senile (amyloid) plaques in the spaces between nerve cells. Excess formation of these two abnormalities is commonly seen in Alzheimer's disease.**

the more superficial layers of the cerebral cortex, where connections between different parts of the cerebral cortex are made. Synapses in the deeper parts of the cerebral cortex, where nerve cells are more concerned with sending information to lower parts of the brain and spinal cord, are less affected. Excitatory synapses, which increase cerebral cortex activity, also appear to be more affected than the inhibitory synapses that tone down cerebral activity.

Keeping your brain healthy into old age

Some decline in brain function is inevitable in old age, but there are many positive steps you can take to keep your brain healthy for as long as possible. These should be followed from the beginning of adult life to have the best chance of slowing the ageing process, but can be applied at any age for some benefits.

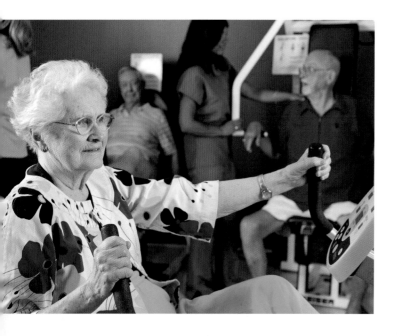

↑ **Gentle, but extending, age-appropriate physical exercise is vital for maintaining brain health.**

The brain stays at its healthiest when all its functions are given exercise throughout life. Research has shown that people who regularly stimulate and challenge their brain with complex mental activities (such as crossword puzzles or learning a new language) are on average more likely to have better cognitive function, less likely to experience cognitive decline with ageing, and less likely to develop dementia.

Physical exercise and brain health
Regular physical exercise is not only important for controlling weight and avoiding cerebral arterial disease (see below), but also helps maintain the nervous system components that control balance, coordination, and motor routines. Studies have also shown that physically active people have less age-related brain shrinkage than do inactive people.

The optimal diet for a healthy brain

Keep your cerebral blood vessels healthy by following the dietary advice of government health authorities, rather than fad diets. Eat a diet that is low in refined sugar and trans- or saturated fats, but rich in fiber; and include two servings of fruit and five servings of vegetables daily. Keep your body mass index within the range of 20 to 25. Reduce your abdominal fat so that your waist circumference is less than half your height. Take regular exercise. Stop smoking and avoid the cigarette smoke of others. Drink only moderate amounts of alcohol (no more than two standard drinks or 0.7 oz (20 ml) of alcohol on any day). Have your blood pressure, blood fats, and fasting blood glucose checked by a health professional and follow the treatment regimes that they recommend.

Healthy cerebral blood vessels

Everyone consuming the excessively energy-rich Western diet risks a serious disease process called atherosclerosis that restricts or completely stops blood flow through arterial vessels throughout the body and in the brain in particular (see pp. 112–13). The most common cause is the formation of fatty deposits (plaques) within the inner lining of the arteries. Apart from a poor diet, risk factors include smoking tobacco, having untreated or poorly controlled diabetes mellitus, drinking excessive amounts of alcohol, and having untreated high blood pressure and elevated blood fats.

Large vessel disease due to atherosclerosis can cause obstruction or rupture of cerebral arteries with a resulting sudden loss of brain function (a stroke), while small vessel disease can cause a slowly progressive, but relentless, loss of cerebral function (microvascular dementia).

Social activity and brain health

Research has shown that people with strong social networks are less likely to develop dementia than those who have weak social networks. Volunteering for community organizations is an excellent way to improve your social contacts and keep mentally alert. Social activity also helps to reduce stress and depression.

Sleep

Sleep is an active process that is essential for brain health. The amount of sleep that each person needs may vary, but is usually seven to eight hours per night. People tend to sleep more lightly as they age, although the same total amount of sleep is needed during the whole of adult life. Sleeping problems are common in several brain diseases, including Alzheimer's disease. Once sleeping problems develop, they can add to a person's impairment and cause confusion, frustration, or depression. Sleep may help the body conserve energy and nutrients that the immune system needs to protect us from infectious disease. Adopt good sleep hygiene: have a schedule, get regular exercise, relax before bed, avoid stimulants like coffee before bedtime, and wake with the sun so that your hypothalamus gets the maximal stimulation at the right time of the day.

↓ **Learning a new language or engaging in mental puzzles is a great way to maintain cognitive flexibility and performance. Activities that require the formation of new connections, rather than relying on old pathways, are the most beneficial.**

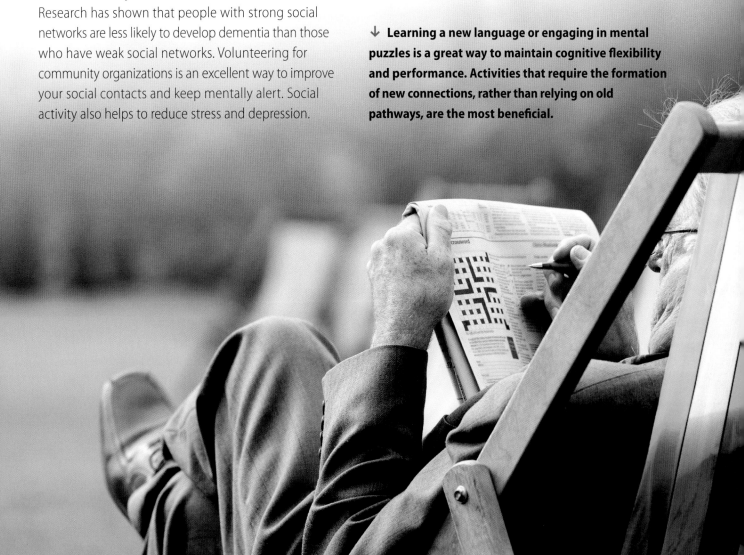

Gender, sexuality, and the brain

Gender differences are apparent in body anatomy, some aspects of sexual behavior, and in the cerebral cortex and its connections. Some claims of gender- or sexuality-related differences in brain structure are based on small-scale studies and are open to dispute.

The most obvious difference between the genders is that the male brain is 10 percent larger than the female brain, but this may simply reflect the need for more nerve cells to control the larger body of men and does not necessarily imply superior intellectual function.

The planum temporale, involved in language processing, is larger in women than men and may be related to better verbal fluency. Women are also reported to have slightly thicker gray matter in the cerebral cortex of the temporal and parietal lobes. Men are reported to have a slightly higher density of nerve cells in the cerebral cortex, which implies women have more nerve cell processes for each nerve cell body. The latter is probably of greater benefit in cognitive function, but these conclusions remain controversial because of the difficulty of obtaining and analyzing a sufficiently large sample of both genders.

Sexual behavior and the brain

The tendency of women to take a receptive posture, appears to be at least partly due to differences within the hypothalamus, although the mechanism is poorly understood. Studies in rats show that males and females have a differently structured hypothalamus and found that these differences emerge during early life from differences in developmental nerve cell death. Studies of the human hypothalamus reveal different nerve cell groups in the two

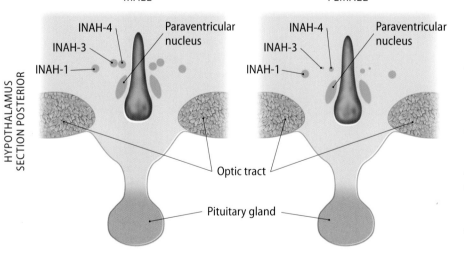

MALE

FEMALE

HYPOTHALAMUS SECTION ANTERIOR

INAH-1

INAH-1

INAH-2

Optic chiasm

MALE

FEMALE

HYPOTHALAMUS SECTION POSTERIOR

INAH-4
INAH-3
INAH-1
Paraventricular nucleus

INAH-4
INAH-3
INAH-1
Paraventricular nucleus

Optic tract

Pituitary gland

← **There are subtle but important differences between males and females in the arrangement of nerve cell groups in the hypothalamus. In particular, the interstitial nuclei of the anterior hypothalamus numbers 2 (INAH-2) and 3 (INAH-3) are bigger in males than females. The INAH-3 is also reported to be larger in heterosexual compared to homosexual men.**

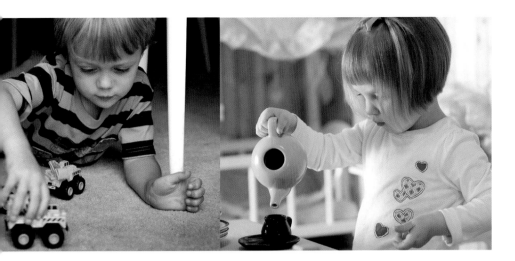

← While patterns of play may be partly determined by adult influence, gender-specific differences in behavior and interests emerge at a very young age, perhaps due to hormone-related differences in brain structure.

genders, with two nerve cell groups (the interstitial nuclei of the anterior hypothalamus) being larger in men than women. These human studies are based on small populations of each gender and remain controversial. Claims that there are structural brain differences associated with sexual orientation (homosexual versus heterosexual) and gender identity (a person's subjective sense of being male or female) are also open to dispute.

Gender differences in cortical function

Functional differences between men and women are recognized on the basis of rigorous psychometric testing. Men perform better than women on visuo-spatial tasks, such as imagining the rotation of a three-dimensional figure in space. One noticeably robust sex difference is that boys outnumber girls 13:1 in advanced mathematical reasoning ability. On the other hand, women perform better than men on verbal fluency tasks, perceptual speed, and some fine-motor skills. Although these differences are statistically significant, they often emerge only from study of a

large number of people. There is therefore substantial overlap between the sexes and average intellectual differences between the sexes are much smaller than the variability within each sex.

Brain function in men may also be more lateralized than in women, but this remains a controversial area. Some reports have claimed that women have a larger corpus callosum than men, consistent with better transfer of information between the two sides of the brain, but other scientists have argued that smaller brains (as seen in women) would tend to have a proportionally larger corpus callosum regardless of function. In a clinical setting it has been noted that women are more likely to recover speech after a stroke that damages cortical speech areas, suggesting that they are better able to press the non-dominant hemisphere into service when required.

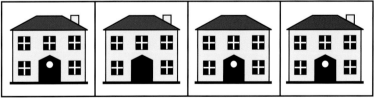

Female—perceptual speed: which two houses are an exact match?

→ Women perform slightly better (on average) at tasks requiring the matching of images, whereas men perform slightly better at tasks that involve the mental rotation of three-dimensional objects.

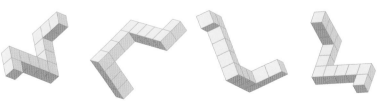

Male—spatial tasks: which two objects are identical (but seen from different angles)?

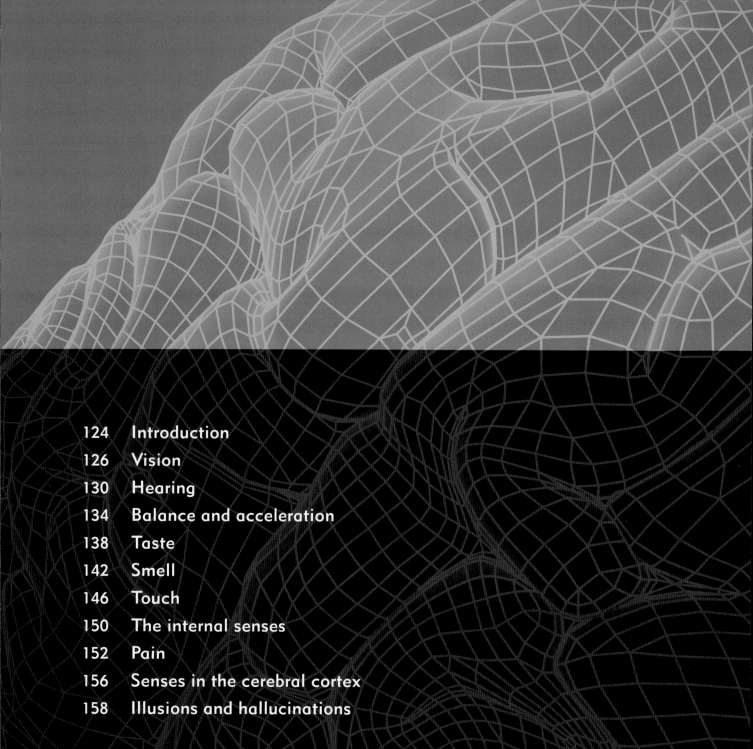

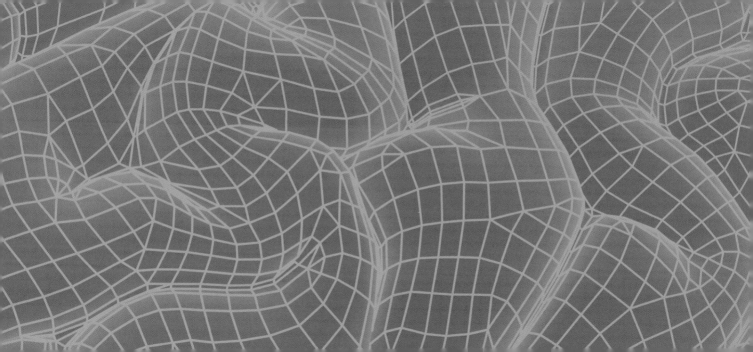

Introduction

Our perception of the world around us is the product of a constant stream of sensory input from specialist cells throughout our body. Our primary senses are vision and hearing, with contributions from chemical senses like smell and taste, detection of stimuli at the skin surface (touch, pain, and temperature), and less familiar but vital senses including our vestibular sense and the senses that regulate our internal body environment.

There are fewer than 30 million sensory nerve cells in the human body (compared with 80 to 90 billion nerve cells in the brain). Most of these are attached to the spinal cord. Much of the raw information received by our senses must be processed before it can usefully influence our conscious and unconscious actions. This work is done by complex networks of intermediate neurons (interneurons), located at the site of sensory input (such as the spinal cord) and higher in the brain.

Sensory nerve cells

Sensory nerve cells are the first components in most sensory pathways. These cells are either directly sensitive to stimuli, such as the cells that detect pressure and temperature changes, or are in close contact with receptor cells that are not nerve cells themselves. The basic task for the receptors and sensory nerve cells is to convert information carried in external energy sources (light, heat, sound, touch, or vibration) or environmental chemicals (odors, pheromones, flavors) into nerve impulses.

This process of converting one form of energy or chemical stimulus into another is called transduction. Transduction is often achieved by means of specially gated ion channels in the membranes of receptors. Some of these are mechanically gated channels that open in response to the bending of fine hairs on the receptor cell's tip. Detection of pressure waves in the inner ear is a good example of this. Others are ligand-gated (molecule-binding) channels that open when a particular chemical becomes lodged in a matching protein molecule on the cell surface. Chemical senses like taste and smell are examples of this. Yet other ion channels are thermally gated and open in response to changes in temperature.

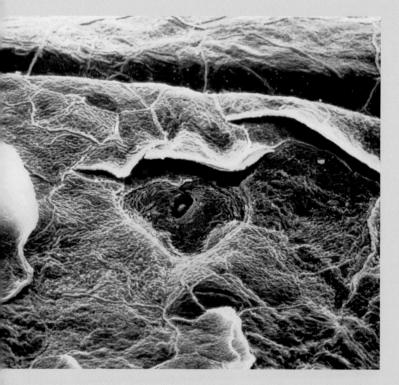

← **The pink form near the center of this micrograph is a taste bud on the upper surface of the tongue. Taste buds are chemically activated sense organs.**

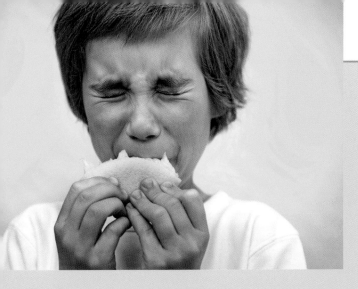

↑ **The acid in citrus fruits like lemons is detected by a subset of taste buds on the tongue and is perceived as sour—one of the five basic tastes.**

The end result of opening ion channels is a change in the electrical properties of the receptor cell; this change is then used to activate sensory nerve fibers.

Making sense of sensory impulses

None of the transduction process has any value unless sensory information is processed to extract behaviorally important data. Naturally, those aspects of the senses to which we are most attuned are those that were most important to our ancestors' survival. This is why our vision is specialized to judge distances to objects and to pick out colored objects like ripe fruit from a uniform leafy back-ground, characteristics inherited from our tree-dwelling, branch-swinging primate ancestors. This requires complex analysis of a flood of visual data from parallel information channels. The large sensory areas of the cerebral cortex are the main sites for such complex analysis.

Our sensory isolation

Although we can guess at what another person may be sensing if, for example, they stub their toe, sensory experience is private. It is impossible for us to know exactly how another person experiences their sensory world, let alone the many senses that other animals perceive. We cannot share the continual pain experienced by another person when they suffer from chronic disease, and it is impossible to adequately describe the colors of a sunset to a person who has been born blind.

Superhuman senses

Across all vertebrate animals there are as many as 20 different senses. Some of these seem quite strange and lie well outside human experience. The ability to detect electrical fields is found in jawless fish, sharks, some ray-finned fish, some amphibians, and monotreme mammals (platy-puses and echidnas). Other vertebrates can detect infrared (heat) radiation almost with the acuity of vision (some snakes) and use this to hunt small, warm mammals in total darkness. Many aquatic animals (fish, amphibian larvae, and some adult amphibians) can detect low frequency pressure waves in the surrounding water. Finally, some fish, amphibians, and birds can detect magnetic fields and use this sense to orient themselves against Earth's magnetic field during migration.

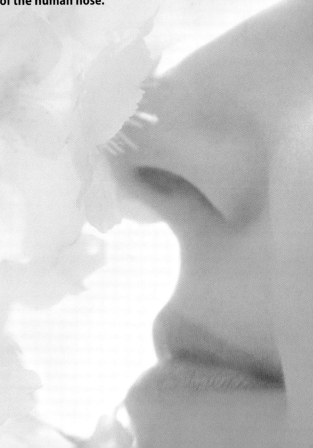

↓ **Smell is a chemical sense, like taste. The nectar of some flowers contains volatile chemicals called odorants that are detected by the olfactory areas of the human nose.**

Vision

Our eyes can perceive images over a one billion-fold range of illumination, from faint starlight to bright sunlight, and distinguish lines just 0.008 inches (0.2 mm) apart at a distance of 12 inches (30 cm). The eyes develop as outgrowths of the embryonic brain, and the retina—the light-sensitive area of each eye—is an integral part of the tissue of the brain.

Two structures within the human eye bend light to form an image on the retina at the back of the eye. The first of these is the transparent cornea at the front of the eye. The cornea actually does most of the task of forming the image, but it cannot change its shape to focus on near or distant objects. Behind the cornea is the lens, a transparent structure whose shape can be adjusted by a system of muscles and ligaments arranged around its rim. The lens is more spherical in shape when focusing on a near object and flatter when focusing on a distant object.

The retina

The cornea and lens project an inverted image of the world onto the retina. The retina converts light into electrical signals that exit the retina through the optic nerve. The place on the retina where optic nerve axons converge before leaving the retina is known as the optic disk. It is not sensitive to light and corresponds to a blind spot in the visual field. The internal surface of the human retina has a rich blood supply.

The most sensitive visual pathways in the retina are concentrated directly behind the center of the lens.

→ **Eye muscles reshape the lens according to whether the object in sight is near or far. Light rays are refracted by the cornea, crossing over to create an upside-down image on the back of the retina.**

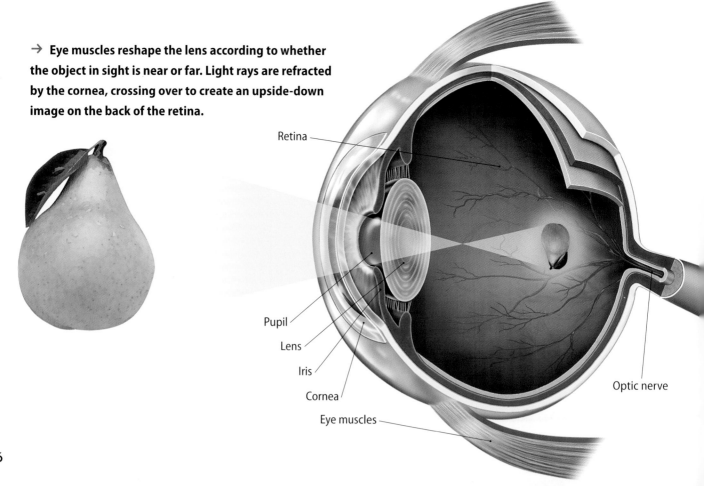

Retina

Pupil

Lens

Iris

Cornea

Eye muscles

Optic nerve

At this point there is a 0.06 inches (1.5 mm) diameter depression called the fovea. This region is specialized for very fine detailed vision and has a rich population of light-sensitive cells (cone photoreceptors) specialized for color vision. A yellowish region about 0.2 inches (5 mm) wide called the macula lutea (from the Latin for "yellow spot") surrounds the fovea. It contains a pigment that absorbs blue light, to reduce scattering of light in the fine vision area. Eye movements can bring the fovea to bear on objects of interest in the world around us.

The periphery of the retina is mainly used to detect motion and to signal the brain to turn the eyes so that objects in the visual periphery can be examined with the fovea.

Circadian rhythms

A special type of retinal ganglion cell contains a light-sensitive protein called melanopsin. These cells synchronize our circadian rhythms with daylight and darkness via pathways from the retina to the suprachiasmatic nucleus of the hypothalamus and on to the pineal gland to regulate melatonin production.

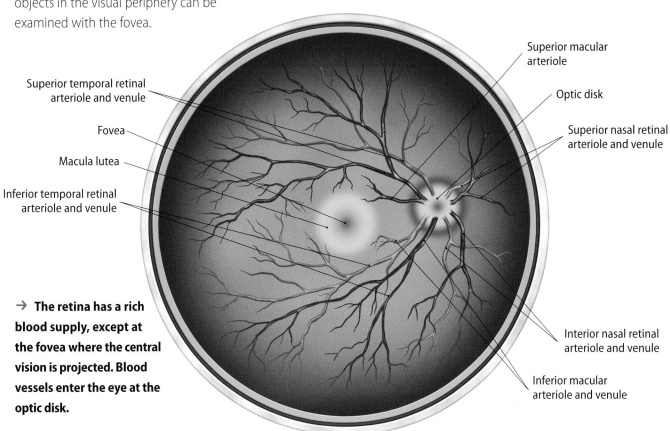

Superior temporal retinal arteriole and venule

Fovea

Macula lutea

Inferior temporal retinal arteriole and venule

Superior macular arteriole

Optic disk

Superior nasal retinal arteriole and venule

Interior nasal retinal arteriole and venule

Inferior macular arteriole and venule

→ **The retina has a rich blood supply, except at the fovea where the central vision is projected. Blood vessels enter the eye at the optic disk.**

Photoreceptors

There are two types of photoreceptors in the eye—rods and cones. The 120 million rod photoreceptors are sensitive to dim light, but not to color; whereas the 6 million cone photoreceptors are sensitive to color, but not to dim light. The sensitivity of the photoreceptors to particular wavelengths of light depends on the type of visual pigment they contain. Rod photoreceptors contain rhodopsin pigment while the cones contain one of three opsin pigments.

Each pigment contains a light-sensitive molecule called retinal that changes shape when struck by a packet of light energy (photon). Dark-adapted rods are so sensitive that they can detect the strike of a single photon. When retinal changes shape, the electrical properties of the photoreceptor are altered,

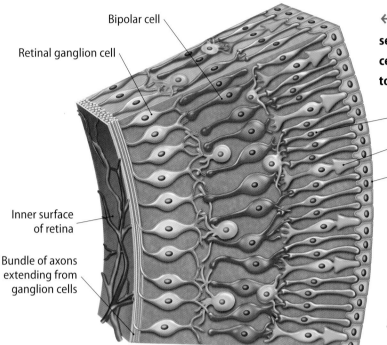

Bipolar cell

Retinal ganglion cell

Inner surface of retina

Bundle of axons extending from ganglion cells

← **This illustration shows the retina in cross section. Light must pass through two layers of cells (the retinal ganglion cells and bipolar cells) to reach the photoreceptors (rods and cones).**

Rod cell

Cone cell

Back of retina

which then triggers the release of glutamate where the photoreceptor is in contact with bipolar cells.

Cones are densely concentrated in the fovea reaching about 130 million per square inch (200,000 per sq mm). Rods are absent from the center of the fovea but reach densities of about 97 million per square inch (15 million per sq cm) in the periphery of the retina.

Visual processing in the retina

The pathway from the photoreceptors through bipolar cells to retinal ganglion cells begins a process by which the pattern of rod and cone activation is broken down into its behaviorally important visual components: areas of motion for the peripheral retina and the boundaries between different colors and levels of illumination for the central retina.

The detection of borders between light and no-light begins in the bipolar cells. The activity of these cells is more sensitive to the presence of a visual border rather than to the overall light level. This means that objects remain clear to us even while illumination changes.

Retinal ganglion cells respond to the contrast between illumination of the center of their sensitive area and their edges. Some retinal ganglion cells respond to light in the center of their receptive area

by increasing the firing rate of impulses (ON center cells), others respond by decreasing their firing rate (OFF center cells). Different types of retinal ganglion cells have different sized receptive areas, different color sensitivity, and respond over different time scales.

In the central part of the retina, both bipolar and retinal ganglion cells are very small (midget cells) and packed tightly together. This allows information from a single cone to activate only two midget bipolar cells with each in turn activating a single midget retinal ganglion cell. One of the retinal ganglion cells fires faster in response to increased light and the other fires faster in response to reduced light and this information is passed on to the brain. It is this dense packing and minimal convergence of connections in the central retina that allows the detection of fine visual detail at this region.

Color vision

The retina contains three different types of cone photo-receptors: "blue" S-cones are most sensitive to blue light (peak sensitivity to light at wavelengths of 420 nano-meters); "green" M-cones are sensitive to green light (531 nanometers); and L-cones, which, although also known as "red" cones, are actually most sensitive to yellow-green light (559 nanometers). Any color in the spectrum can be matched by a combination of the three primary colors that stimulate the three sets of cones.

The proportion of the three cone types varies across the population. Even in people with normal color vision, the ratio of L- to M-cones can vary from about equal to 15 to 1. S-cones make up about 5 percent of the total cone population in all people.

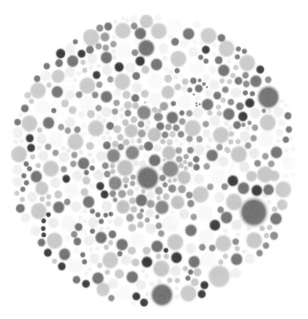

↑ **A person with normal color vision will see a "6" in this color blindness test image, but someone with red-green color blindness will see only dots.**

↓ **The eyes have overlapping fields of vision. Images are inverted, transposed, and converted into nerve impulses which are sent via the optic chiasm to the visual cortex, where they are combined and interpreted.**

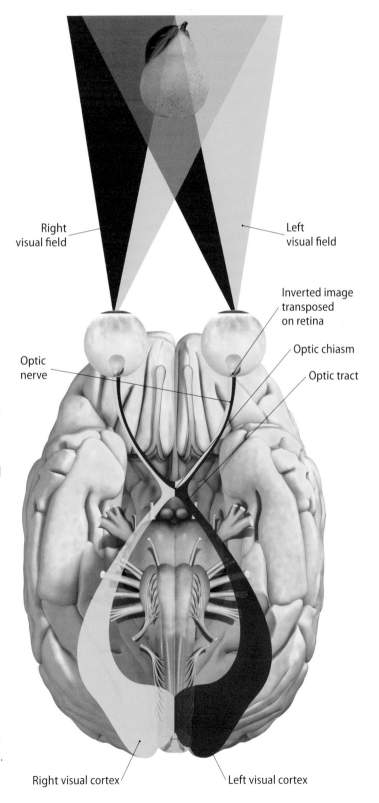

Right visual field

Left visual field

Inverted image transposed on retina

Optic chiasm

Optic tract

Optic nerve

Right visual cortex

Left visual cortex

About 2 percent of the male population have red-green color blindness because they lack either the red or green pigment in their photoreceptor cells (conditions called protanopia or deuteranopia, respectively). These males have difficulty distinguishing red from green hues.

The genes for the red and green visual pigments are carried close together on the X chromosome, so color blindness is usually seen only in males, who have one X chromosome. Females have two X chromosomes and are unlikely to be color-blind because it would be very rare to have abnormal genes on both X chromosomes.

Blue color blindness (tritanopia) is very rare in both sexes because the gene for the blue pigment is on chromosome 7, of which both sexes have two copies.

The optic chiasm

Because they are positioned a few inches apart, each of our eyes has a slightly different view of the world. The ability to compare inputs from the two eyes allows us to judge distances accurately. The axons of retinal ganglion cells are distributed at a crossing point called the optic chiasm. From there, information from the side of the retina nearest the nose crosses over to the other side of the brain. Images are combined and interpreted in the visual cortex.

Hearing

The sensory organs for hearing are located in the dense temporal bone of the skull. A delicate membrane (the eardrum) and a chain of tiny bones transmit vibrations from the external environment to the inner ear where pressure waves are converted to electrical signals for the brain.

↓ **The ear is divided into an outer ear that channels sound to the eardrum, a middle ear with three tiny bones, and an inner ear that contains the sensory hair cells for hearing, balance, and acceleration.**

The human ear can detect sound waves in the range of pitch (frequencies) from 20 to 20,000 cycles per second (Hz). In the pitch range where the ear is most sensitive (about 1,000 to 3,000 Hz), a range corresponding to the pitch of speech, we can hear sounds softer than the faintest whisper (less than 10 decibels for young ears). The sound pressure level of a loud orchestra (about 100 decibels) is about 50,000 times greater than the softest sound that can be heard.

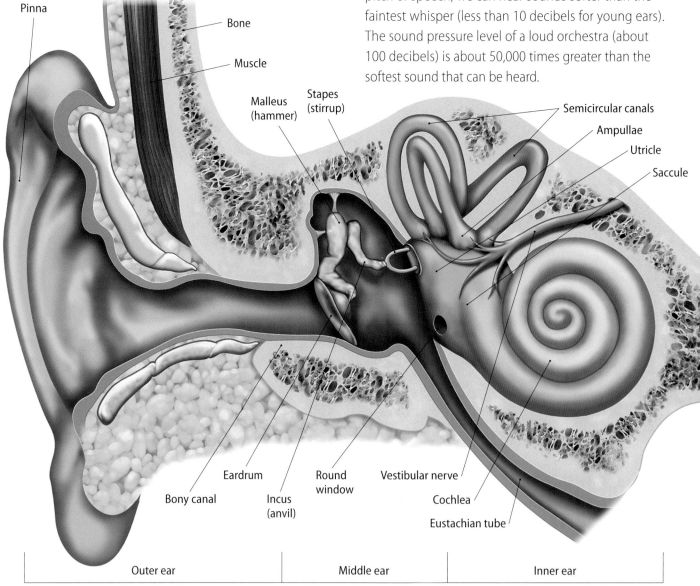

Pinna

Bone

Muscle

Malleus (hammer)

Stapes (stirrup)

Semicircular canals

Ampullae

Utricle

Saccule

Eardrum

Bony canal

Incus (anvil)

Round window

Vestibular nerve

Cochlea

Eustachian tube

| Outer ear | Middle ear | Inner ear |

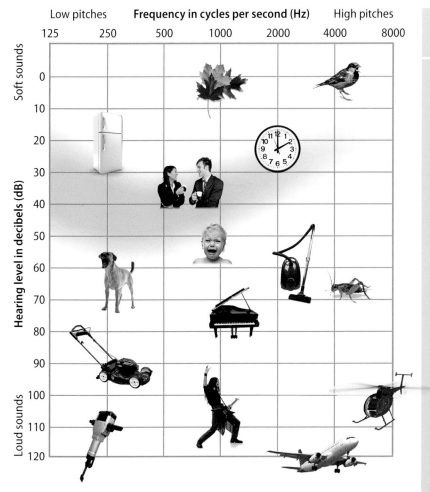

Low pitches Frequency in cycles per second (Hz) High pitches

↑ **The human ear can detect sounds from 20 to 20,000 Hz but most heard sounds are between 150 and 8,000 Hz. The blue shaded zone in this graph corresponds to the range of normal speech.**

Essential amplifiers

Within the inner ear's organ of Corti are two types of hair cells—inner and outer. Most auditory sensory fibers to the brainstem (about 90 to 95 percent) come from the inner hair cells, but if outer hair cells are destroyed and we are forced to rely solely on the inner hair cells our hearing is very poor, barely good enough to hear a loud conversation. Even though they give rise to very few sensory fibers to the brainstem, the outer hair cells serve a critical amplifying role. Whenever a pressure wave triggers the outer cells, the resulting electrical changes give rise to a vigorous change in the length of the cells. Because the outer hair cell stereocilia are embedded in the tectorial membrane (see illustration next page), these changes produce movement of the membrane and the fluid of the inner ear which in turn stimulates the inner hair cells.

The external and middle ear

Sound waves are channeled down the tube of the external ear where they cause the eardrum to vibrate. These vibrations are transmitted across the middle ear by a series of tiny bones (auditory ossicles) called the hammer, anvil, and stirrup (malleus, incus, and stapes). The foot-plate of the stirrup sits on a membrane-covered opening called the oval window. It is here that vibrations are transmitted to the fluid of the inner ear.

The eardrum has an area much larger than the oval window. This, along with the combination of fixed and freely moving pivots along the ossicle chain, amplifies sound vibrations by about three times.

From pressure waves to nerve impulses

The hearing part of the inner ear is a coiled structure called the cochlea (Latin for "snail"). The cochlea has 2.75 turns from its base to its tip and contains three fluid spaces: the scala vestibuli; scala media (also known as the cochlear duct); and scala tympani. Pressure waves from vibrations of the foot-plate of the stirrup on the oval window pass up the spiral of the cochlea through the scala vestibuli. The vibrations cross the scala media to the scala tympani to produce pressure waves that pass back down to the cochlea base and induce vibrations of another window to the middle ear, the round window.

The scala media contains the auditory sense organ of the inner ear, a structure known as the organ of Corti. This contains a single row of about 3,500 inner hair cells and a three- to five-cell-wide band of approximately 15,000 outer hair cells, both spiraling up the cochlea. The hair structures of the sensory cells are called stereocilia. Those for the outer hair cells are embedded in an overlying gelatinous structure called the tectorial membrane, while those for the inner hair cells are not. Movements of the surrounding fluid bend the stereocilia of the inner hair cells, whereas vibrations of the underlying basilar membrane flex the stereocilia of the outer hair cells. The insertion of the outer hair cell stereocilia into the tectorial membrane also allows them to act as amplifiers (see "Essential amplifiers," previous page). The tiny movements of the stereocilia open mechanically gated ion channels in the tips of the hair cells, producing electrical changes in the receptor cells that are transmitted to the brainstem as nerve impulses.

→ **This false-color micrograph reveals the sensory hairs of the inner ear. Each crescent-shaped arrangement of hairs lies atop a single cell.**

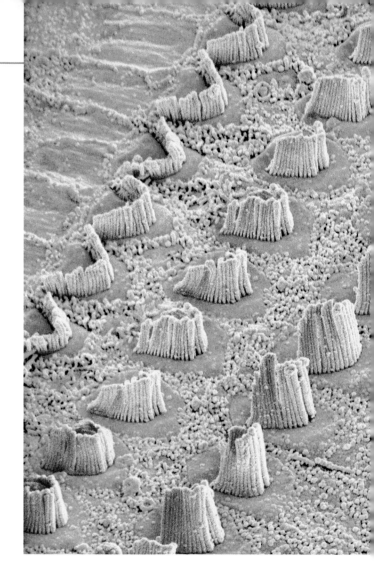

↓ **Movements of the tiny hairs within the organ of Corti provide the brain with information on the intensity and pitch of sound.**

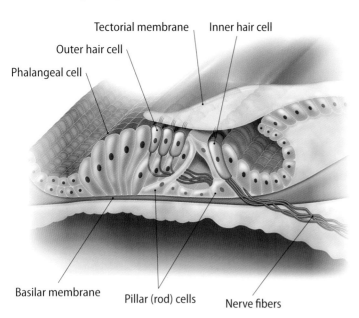

Tectorial membrane
Inner hair cell
Outer hair cell
Phalangeal cell
Basilar membrane
Pillar (rod) cells
Nerve fibers

The auditory pathway

Impulses from the auditory part of the inner ear pass along the cochlear part of the vestibulocochlear nerve through a series of nerve cell groups on both sides of the brainstem leading to the inferior colliculi of the brainstem. The inferior colliculi then send impulses to the medial geniculate nucleus of the thalamus, which in turn channels the information to the primary auditory cortex. The auditory cortex on each side gets most of its information from the opposite ear, although some comes from the ear on the same side.

Coding and transmitting sound information

A sound wave has several features that must be conveyed along the auditory pathways: pitch or frequency; loudness; and the relative mix of frequencies (timbre).

Two types of neural signaling (known as "coding") are used in the auditory system to convey pitch: place

↓ **Information from each ear is passed by the cochlear division of the vestibulocochlear nerve (orange lines) to the cochlear nuclei of the brainstem and then through a series of brainstem nuclei to the inferior colliculus and medial geniculate nucleus of the thalamus (purple, green and red lines) before reaching the auditory areas of the cerebral cortex on both sides (blue lines).**

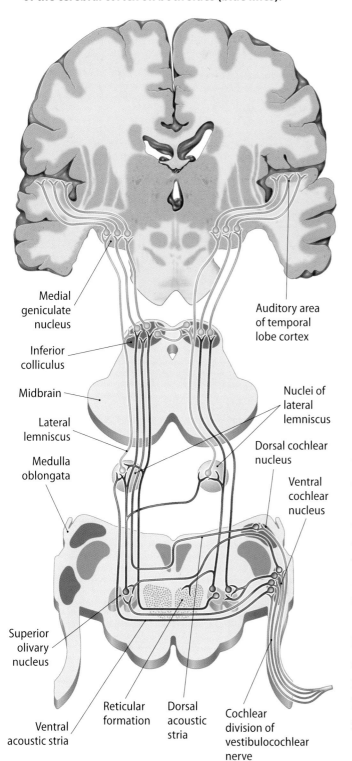

Medial geniculate nucleus

Inferior colliculus

Midbrain

Lateral lemniscus

Medulla oblongata

Superior olivary nucleus

Ventral acoustic stria

Reticular formation

Dorsal acoustic stria

Cochlear division of vestibulocochlear nerve

Auditory area of temporal lobe cortex

Nuclei of lateral lemniscus

Dorsal cochlear nucleus

Ventral cochlear nucleus

and rate coding. Place coding works via the activation of hair cells in a specific part of the organ of Corti when a specific frequency is heard. For example, high-frequency sound initiates vibration of the basilar membrane at the base of the cochlea, thus causing nerve impulses only from that part of the organ of Corti. Rate coding is useful for moderate- to high-frequency sounds and depends on the firing of cells in synchrony with the movements of the basilar membrane. Thus, rate coding nerve activity closely corresponds to the timing pattern of the sound waves.

Loudness, or amplitude sound detection, is achieved by the recruitment of increasing numbers of auditory axons. In other words, as sound increases in intensity, more axons in the cochlear nerve become active.

Detection of timbre depends on the auditory system's ability to analyze the different fundamental frequencies of complex sounds and occurs only at the level of the auditory cortex.

Detecting the direction of a sound

The auditory system can localize the source of a sound by using a combination of clues. The external ear is shaped to preferentially channel sounds from in front, and a little to the side of, the head.

The two ears are separated by between 4 and 7 inches (10 and 18 cm), depending on age and gender, so sound coming from one side of the head arrives a little earlier in the nearside ear. Sound is also a pressure wave, meaning that it is a sequence of compressions and rarefactions of the air. Detecting the direction of low-frequency sounds is based on differences in the arrival time and the phase (i.e., comparing the timing of air compressions) between the two ears. For high-frequency sounds the brain uses intensity differences between the two ears to determine whether the sound is on one side of the head or the other.

The superior olivary cluster of nerve cells in the brainstem plays a vital role in judging the direction of sound. Nerve cells in the medial superior olivary nucleus detect sound location by differences in intensity; those in the lateral superior olive detect sound location by differences in phase or arrival time.

Balance and acceleration

The vestibular sense allows us to maintain a sense of balance, body position, and acceleration, whether we are perfectly still, walking a tightrope or hurtling along on a rollercoaster.

The body's vestibular sense organs are located in the fluid-filled spaces of the inner ear. Our perception of body position also closely depends on our vision, along with sensors in the joints and muscles that transmit messages to the brain.

Sensing gravity and linear acceleration

The pull of gravity stimulates sensory structures in the inner ear that also respond to acceleration in a straight line, so the perception of these two are linked. Both sensory structures (the macula of the saccule and the macula of the utricle) have a field of receptor cells with fine hairs called kinocilia at their tips. The ends of the

kinocilia are embedded in an overlying gel. Minute crystals of calcium carbonate give the gel extra mass, so changes in movement of the head bend the kinocilia and open mechanically gated ion channels in the receptor cells. The changes in conduction across the cell membranes of the hair receptors are converted into signals that travel along the vestibular part of the vestibulocochlear nerve to the brainstem. The part of the vestibulocochlear nerve carrying this type of information is only a few thousand axons.

The two macular organs of each inner ear are oriented at approximately a right angle to each other and detect different types of linear acceleration. The macula of the utricle is oriented mainly in a horizontal plane, so movement of the head forward and backward, or from side to side, produces the most movement of the hair cell tips. It is not particularly sensitive to vertical movements of the head or the pull of gravity. The macula of the saccule is oriented in a vertical plane parallel to the midline of the head, so it is most sensitive to forward and

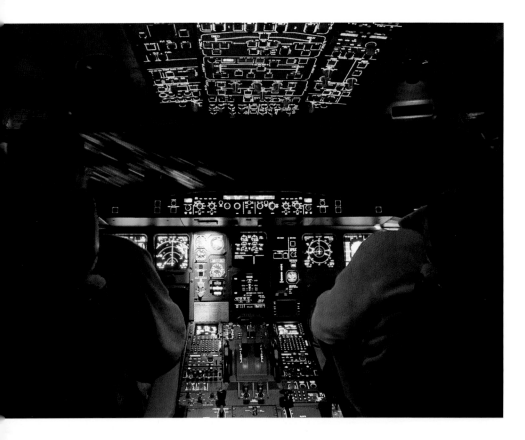

← **Our vestibular sense is easily confused when moving through space in the absence of visual clues. Pilots are taught to trust their instruments absolutely even when they seem at odds with their sensory reality.**

→ **The two macular organs and the three semicircular canals of the inner ear are oriented at right angles to each other. Together they give us a sense of position and movement corresponding to the three planes of space.**

↓ **The vestibular apparatus of the inner ear detects rotation and linear acceleration when fluid within them flows past sensory hair cells. Rotation is detected within the semicircular ducts (inside canals of the same name). The utricle and saccule detect gravity and movement in a straight line.**

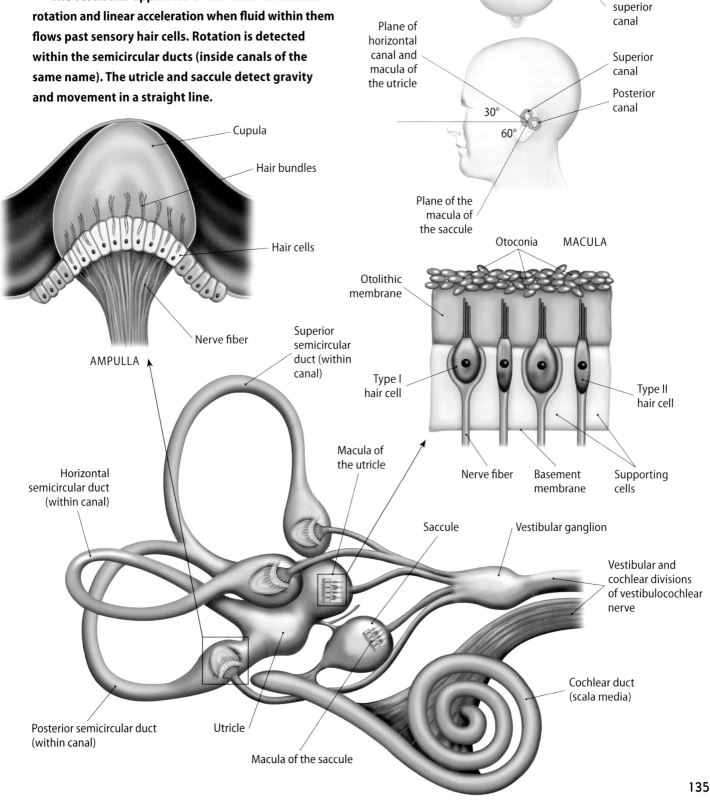

Posterior

Horizontal

Superior

Plane of posterior canal

90°

Plane of superior canal

Plane of horizontal canal and macula of the utricle

Superior canal

Posterior canal

30°

60°

Plane of the macula of the saccule

Cupula

Hair bundles

Hair cells

Nerve fiber

AMPULLA

Otoconia   MACULA

Otolithic membrane

Type I hair cell

Type II hair cell

Nerve fiber   Basement membrane   Supporting cells

Superior semicircular duct (within canal)

Macula of the utricle

Saccule   Vestibular ganglion

Vestibular and cochlear divisions of vestibulocochlear nerve

Horizontal semicircular duct (within canal)

Cochlear duct (scala media)

Posterior semicircular duct (within canal)

Utricle

Macula of the saccule

World in a spin

Ageing or a blow to the head may detach the tiny crystals from the gel over the macula of the utricle and these may enter a semicircular duct, a condition known as benign paroxysmal positional vertigo. The posterior semicircular duct is most often involved because it lies below the utricle when the head is upright. The crystals can shift during head movements such as rolling over in bed, causing surges of fluid in the semicircular duct and a disturbing illusion of movement called vertigo. Symptoms improve when the crystals work their way out of the duct. If symptoms are persistent, a clinician may assist with a sequence of head positioning movements to return the crystals to the utricle.

backward, or up and down movements of the head, and is sensitive to the pull of gravity in the normal head position.

The sensitivity of each macula is further enhanced by the fine-scale anatomy of each. Both maculae have groups of hair cells that are oriented in different directions, so even the slightest tilt of the head can stimulate unique responses from very specific parts of each macula, giving a distinctive pattern of nerve impulses in the vestibular nerve for any head position. These unique patterns of nerve impulses allow us to detect head tilts of as little as a few degrees.

→ **Almost all mammals have vestibular apparatuses very similar to our own. However, climbing animals such as cats have a far superior sense of balance and faster vestibular reaction speeds.**

Sensing head rotation

In each inner ear there are three semicircular ducts (horizontal, superior, and posterior). Pairs of ducts on the two sides of the head act together to detect rotation of the head around one of three spatial axes arranged at right angles to each other. The two horizontal ducts detect rotational movement around an axis tilted about 30 degrees back from the vertical. The superior duct of one side works with the posterior duct of the other as a functional pair to detect rotation around an axis oriented at 45 degrees to the midline.

Each semicircular duct contains fluid with inertial mass that resists rotational movement. Just as the water in a glass tends to stay still as we rotate the glass, the fluid in these semicircular ducts tends to stay still when the head rotates. Of course, the fluid is moving relative to the interior of the rotating duct, so head rotation induces a flow of fluid past the duct wall and the hair cells convert this movement into nerve impulses. Each semicircular duct has a sensory region called the ampulla. The internal structure of these is similar to the maculae of the utricle and saccule in that there is a cluster of mechanically sensitive hair cells with tiny hairs called stereocilia embedded in an overlying gel called a cupula. Movement of fluid in each duct bends the cupula gel and the embedded cilia, stimulating the firing of increased numbers of impulses from the sensory hair cells. These pass along the vestibular part of the vestibulocochlear nerve to the brainstem.

Vestibulo-ocular reflexes

The photoreceptors of the retina convert light into electrical signals at quite a slow rate, so if we are to maintain a stable image on the retina during head rotation we must move our eyes with great accuracy. The vestibulo-ocular reflex makes this possible and is the most important function of the vestibular system.

This reflex works even in complete darkness and is controlled entirely from the brainstem and cerebellum. It depends on groups of nerve cells in the brainstem called the vestibular nuclei

→ **Information about the orientation and acceleration of the body can be used unconsciously by the cerebellum and vestibular nuclei, as well as being perceived consciously through a pathway to the cerebral cortex. Incoming signals are shown in blue; outgoing in red.**

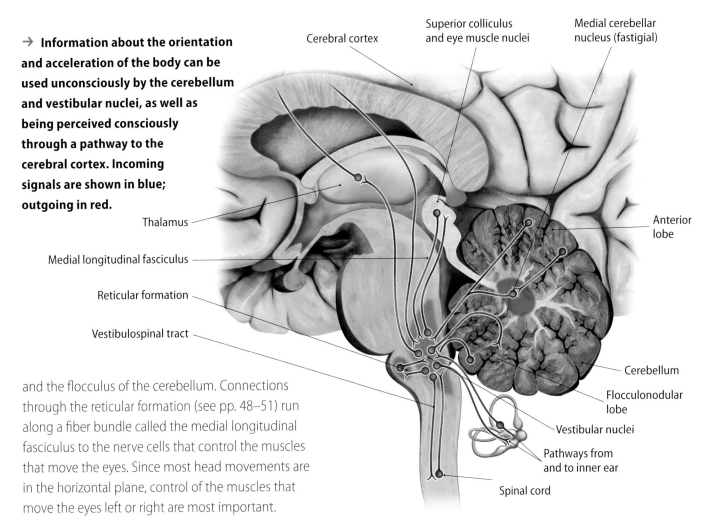

Cerebral cortex

Superior colliculus and eye muscle nuclei

Medial cerebellar nucleus (fastigial)

Thalamus

Anterior lobe

Medial longitudinal fasciculus

Reticular formation

Vestibulospinal tract

Cerebellum

Flocculonodular lobe

Vestibular nuclei

Pathways from and to inner ear

Spinal cord

and the flocculus of the cerebellum. Connections through the reticular formation (see pp. 48–51) run along a fiber bundle called the medial longitudinal fasciculus to the nerve cells that control the muscles that move the eyes. Since most head movements are in the horizontal plane, control of the muscles that move the eyes left or right are most important.

Staying upright

Information about the position of the head in space is processed in the vestibular nuclei of the brainstem. The most lateral of these nerve cell groups acts through an axon pathway called the lateral vestibulospinal tract to

control motor nerve cells of the spinal cord that drive the "antigravity" muscles. These are muscle groups down the midline of the body that resist the pull of gravity and maintain posture.

Closer to the midline of the brainstem, groups of vestibular nerve cells control the muscles of the neck to stabilize head position and to help coordinate eye and head movements.

Vestibular consciousness

At almost all times we stay balanced without having to give it any thought. But it is not true to say that vestibular sensation is completely closed off to our conscious experience. Some information reaches conscious awareness through pathways to the thalamus and on to the cerebral cortex. Areas of the cerebral cortex that are involved in balance include the posterior insula near the auditory cortex and a small region of parietal lobe cortex near the head area of the somatosensory cortex.

Ménière's disease

Affecting about two people in every thousand, Ménière's disease is due to excess fluid in the inner ear. Causes may include excess salt intake, middle ear or respiratory tract infection, or head trauma. The resulting inner ear swelling gives the patient bouts of feeling as if the world is spinning (rotational vertigo), ringing in the ear (tinnitus), and fluctuating, but progressive, hearing loss.

Taste

Our sense of taste allows us to enjoy the flavors of food and drink, and also warns us against toxins. Taste includes very specific sensations from receptor cells on the tongue, as well as related input from nerve endings in the mucous membranes of the mouth, and textural feelings provided by touch receptors on the tongue or in the jaw.

The tongue is covered by bumps called papillae, many of which contain special clusters of sensor cells called taste buds. Three types of papillae are found on the tongue: 200 to 300 mushroom-like fungiform papillae on the front two thirds of the tongue with three to five taste buds each; 15 tiger-stripe-like foliate papillae on the side of the tongue with 100 to 150 taste buds; and about nine castle-and-moat-like circumvallate papillae with about 250 taste buds each, arranged in a "V" shape two thirds back from the tongue tip.

   Altogether there are on average about 5,000 taste buds on the entire tongue, but there are large variations between individuals.

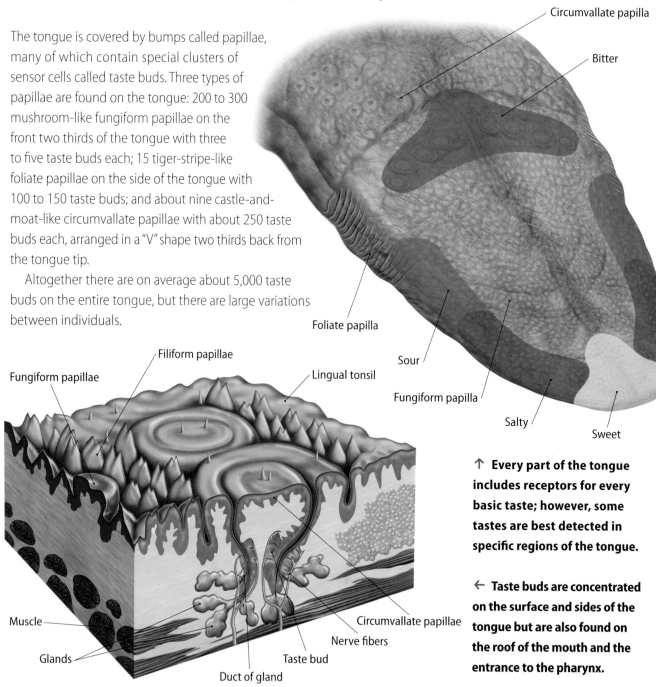

Circumvallate papilla

Bitter

Foliate papilla

Sour

Fungiform papilla

Salty

Sweet

Fungiform papillae

Filiform papillae

Lingual tonsil

Muscle

Glands

Duct of gland

Taste bud

Nerve fibers

Circumvallate papillae

↑ **Every part of the tongue includes receptors for every basic taste; however, some tastes are best detected in specific regions of the tongue.**

← **Taste buds are concentrated on the surface and sides of the tongue but are also found on the roof of the mouth and the entrance to the pharynx.**

Taste bud structure and function

Each taste bud consists of sensory and supporting cells, clustered together like cloves of garlic in a bulb. Taste sensory cells have fine processes at their top that extend through a tiny pore into the fluid of the mouth. The membranes of these processes have embedded in them very specific receptors that are designed to receive molecules of only a particular shape. Taste molecules (tastants) dissolved in saliva come into contact with these processes and, if the tastant has the correct shape, will dock with a receptor. Docking tastants stimulate an electrical change in the receptors that is transmitted to the brainstem along the facial, glossopharyngeal, or vagus nerves.

Taste receptor cells are constantly exposed to the potentially damaging environment of the mouth and last only 10 to 14 days. Cells at the base of each taste bud replenish the receptor cell populations throughout life, although this process declines in old age.

How many flavors are there?

The traditional four basic flavors of sweet, salt, sour, and bitter do not cover the full range of flavors that humans can perceive. Another important flavor is umami (from the Japanese for "delicious"), which is the perception of "savoriness" from the flavor-enhancing effects of the amino acid glutamate. Other receptors are sensitive to fatty acids, one reason why fatty foods are often more flavorsome than other foods.

Taste has a life-saving function

A taste for sweet foods is beneficial in the natural world because these are rich in energy and are less likely to be toxic, but can be harmful when eaten in excess. The salty taste of food is most often due to the presence of sodium chloride, but it can also be due to potassium chloride. A predilection for salty flavor reflects the importance of salt for maintaining health. Salt can be rare in a natural diet, however it is hazardous when available in excess in processed foods. Sour foods contain acids, usually the weak food acids in fruits. The ability to detect a bitter flavor is life-saving in the natural world because bitterness often indicates

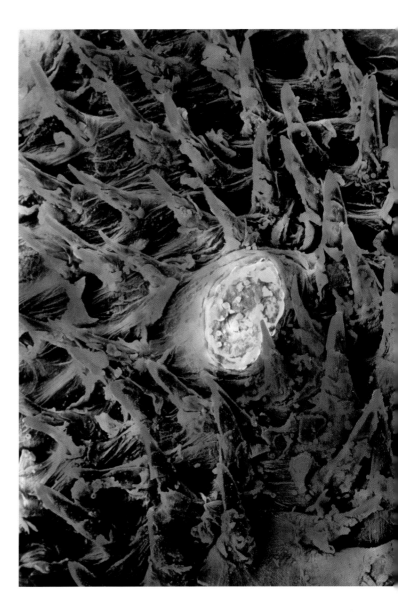

↑ **The taste pore seen in blue at the center of this micrograph is an opening in the tongue surface that leads to a barrel-shaped taste bud underneath.**

toxicity. However, we can overcome the distaste induced by bitterness and come to enjoy it in some foods, such as with quinine in bitter lemon drinks.

Other oral sensations

In addition to the very specific perception of flavor by taste receptors, some food and drink contains molecules that stimulate nerve endings in the lining of the mouth. This information includes the sensation of burning from hot chili, and the feeling of coolness from spearmint. Chili in food burns the mouth because it contains a molecule called capsaicin that activates pain fibers.

There are also a host of other sensations that accompany food and contribute to our dining pleasure. For example, the temperature of food strongly influences the enjoyable aspects of eating and profoundly enhances flavors. Similarly, many flavors are only properly sensed when volatile chemicals rise to the olfactory area of the nose. People who have lost their sense of smell often complain that food tastes bland and uninteresting.

Food manufacturers know that the crunch and texture of food ("mouth feel") contributes to our enjoyment of many foods such as breakfast cereals and snack foods. These physical aspects of food are detected by touch receptors located in the wall of the mouth and pressure sensors in the teeth and the joint between the jaw and skull.

Taste perception and pathways

Some taste information triggers reflexes that originate in the brainstem (salivation, swallowing, and coughing), but most of the information reaches the higher parts of the brain for conscious awareness. Taste is important for influencing behavior, causing us to seek out some foods and avoid others, so taste information must be able to influence memories and motivations in the cerebral cortex and limbic system.

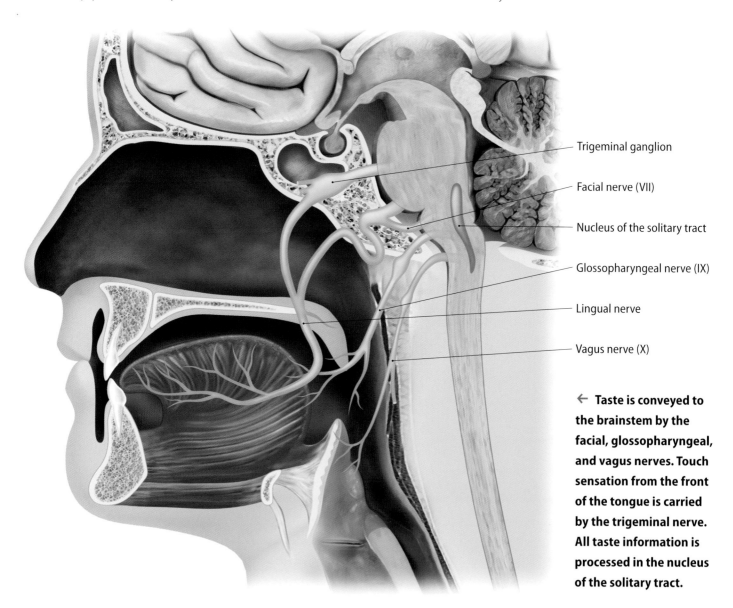

Trigeminal ganglion

Facial nerve (VII)

Nucleus of the solitary tract

Glossopharyngeal nerve (IX)

Lingual nerve

Vagus nerve (X)

← **Taste is conveyed to the brainstem by the facial, glossopharyngeal, and vagus nerves. Touch sensation from the front of the tongue is carried by the trigeminal nerve. All taste information is processed in the nucleus of the solitary tract.**

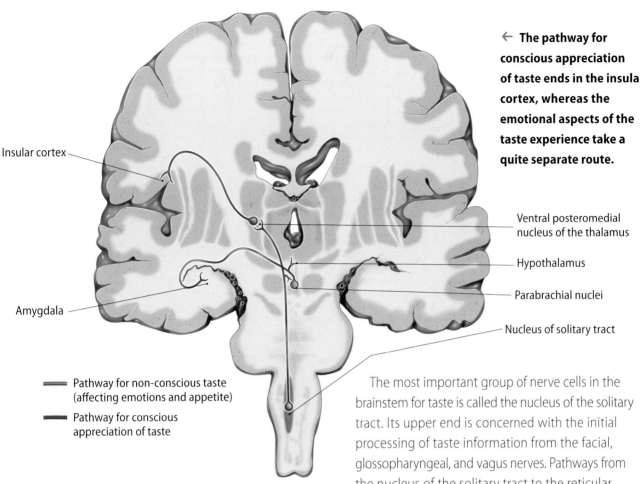

Insular cortex

Amygdala

Ventral posteromedial nucleus of the thalamus

Hypothalamus

Parabrachial nuclei

Nucleus of solitary tract

← **The pathway for conscious appreciation of taste ends in the insula cortex, whereas the emotional aspects of the taste experience take a quite separate route.**

━━━ Pathway for non-conscious taste (affecting emotions and appetite)

━━━ Pathway for conscious appreciation of taste

Supertasters

Supertasters are people who experience taste with a much greater intensity than the average person. The heightened sensitivity of supertasters is due to a high number of fungiform papillae on their tongues. Women and people of Asian or African descent are more likely to be supertasters.

While supertasters usually take great pleasure in food, they can taste bitterness in foods that most people cannot detect and may be dismissed as "picky eaters." They have a reduced preference for some alcoholic beverages, coffee, bitter fruit juices, chili, and some vegetables (Brussels sprouts, kale, spinach, broccoli). Supertasting is potentially protective because these people have a decreased liking for fat and are better equipped to avoid obesity in a junk-food saturated world.

The most important group of nerve cells in the brainstem for taste is called the nucleus of the solitary tract. Its upper end is concerned with the initial processing of taste information from the facial, glossopharyngeal, and vagus nerves. Pathways from the nucleus of the solitary tract to the reticular formation control reflexes that increase the secretion of saliva, stimulate swallowing, or trigger coughing (if a damaging substance is ingested that might cause swelling and blockage of the airway).

Pathways from the nucleus of the solitary tract carry taste information up to the medial part of the ventral posterior thalamic nucleus and from there to the gustatory (taste) part of the cerebral cortex. This region is in the insula (a hidden part of the cortex deep inside the lateral fissure) and the nearby cortex of the frontal lobe. The gustatory cortex then channels information on to the cortex on the underside of the frontal lobe (orbital cortex) where taste and smell information are combined, or to the amygdala, by which taste information reaches the parts of the brain concerned with emotions and the control of appetite. These aspects of taste are below the level of normal consciousness but are linked to memory and give us the feelings of pleasure when we eat delicious food or revulsion when we encounter foods that have made us sick in the past.

Smell

The sense of smell is not as important for humans as for most other mammals, but trained humans can detect many thousands of different odors. Smell and taste often act in unison, even though their pathways in the brain are quite separate until the cerebral cortex.

Our sense of smell—the olfactory sense—responds to the chemical nature of airborne substances breathed through the nose, and also to odors from food and drink that reach the olfactory receptors in the nasal cavity from the mouth and pharynx. Smell has the most direct pathway to the brain of all the senses.

Olfactory receptor cells

The olfactory or smell system begins with an area of receptor cells at the top of the nasal cavity. Known as the olfactory region, it is perfectly positioned to receive odors inhaled through the nose or risen through the pharynx (upper throat) from food in the mouth. The olfactory region is about a quarter of a square inch

(1–2 sq cm) and contains about three million receptor nerve cells. Each receptor nerve cell has a single dendrite capped by a knob-like end. Between 10 and 30 fine processes called cilia radiate from each of these knobs across the surface of the olfactory area. Odor molecules (odorants) must dissolve in the mucus on the surface of the olfactory area, or bind to special odorant binding proteins, before they can be brought into contact with the cilia of the olfactory nerve cells. Special Bowman's glands beneath the olfactory area produce the secretions that maintain this essential layer of fluid.

Each olfactory receptor cell has a specific type of olfactory receptor protein. Humans have about a thousand genes for olfactory receptor proteins. Considering that

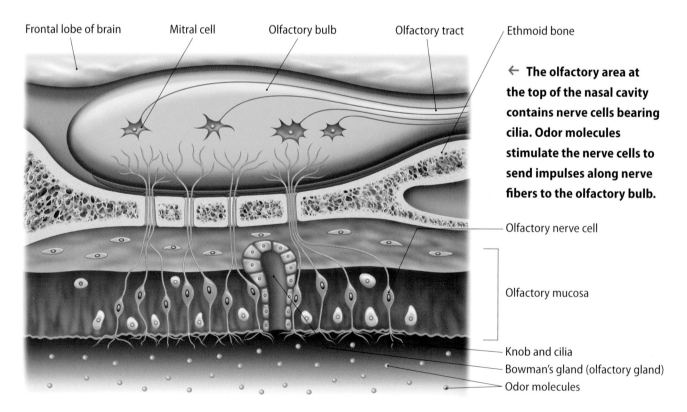

Frontal lobe of brain   Mitral cell   Olfactory bulb   Olfactory tract   Ethmoid bone

← **The olfactory area at the top of the nasal cavity contains nerve cells bearing cilia. Odor molecules stimulate the nerve cells to send impulses along nerve fibers to the olfactory bulb.**

Olfactory nerve cell

Olfactory mucosa

Knob and cilia
Bowman's gland (olfactory gland)
Odor molecules

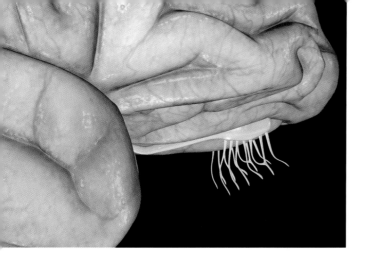

↑ **The olfactory bulb lies immediately beneath the frontal lobe of the brain and receives dozens of tiny axon bundles from olfactory nerve cells (visible here as white appendages) in the top of the nose.**

smell is not a very important sense for humans, these genes make up an amazing 1 percent of the human genome. Not all genes are functional, so there are about 300 different types of olfactory receptor cells in the human nose. Each receptor protein type may bind and respond to a group of odorants, but this array of molecules partially overlaps with that for other receptor proteins. The balance of responses from different receptor types can be used to detect a wide range of different odors, well in excess of the 300 you would expect if each receptor type bound to only one odorant.

When an odorant binds to an olfactory receptor, it triggers a series of impulses in the axon of the cell. These impulses pass along the nerve fibers through the roof of the nasal cavity. Receptor cells become less responsive with time, even if the odorant remains at the same concentration, which is why we quickly acclimatize to long-standing odors.

Ever-growing axons

Olfactory receptor nerve cells are in an unusually vulnerable position for nervous system cells. Their position at the top of the nasal cavity brings them into contact with dust, microbes, and the dry air, so olfactory receptors last only a few months and must constantly be replenished. Not only must the receptor cells be replaced, their axons into the brain must grow anew with each generation of receptors. The special properties of their supporting cells (the olfactory ensheathing cells or OEC) make this continuing axon growth possible. Some neuroscientists have used this property to assist axon growth after spinal cord damage, by injecting OEC into the injured spinal cord.

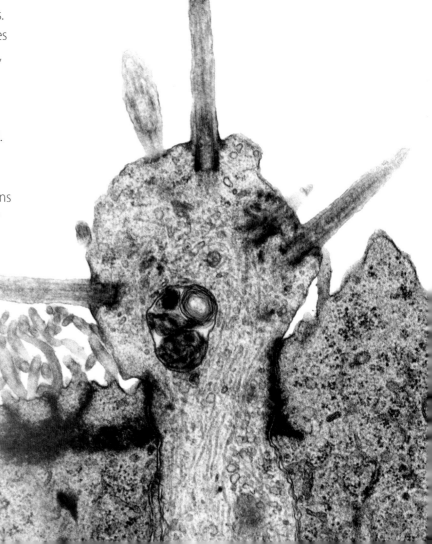

→ **This artificially colored micrograph shows cilia projecting from an olfactory nerve cell. There are millions of olfactory receptor nerve cells in a human nose.**

Pathways for smell

Olfactory receptor cell axons run through the roof of the nose into the olfactory bulb, a part of the forebrain. The olfactory bulb is made up of several layers and contains special globular structures called glomeruli that are penetrated by olfactory axons. Within each glomerulus, axons from olfactory receptor cells contact the dendrites of neurons called mitral cells. The axons from all those receptor cells that have a particular type of receptor protein converge on only a few glomeruli, so different odorants activate different sets of glomeruli in patterns that map out the chemical properties of the odorant across the bulb.

The olfactory bulb also receives axons from other parts of the brain, indicating that our sense of smell can be influenced by conditions in other brain regions. Axons coming from the brainstem use noradrenaline (norepinephrine) or serotonin as their neurotransmitter and probably help to focus or tune sensitivity to particular odors.

Olfactory pathways to memory and emotion

The output from the olfactory bulb is via the axons of mitral nerve cells that run into the rest of the forebrain by a pathway called the lateral olfactory tract. This pathway reaches a region called the primary olfactory cortex in the temporal lobe. From here information is channeled to limbic system structures including the hippocampus and the amygdala. This allows the sense of smell to influence and tag our memories and emotions. Other pathways from the olfactory cortex to the hypothalamus control the timing of reproductive cycles (see "Pheromone sense?," opposite) and may influence appetite.

Smell and taste meld

The primary olfactory cortex channels information about aromas to the dorsomedial nucleus of the thalamus and from there to the region on the underside of the frontal lobe called the orbital cortex. The convergence of taste and aromas at this region make it an association cortex for flavor. The nerve cells in this region may be quite

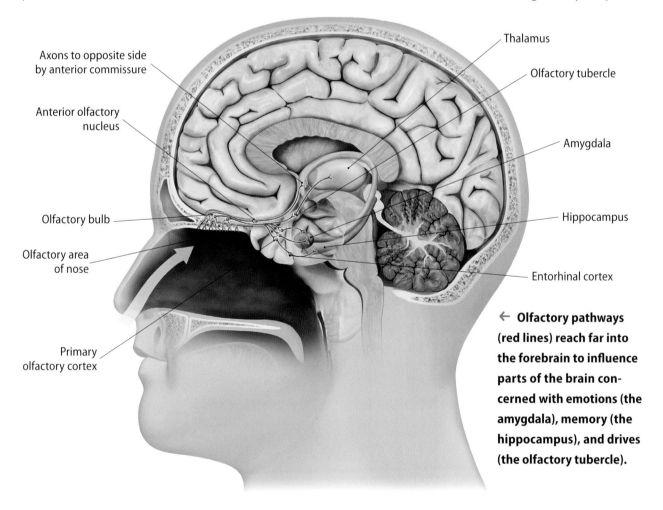

Axons to opposite side by anterior commissure

Anterior olfactory nucleus

Olfactory bulb

Olfactory area of nose

Primary olfactory cortex

Thalamus

Olfactory tubercle

Amygdala

Hippocampus

Entorhinal cortex

← **Olfactory pathways (red lines) reach far into the forebrain to influence parts of the brain concerned with emotions (the amygdala), memory (the hippocampus), and drives (the olfactory tubercle).**

→ **Our sense of smell is intimately linked with our emotions and memories. Well-trained experts such as this perfumer in Grasse, France, can distinguish up to 10,000 different scents.**

complex in their responsiveness, such that single nerve cells may respond to not just the smell and taste, but also the texture and sight of a particular type of food. In other words, information from four different senses about a very specific food type has come together in the one nerve cell. Nerve cells here also play an important role in the reward value of food and drink.

Loss of smell

Although smell is not the most important sense for humans, its loss can reduce our enjoyment of life, especially by depriving us of the aromas of food. Head injury can tear the delicate olfactory receptor axons as they run from the nose to the forebrain. Degenerative nervous system diseases like Parkinson's and Alzheimer's can cause a loss of smell when nerve cells in the olfactory pathways degenerate, or are deprived of noradrenaline-containing axons from the brainstem.

Tumors in the temporal lobe may affect the sense of smell, and the perception of unpleasant odors may be the only sign that a life-threatening malignant tumor is growing. Epileptic seizures arising in the temporal lobe can cause strange odors along with lip-smacking, and chewing movements.

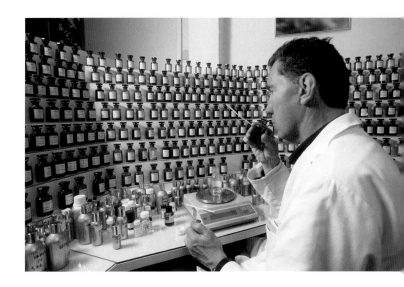

Pheromone sense?

Pheromones are chemicals produced by an animal that have very specific effects at low concentrations on other members of the same species. Many mammals use pheromones in their urine, glandular, or vaginal secretions to influence the sexual behavior and hormonal cycles of members of the same or opposite sex. Most pheromones act through an organ called the vomeronasal organ in the midline of the nasal cavity, but its role in human behavior is open to question. In humans, the vomeronasal organ and the accessory olfactory nerve pathways from it degenerate during development, so whatever pheromonal effects occur in humans must be through the main olfactory pathway. Secretions from women's armpits can influence the menstrual cycles of women around them, accounting for the synchronization of reproductive cycles that often occurs in women who live together closely in dormitory conditions.

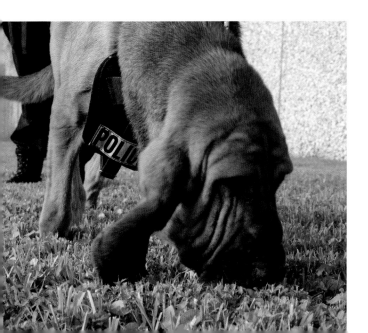

← **Humans have a relatively poor sense of smell compared to most mammals. Dogs have a sense of smell about 100,000 to ten million times more sensitive (depending on the breed) than ours.**

Touch

This sense is more complex than it first seems. Touch is not only our capacity to detect light skin contact such as with a feather (simple touch), but also includes the ability to detect pressure (pressure sense), to tell whether we have been touched at two points close together (two-point discrimination), and the capacity to assess surface textures.

On the surface of the skin and a little way below are thousands of sensory nerve endings that provide us with our tactile sense. These can detect different levels of pain, pressure, and vibration. (Pain is discussed in detail on pp. 152–5.)

Touch and vibration receptors

These types of receptors are collectively called mechano-receptors because they detect mechanical changes in the skin. Most of these receptors are located at the boundary between the epidermis and dermis of the skin, but some are deeper in the dermis, close to the underlying connective tissue and muscles.

Some mechanoreceptors have thick wrappings of elastic connective tissue that serve as mechanical filters, changing and spreading the mechanical stimulus before it reaches the sensory nerve ending deep inside. This ensures that mechanical stimuli that change with time, e.g., cyclical changes in the indentation of the skin as produced by vibrating objects, produce the most

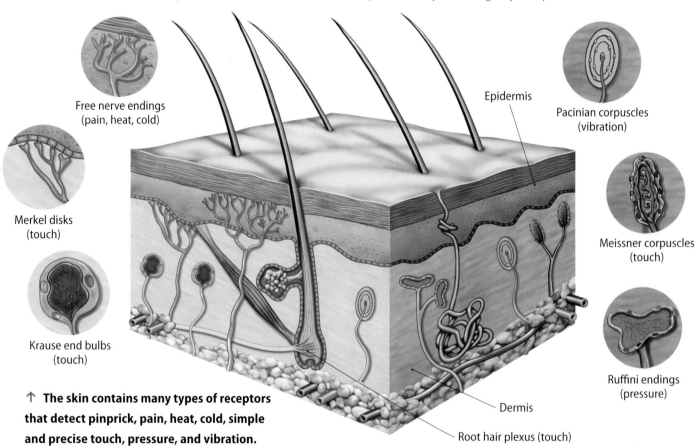

Free nerve endings
(pain, heat, cold)

Merkel disks
(touch)

Krause end bulbs
(touch)

Epidermis

Pacinian corpuscles
(vibration)

Meissner corpuscles
(touch)

Ruffini endings
(pressure)

Dermis

Root hair plexus (touch)

↑ **The skin contains many types of receptors that detect pinprick, pain, heat, cold, simple and precise touch, pressure, and vibration.**

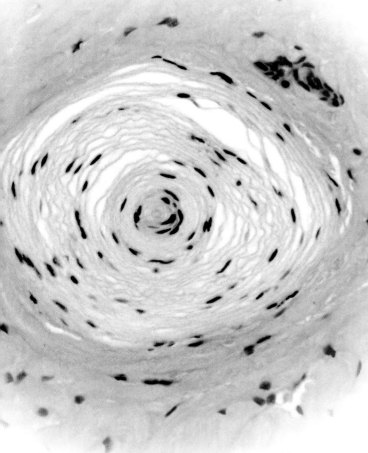

← **Pacinian corpuscles detect vibration and are used to assess texture. Each contains a single nerve ending surrounded by concentric rings of connective tissue.**

The hands have it

The fingertips and skin of the lower face are exquisitely sensitive to touch. Touch receptors in the very tips of the fingers are present at densities of 500 to 1,000 per square inch (several hundred per sq cm) and we can detect two objects as separate stimuli even if they are as close as 0.04 inches (1 mm) apart. By contrast, touch receptors on the skin of the abdomen have densities of only five to ten per square inch (one or two per sq cm) and we are unable to detect two stimuli there as being separate unless they are at least 0.4 inches (1 cm) apart when they touch us.

impulses from the sensory ending. These thickly encapsulated types of mechanoreceptors are called rapidly adapting, because they quickly "adapt" to a sustained stimulus like pressing a blunt object into the skin and cease to send impulses.

By contrast, other mechanoreceptors either have a thin capsule, or no capsule at all. These are slowly adapting mechanoreceptors that are most sensitive to sustained mechanical forces. The thinly encapsulated receptors respond best to unchanging pressure pushing into the skin. The unencapsulated receptors respond best to ongoing light touch of the skin surface.

Other receptors consist of nerve endings around hair roots. Bending the hair deforms the sensory ending and triggers nerve impulses, but this type of receptor responds best to something brushing across the skin and not to steady bending of the hair.

Fine touch detection

Our ability to detect fine details by touch depends on input from an array of receptors across the skin surface. By conveying the signals from many receptors through separate channels up to the cerebral cortex and comparing the inputs with a virtual map in the cortex, our brain is able to perceive the shape, size, texture, and

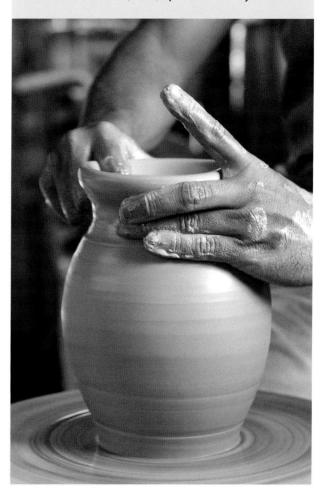

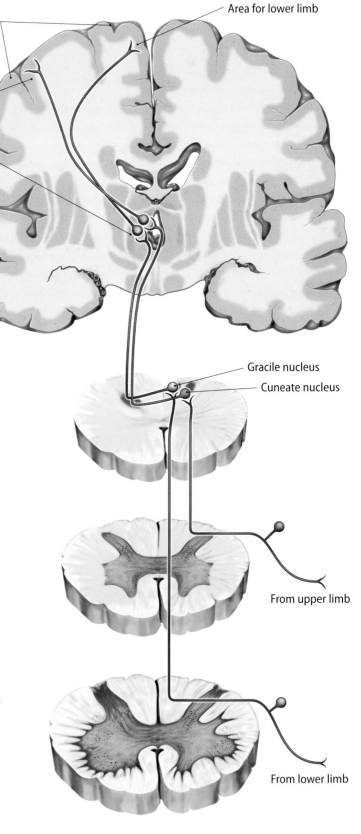

Primary somatosensory cortex

Area for lower limb

Lower limb pathway
Upper limb pathway

Area for upper limb

Ventral posterior nucleus of the thalamus

Gracile nucleus
Cuneate nucleus

From upper limb

From lower limb

location of what has touched the skin. The closer together the receptors are in the skin surface, the finer the scale of the virtual map. The density of receptors in the skin therefore is vital for fine touch and is highest where feedback is important for fine muscle control, such as the lower face and the hands.

Touch pathways

Activation of mechanoreceptors in the skin produces nerve impulses in the peripheral nerves. The sensory axons in these nerves form part of dorsal root ganglion cells. The other process of these cells runs into the dorsal horn of the spinal cord. Some of these axons make contact with nerve cells in the spinal cord for the use of touch in local reflexes.

Other axons pass through the spinal cord without contacting any nerve cell. These are the axons carrying information related to fine touch, vibration, and limb position and run in the white matter at the back of the spinal cord (dorsal or posterior columns). These axons run in isolation from other nerve cells until they reach the medulla, where they contact nerve cells of the dorsal column nuclei. Nerve cells in the dorsal column nuclei pass these signals up to the lateral part of the ventral posterior thalamic nucleus.

Some central axons make contact with a chain of two nerve cells that give rise to axons that run directly from the spinal cord to the thalamus. This spinothalamic pathway is mainly for conveying information about pain and temperature, but also contains some axons carrying information about simple touch.

Yet other pathways carry information about the movement of hairs and some other touch receptors to the lateral cervical nucleus in the spinal cord of the neck and from there to the thalamus.

↑ **Fine touch is conveyed to the primary somatosensory cortex on the opposite side of the brain from where the sensation originated.**

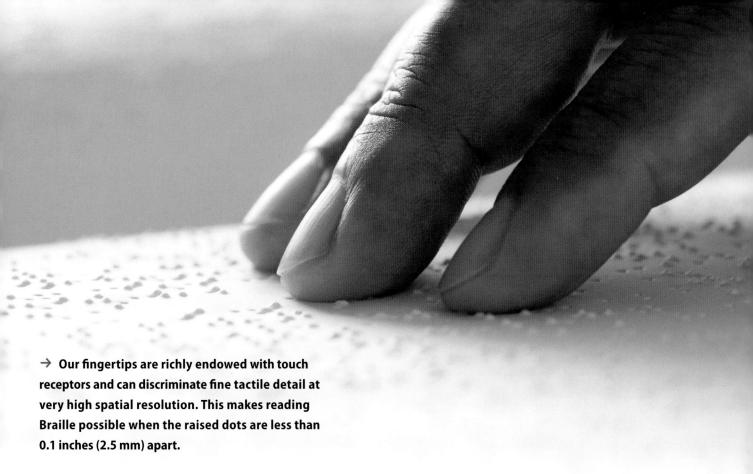

→ **Our fingertips are richly endowed with touch receptors and can discriminate fine tactile detail at very high spatial resolution. This makes reading Braille possible when the raised dots are less than 0.1 inches (2.5 mm) apart.**

Sensing texture

When we wish to judge whether a surface is smooth or rough we pass our fingertips across it. Tiny projections on the surface indent the skin and movement of these projections across the skin activates the thickly encapsulated endings called Pacinian corpuscles that respond best to vibration. Pacinian endings can respond to microscopic indentations of the skin—as little as 0.00004 inches (0.001 mm), about a hundredth the width of a sheet of photocopy paper.

Axons carrying information from different parts of the body are kept separate at many levels. The spatial arrangement of these axons resembles miniature maps of the body (called homunculi, from the Latin *homunculus* meaning "little man"). These miniature body maps can be found in the axon bundles themselves and in the nerve cell groups processing touch information in the brainstem and thalamus, as well as on the surface of the cerebral cortex.

Unconsciousness feeling

Information about touch and pressure on the skin, as well as data from muscle stretch receptors are used to coordinate movements. This information (which never reaches conscious awareness) is carried up the spinal cord and into the cerebellum by spinocerebellar pathways (for the lower limb) or by the cuneocerebellar pathway (for the upper limb).

The inherited disease called Friedreich's ataxia damages these pathways and leads to poor coordination, because the cerebellum is deprived of both tactile sensation and information about the limbs and their position and is unable to assess whether movements are being made correctly. People with Friedreich's ataxia also tend to have abnormal conscious tactile sensation.

Tactile agnosia

When a tumor damages a person's dorsal columns, their ability to discriminate between two points touching the skin close together is reduced and they will have a poor sense of joint position. But the most profound effect is astereognosis, a loss of the ability, in the absence of vision, to identify everyday objects such as a coin or a pen when held in the palm and fingers.

The internal senses

The state of the internal organs is kept within narrow constraints based on information provided by internal sensors. Sometimes, this information reaches awareness, but often it never surfaces in our conscious experience.

The internal senses are critically important for controlling the life-maintaining functions of the heart, gut, lungs, and urinary bladder.

Monitoring the cardiovascular system

Sensory information about pressure in the arteries and heart chambers regulates the heart and blood vessels. For instance, a sudden rise in blood pressure in the carotid artery and the arch of the aorta stimulates a barrage of nerve impulses along the glossopharyngeal and vagus nerves to the brainstem. The lower parts of the nuclei of the solitary tract on each side of the medulla are the main sites where these nerve fibers end. This information does not reach our conscious awareness, but stimulates pathways along clusters of nerve cells on the front surface of the medulla. The end result of the rise in blood pressure is reduced activity in the nerve cells of the sympathetic nervous system that maintains the tone of smooth muscle in artery walls.

Sensing poison

The dangerous consequences of eating poisonous or contaminated food can be avoided by vomiting the hazardous food up before too much harm is done. The vomiting reflex begins when cells surrounding an irritated part of the digestive tract (esophagus, stomach, or upper bowel) release large amounts of serotonin into the blood. The increased serotonin activates nerve fibers in the vagus nerve. These fibers end in the nucleus of the solitary tract and area postrema of the medulla that control vomiting. Other toxins produced by gut disease may pass through the circulation to the area postrema to induce the feeling of nausea and stimulate vomiting.

Respiratory sense

Control of breathing relies on accurate information about the state of inflation of the lungs and chest wall. Lung inflation is sensed by stretch receptors in the lung wall and larger airways. This information is conveyed to the brainstem along the vagus nerve. Other stretch receptors are located in the joints of the chest wall.

Bladder fullness

The sensation of bladder fullness is not only important for knowing when the bladder has reached capacity, but also plays a critical role in the reflex loops that trigger bladder emptying. Stretch receptors in the wall

Bladder reflex control

Infants empty their bladders by a vesicovesical (bladder to bladder) reflex in the spinal cord when a set volume is reached, but adults can inhibit this reflex for a period of time. In adults, the periaqueductal gray of the midbrain brings together information about bladder distension and the current social situation (from the pre-frontal and limbic cortex) before activating a pontine micturition center in the pons to relax the sphincters that usually prevent urine outflow and activate contraction of smooth muscle in the bladder wall to begin emptying. The ability to inhibit the spinal reflex and make conscious decisions about when to empty the bladder is usually acquired during the second year of life.

of the bladder are activated when bladder volume rises above about half a pint (250 ml). These carry impulses to the sacral levels of the spinal cord and can stimulate an emptying reflex in infants that is inhibited in adults. Sensory pathways run from the sacral spinal cord to the part of the midbrain around the cerebral aqueduct (periaqueductal gray), the hypothalamus, and the medial part of the ventral posterior nucleus of the thalamus. Conscious perception of urinary bladder distension occurs in the insula cortex deep inside the lateral fissure.

↓ **The central nervous system receives a constant stream of information from the internal organs about blood pressure, blood oxygen levels, and lung, urinary bladder, and gut distension. This is used to control the internal environment of the body.**

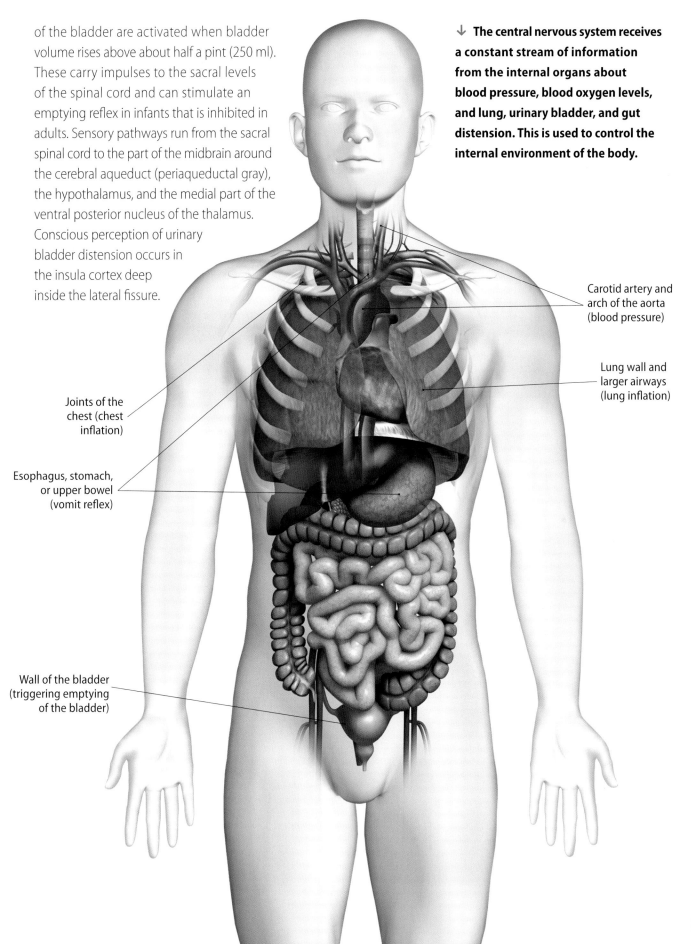

Carotid artery and arch of the aorta (blood pressure)

Lung wall and larger airways (lung inflation)

Joints of the chest (chest inflation)

Esophagus, stomach, or upper bowel (vomit reflex)

Wall of the bladder (triggering emptying of the bladder)

Pain

An unpleasant experience associated with real or potential damage to the body, pain usually signals that tissues are being damaged and also urges rest and recovery from any damage that has been done. Unfortunately, pain may outlast the initial injury and the healing process, or it may have a cause that cannot be removed.

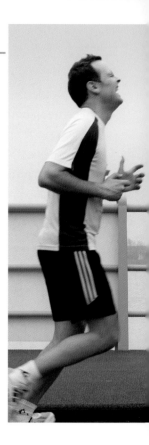

Pain can be a sharp sensation (such as a pinprick)—a warning sign to withdraw a body part rapidly from a potentially dangerous situation—or a sustained ache, which usually indicates a long-standing tissue injury by trauma or inflammation. The pathways for these different pain types may be quite distinct.

→ **Prolonged exercise may both cause pain, by release of lactic acid in muscles, and relieve it, when natural opioid chemicals are released to produce a "high."**

Nociceptors

The group of sensory endings that detect damaged tissue or potentially damaging stimuli are called nociceptors. Nociceptors are activated by intense physical stimuli that can potentially break or rupture

↓ **This PET scan shows active areas of the brain during an attack of cardiac pain. In the top row, the thalamus (at brain centre) is channeling sensory information. In the bottom row, the frontal and parietal lobes are active when conscious pain is being experienced.**

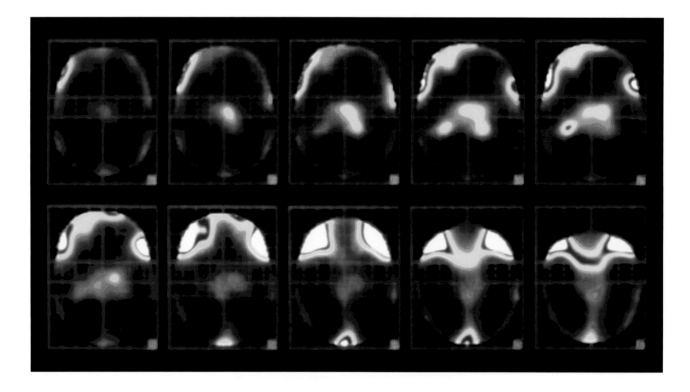

→ **Pain from the body passes up the spinal cord in the spinothalamic tracts before being passed on to the primary somatosensory cortex for conscious awareness.**

The misery of a pain-free life

Pain warns us of tissue damage and encourages us to rest damaged parts of the body, so its absence is a very serious problem. Some people have a selective loss of the unmyelinated fibers that convey pain and temperature, or have a molecular defect in the pain receptors themselves. People who cannot feel pain habitually injure their skin because they cannot detect the initial pinprick or burn that would otherwise cause them to withdraw from the damaging agent. Being unable to detect pain from joints, they may repeatedly misuse the joint and cause permanent damage, or they may be unaware of broken bones and continue to use the affected limb, compounding the damage.

Primary somatosensory cortex

Area for upper limb

Area for lower limb

Ventral posterior nucleus of thalamus

Axons of the spinothalamic tract

Dorsal root ganglion cell

Pain from upper limb

Spinothalamic tract nerve cells

Dorsal root ganglion cell

Pain from lower limb

═══ Lower limb pathway
━━━ Upper limb pathway

the skin, e.g., pinching or cutting; the release of some chemicals in the skin, joints, or muscles; or potentially damaging levels of heat or cold.

Nociceptors consist of simple nerve endings in the tissue of the skin, joints, muscles, or internal organs. In fact, nociceptors are found everywhere, except within the brain itself. Most of the nociceptors of internal organs or muscles are inactive during the normal course of life. It is only during disease or following injury that these silent nociceptors become active.

Pain pathways to consciousness

Information about pain is carried to the spinal cord where it is fed into ascending sensory pathways in the front and side of the spinal cord. The spinothalamic pathway carries information about pinprick, temperature, and simple touch to the ventral posterior nucleus of the thalamus on the opposite side of the body, where contacts are made

with nerve cells that then carry the information further up to the primary somatosensory cortex. This provides the conscious awareness of both the nature of the painful stimulus (burning, stinging, aching) and the precise location of the pain.

There are also descending pathways from the raphe nuclei of the brainstem to the spinal cord that can influence the perception of pain by modifying its transmission at the spinal cord level.

Local anesthesia

The unmyelinated axons that carry the dull ache of pain are more sensitive to the effects of local anesthetics than the myelinated axons that carry sharp pinprick. During the initial stage of local anesthesia, patients lose any dull aching sensation but can still feel a sharp pin applied to the skin surface. Surgical incisions are not made until both types of pain are blocked.

Sharp pain is followed by a dull ache

The initial feeling of sharp pain, such as when we step on a jagged object, is felt rapidly—within a few tenths of a second—after the stimulus. This sharp initial pain is due to impulses carried along myelin-coated fibers to the spinal cord. It may trigger the withdrawal reflex that protects the body part without conscious thought, or be carried up the spinal cord to the thalamus and reach conscious awareness in the cortex.

An aching pain soon follows and may persist long after the damaging stimulus has been removed. This second pain is carried to the spinal cord by slowly conducting axons without a myelin coat.

Itches and scratches

Tissue damage may be on a small enough scale that there is not a complete activation of pain fibers. This is often seen in skin diseases, particularly those that cause the separation of the cells of the epidermis, producing tiny blisters or vesicles. Similar sensations are felt when insects inject small quantities of irritating chemicals into the skin or when skin parasites burrow beneath the skin. This small-scale tissue damage is felt as an itch that stimulates a scratching response.

Local inflammation and swelling

The skin surrounding a wound often becomes red and swollen even though the tissue there has not itself been directly damaged. This is due to an axon reflex that involves the unmyelinated fibers that signal aching pain. These fibers often branch to a wide area of skin, so

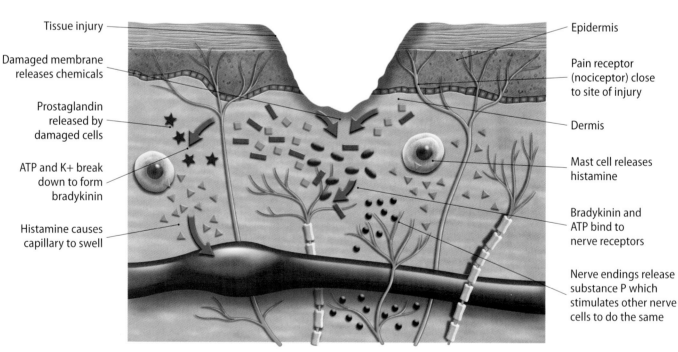

Tissue injury

Damaged membrane releases chemicals

Prostaglandin released by damaged cells

ATP and K+ break down to form bradykinin

Histamine causes capillary to swell

Epidermis

Pain receptor (nociceptor) close to site of injury

Dermis

Mast cell releases histamine

Bradykinin and ATP bind to nerve receptors

Nerve endings release substance P which stimulates other nerve cells to do the same

↑ **Pain is part of the response that occurs when tissue is damaged. Chemicals released during inflammation activate pain receptors in the dermis of the skin.**

★ Prostaglandin ▲ Histamine
● Substance P ▪ K+
🟤 Bradykinin ▬ ATP

activation of the pain fiber by tissue damage in one site spreads throughout the region served by the fiber. The ends of the pain fibers release the neurotransmitter glutamate and neuropeptides into surrounding tissue, leading to the dilation of blood vessels (causing redness) and the leaking of fluid from the vessels (causing tissue swelling, or edema).

Swelling in a body part, such as a thumb after being hit with a hammer, compresses the nerve endings passing through the body part. This pressure blocks myelinated pain fibers that carry pinprick pain, but leave the unmyelinated fibers that carry dull ache unaffected. This accounts for the unpleasant disordered sensations from swollen injured body parts; the part feels numb to the touch, but nevertheless aches incessantly.

Chronic pain and inflammation

Pain is useful when it brings damaging events or agents to our attention, but it can become a merciless tormenter in cases of chronic disease.

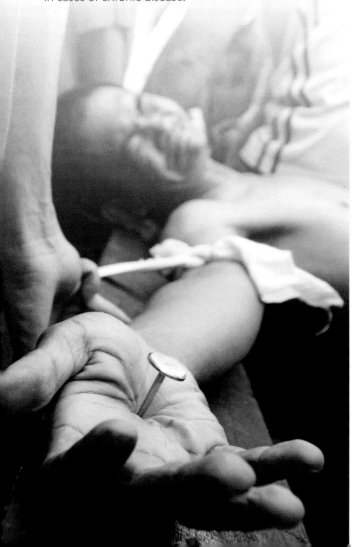

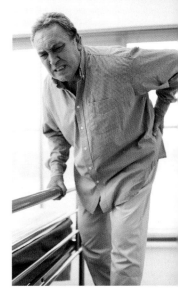

→ **Chronic back problems can cause relentless pain that overwhelms the ability of medication to provide relief.**

The perception of pain and other tactile senses may be distorted when chronic inflammation affects a part of the body. Stimuli that are normally perceived as only mildly uncomfortable may become extremely unpleasant (hyperalgesia) and even light touch may be perceived as painful (allodynia). Chemicals released in damaged tissue, including potassium ions from injured cells, serotonin from platelets that enter from the blood, and an array of inflammatory chemicals such as bradykinin and histamine, all act to sensitize pain endings in the area of damaged tissue. Glutamate released from pain nerve endings may also act to sensitize surrounding nerves.

Reorganization of pain pathway connections inside the spinal cord may also lead to increased pain sensitivity in the areas of the body surrounding the site of injury.

Pain and malaise

Pain is often accompanied by unpleasant sensations that are not localized to a particular part of the body. These feelings may only partially reach conscious awareness and give rise to a general feeling of being unwell without being able to precisely locate the cause. Pain also has the ability to induce changes in the autonomic nervous system that controls blood pressure, heart rate, and the activity of the gut. These aspects of pain depend on information carried along pathways from the spinal cord to the reticular formation of the brainstem, the hypothalamus, and the midbrain.

← **Religious fervor can induce a state in which penitents ignore the pain of serious tissue damage, as when being crucified in this annual Easter ritual in the Philippines.**

Senses in the cerebral cortex

Locations throughout the brain help process the vast amounts of sensory information that come from all over the body every second, but it is the cerebral cortex that is the ultimate destination for most sensory pathways in our bodies.

Each of the senses has a corresponding area of the cerebral cortex devoted to analysis of that type of sensory information. These cortical areas are usually organized or mapped out according to the most important aspect of the sense that they process.

The visual cortex as a parallel processor

The primary visual cortex is organized into a point-by-point map of the visual world on the opposite side of the body. In other words, if you are looking at a cross "+" or letter "A" in visual space, the pattern of nerve cells activated in your visual cortex will also be in the form of a cross "+" or letter "A." This map can be inverted or stretched slightly, but each point on the object in visual space will have its own matching point on the visual cortex. Within this visuotopic map there is an array of functional columns that begin to draw out the separate components of the image (orientation of edges, color, depth, and motion) for further analysis. These components of the image are channeled along parallel pathways to other areas around the primary visual cortex. This simultaneous or parallel processing of the different elements of an image allows a much faster appraisal of the visual world than if each element of the image were analyzed in a sequence.

As part of the simultaneous processing, information about color and depth are processed in parallel with size and shape. The analysis of the color and form of objects (the "what" of visual objects) is achieved by channeling information through a series of secondary or association visual areas toward the back and underside of the temporal lobe (ventral visual stream). On the other hand, the analysis of position and movement of objects (the "where" of visual objects) occurs in a group of association visual areas extending up to the parietal lobe (dorsal visual stream).

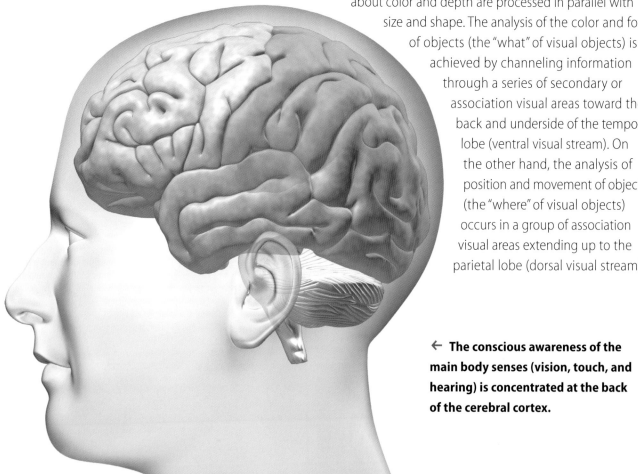

← **The conscious awareness of the main body senses (vision, touch, and hearing) is concentrated at the back of the cerebral cortex.**

→ **The auditory cortex is organized according to the pitch of the sound. High-frequency sounds (detected by sensory cells near the base of the cochlea of the inner ear) are processed in the back and medial auditory cortex, while low-frequency sounds (detected near the apex of the cochlea) are processed in the front and lateral auditory cortex.**

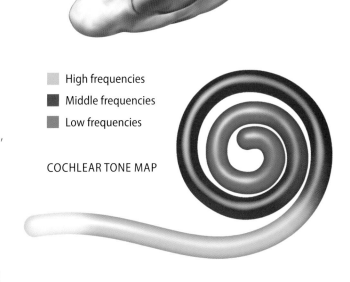

The somatosensory cortex

Information about touch and pain reaches the cerebral cortex at the primary somatosensory cortex, a strip of the brain surface at the front of the parietal lobe. Each side of this strip has a map of the opposite side of the body, with the face lowermost and the upper limb, trunk, and lower limb arranged in a sequence over to the cortex surface near the midline.

Three parallel strips of cortex make up the primary somatosensory cortex. Particular types of receptors (e.g., touch or pain) activate nerve cells in the front strip, but more complex touch information like limb position or the shape of an object held in the hand activates nerve cells in the other two strips.

Nearby areas of cortex (secondary somatosensory cortex) process more complex aspects of touch information. In particular, areas of the cortex on the side and depths of the lateral fissure (insular cortex) are concerned with pain from the skin or internal organs.

■ High frequencies
■ Middle frequencies
■ Low frequencies

COCHLEAR TONE MAP

Prosopagnosia

People who have strokes affecting the underside of the temporal lobe may have a profound difficulty recognizing the faces of family members or famous people, or other categories of visual objects (such as types of animals), due to damage to the components of the ventral visual stream. This condition is called prosopagnosia.

The primary auditory cortex

Information about sound from both ears is directed to the primary auditory cortex on the upper temporal lobe of both sides. The primary auditory cortex is organized by pitch or frequency, with high pitch sounds activating nerve cells in the back of the cortex and low pitch sounds activating nerve cells in the front part. The primary auditory cortex is surrounded by a group of higher auditory areas that are involved in the perception of complex aspects of sound like harmonic complexes. A ventral stream of cortical regions is concerned with converting sound to meaning (the "what" stream), whereas a dorsal stream is concerned with the location of sound (the "where" stream).

Illusions and hallucinations

Over millions of years our senses have evolved to give us the best chance to survive and thrive. They provide us with a richly detailed awareness of the world outside and within our bodies. But can they always be trusted?

Particular types of stimuli can lead us to misinterpret the nature, position, or even the existence of the source of sensation. These illusions depend on peculiar features of sensory pathways. By contrast, hallucinations are complex misperceptions that usually arise from disordered function in the sensory areas of the cortex.

Tactile illusions

Some simple illusions arise because of the limitations of sensory pathways. An example is Green's thermal illusion. Take three coins, place two in a freezer to cool, and then arrange the three coins on a flat surface with the room temperature coin in the middle. Place the index and ring fingers of your hand on the two cold coins and the middle finger on the room temperature coin. The room temperature coin will feel just as cold as the other two because the temperature pathways from the skin have a limited ability to distinguish temperature between objects close together in space.

Vibrating stimuli applied to the wrists also mislead the pathways that convey information about the position of body parts, giving rise to the illusion that the limbs are shrinking.

Visual illusions

Visual illusions may be simple or complex. A simple illusion is the way that the visual cortex "fills in" the part of visual space that corresponds to the blind spot, so that we are not consciously aware of this defect in our visual fields (see "Find your blind spot," opposite).

Other visual illusions arise from the way that the visual system preferentially analyzes visual form on the basis of borders between dark and light. The Kanisza triangle is an illusory white triangle that appears in the foreground of a group of bordering shapes that define the corners of the triangle.

In the Müller-Lyer illusion, lines of equal length may be misperceived depending on whether angled lines at each end of the line are pointing inward or outward. The length of a line may also be misjudged if an apparently three-dimensional object is used as a background and gives the misperception of perspective.

Even more complex visual illusions arise in those parts of the visual cortex in the temporal lobe that are concerned with the extraction of recognizable shapes, such as faces or animal shapes, from borders between light and dark areas.

→ **The visual cortex is good at detecting contrasting borders between objects and their surroundings as well as making spatial judgments based on rules of perspective. These illusions take advantage of these cognitive tendencies.**

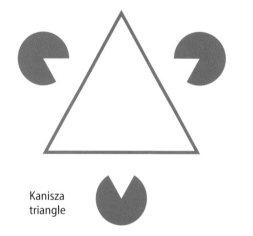

Kanisza triangle

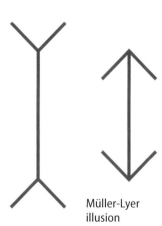

Müller-Lyer illusion

Hallucinations

Hallucinations are complex in nature—for instance, an entire human figure may be seen or whole spoken sentences heard. This complexity indicates that they must arise from abnormal activity in higher sensory or language areas of the cortex rather than those parts of the brain that deal with the simple aspects of sensory data.

Auditory hallucinations, such as hearing a disembodied voice, are a common feature of schizophrenia. Often the voice is insulting, or accusatory, in keeping with the paranoid feelings that the patient experiences. The voices appear to arise from areas in the right hemisphere concerned with the emotional content of language.

Olfactory hallucinations, such as an inexplicable unpleasant odor, may accompany the early stages of an epileptic seizure in the front of the temporal lobe, where the olfactory cortical areas are located. They may also be the first sign of a malignant tumor in that region.

Hallucinations may also be induced by experimental transcranial magnetic stimulation of the higher sensory regions or arise as a result of disordered blood supply to the cortical surface in the prelude to migraine headaches. Many people experience "fortification lines," a series of zig-zagging lines, in the visual field on the opposite side of the body as part of the aura that precedes the migraine headache. Some migraineurs even see whole human figures.

→ **Hildegard of Bingen was an 11th century abbess who experienced mystical visions, which she later illustrated. Featuring scintillating points of light, these visions were likely hallucinations brought on during migraine headaches.**

Find your blind spot

Cover your right eye and focus on the red cross with your left eye at a distance of about 12 inches (30 cm) from this page. You can vaguely see the black dot in the periphery of your visual field. Move the page slowly closer, still focusing on the cross. At a certain distance, the black dot will disappear (when its image falls on the blind spot). With both eyes open, we see no blind spot as objects falling on the blind spot of one eye do not fall on the blind spot of the other eye.

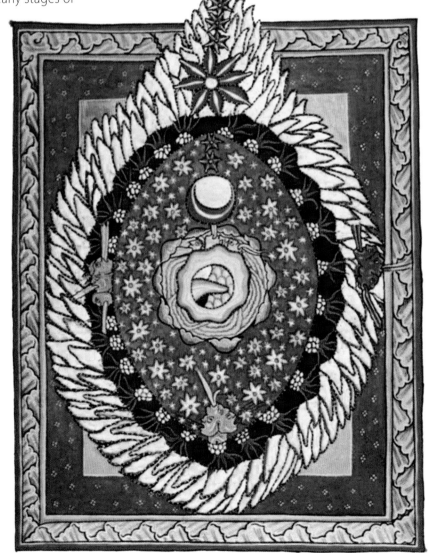

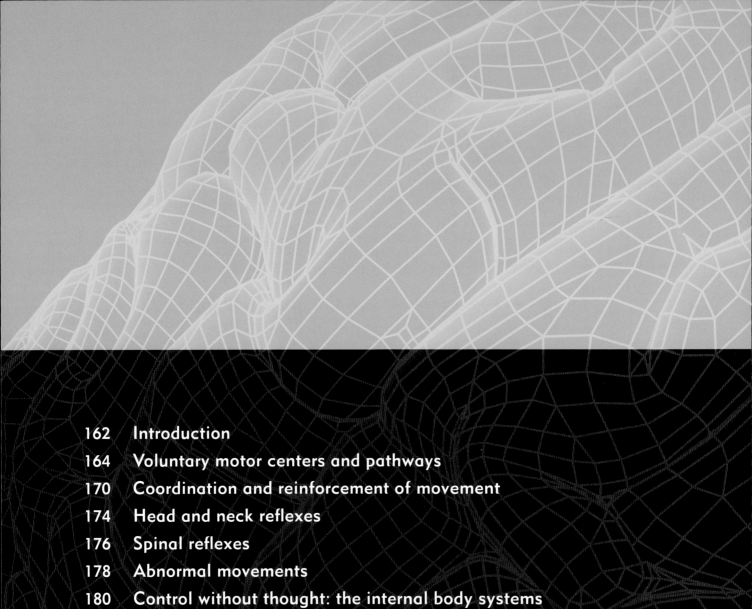

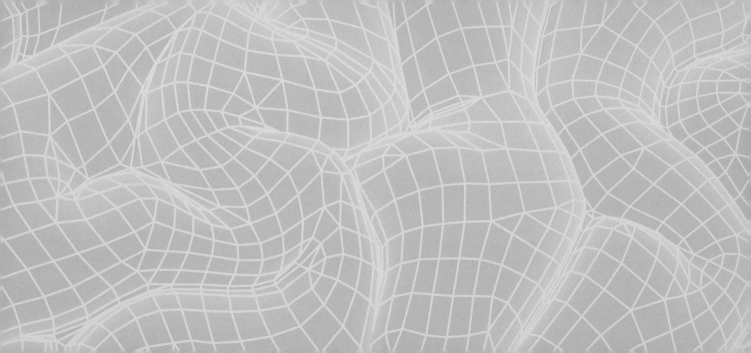

Introduction

There are only a million or so motor nerve cells that directly control our voluntary muscles, but upstream of those motor nerve cells are large areas of the cerebral cortex devoted to motor programs for our common movements, as well as nerve cell networks in the basal ganglia and cerebellum that ensure that every movement is performed smoothly and reliably.

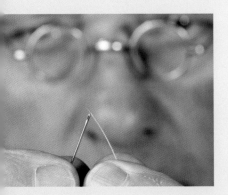

← Fine motor actions like threading a needle require the precise coordination of many tiny muscles in the hand. This is critically dependent on circuits that involve both the basal ganglia and cerebellum.

Each side of the primary motor cortex incorporates a map of the opposite side of the body. Some parts of the body have more behavioral significance than others and these have a more extensive representation. Fine motor control of the small muscles of the face is essential for verbal and nonverbal communication, and precise control of fingers and thumbs is one of our greatest advantages as a species. Both the face and hand have large representations on the primary motor cortex, with particular emphasis on the lips, fingers, and thumbs. The larger cortical area allows individual cortical nerve cells to control quite small groups of muscle fibers, providing fine control.

A hierarchy of motor control

We use our cerebral cortex whenever we consciously plan or imagine the sequence of actions that make up a movement, and it is the cerebral cortex that ultimately directs the brainstem and spinal cord to activate muscles in the correct sequence and duration.

Any voluntary movement must be continuously monitored to ensure that it is proceeding correctly, so feedback loops through the basal ganglia and cerebellum are essential components of the motor system. This feedback is informed by sensory information from the limbs, joints, and muscles, so the motor system rarely acts in isolation from the sensory system. The cerebellum also contains instructions for how to activate muscles optimally for skilled movements, and these must be accessed before movement begins.

The reticular formation of the brainstem, along with neural networks in the spinal cord that can operate in isolation from the brain (central pattern generators), control routine habitual actions while lower motor nerve cells in the brainstem and spinal cord drive the actual contractions of muscles.

Semiautomatic motor actions

Control of our breathing and eye muscles can be conscious, as when we sing or roll our eyes theatrically; a semiconscious emotional response, e.g., a gasp or widening of the eyes in surprise; or completely unconscious, as when we breath without any conscious thought as we focus on another motor task, or follow a moving object with our eyes. This suggests that different motor centers in the brain can override each other as the specific behavior requires. Voluntary control is initiated in the cerebral cortex, but more automatic responses and actions arise in the brainstem, cerebellum, or spinal cord.

Reflex actions

Many of our unconscious actions are reflexes that protect the body from damaging agents or actions. These are hard-wired into the nervous system and do not change in the light of experience. Some reflexes can be overridden by concentrated voluntary control, but only with considerable effort.

Reflex circuitry can be quite simple, such as the axon reflex of pain fibers or the deep tendon reflexes, but usually the circuits include networks of interneurons to coordinate the reflexive response.

Internal control systems

The maintenance of a constant internal environment is essential for survival. Several internal systems tirelessly maintain optimal conditions without any thought or conscious intervention. It is only when we are subjected to the consequences of abnormal function in these complex reflex pathways that they come to our attention.

↑ **Large-scale motor actions require rapid transmission of information about joint, limb, and trunk position and speedy information processing in the brain's motor centers.**

Sleepwalking

Sleepwalking happens mostly in childhood and adolescence and is a complex set of automatic behaviors. It is not associated with the REM stage of sleep when our bodies are effectively paralyzed to keep us from acting out our dreams. Sleepwalkers get out of bed and walk slowly in an automatic way. They may engage in activities such as eating or getting dressed, even playing musical instruments, sending emails, or driving, but their actions are automatic and ungainly. The causes of sleepwalking are still poorly understood, but it is often associated with stress, sleep deprivation, noise, or medication.

Voluntary motor centers and pathways

Control of movement depends on a hierarchy of brain regions in the cerebral cortex that select and initiate motor programs, as well as a series of looped circuits that reinforce, regulate, or coordinate the activation of muscles. Some motor tasks of particular behavioral importance have special circuitry.

To perform even the simplest motor task, different parts of the brain must be activated in the correct sequence.

When we make the decision to perform a motor action, such as to reach out and pick up an object from a desk, the first part of the brain to activate is the prefrontal cortex. This region commands the premotor cortex to devise a plan for the movement and to access the motor routines or programs that will be required for the action. These routines are stored in the lateral parts of the cerebellum (cerebrocerebellum) so the loops that connect the cerebral cortex and cerebellum are activated even before movement begins. If the movement involves both sides of the body, emotional vocalization, or the mental rehearsing of a series of movements before the action, the supplementary motor cortex will also be involved.

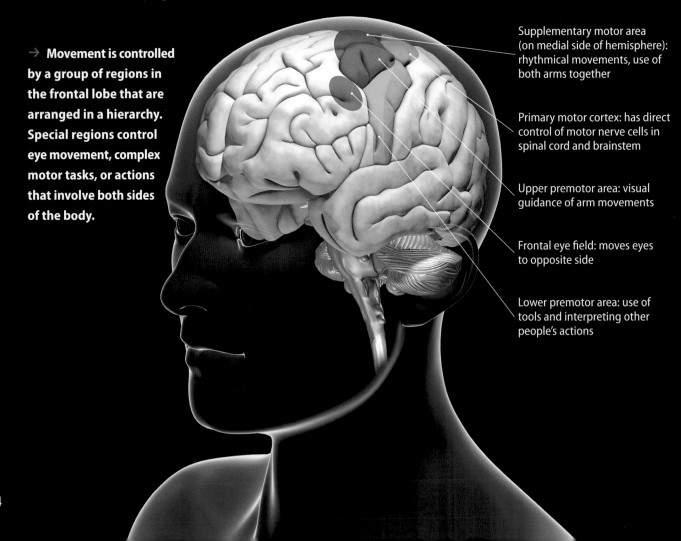

→ **Movement is controlled by a group of regions in the frontal lobe that are arranged in a hierarchy. Special regions control eye movement, complex motor tasks, or actions that involve both sides of the body.**

Supplementary motor area (on medial side of hemisphere): rhythmical movements, use of both arms together

Primary motor cortex: has direct control of motor nerve cells in spinal cord and brainstem

Upper premotor area: visual guidance of arm movements

Frontal eye field: moves eyes to opposite side

Lower premotor area: use of tools and interpreting other people's actions

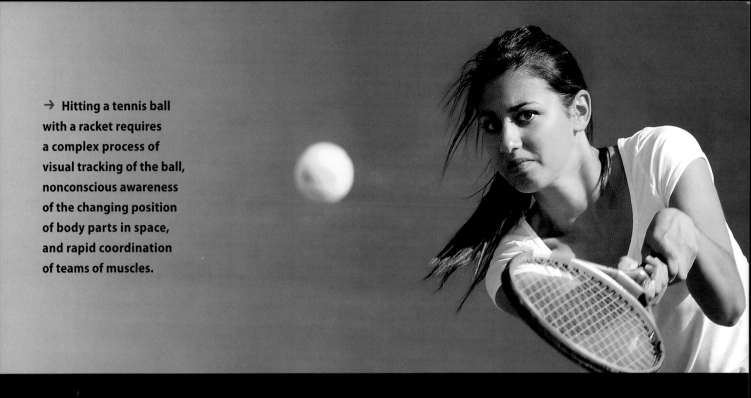

→ **Hitting a tennis ball with a racket requires a complex process of visual tracking of the ball, nonconscious awareness of the changing position of body parts in space, and rapid coordination of teams of muscles.**

The premotor and supplementary motor cortex then direct the primary motor cortex to begin the movement. The primary motor cortex contains large nerve cells called Betz cells that have big axons running to the brainstem or spinal cord. The axons of Betz cells also have branches to other brain regions (including the basal ganglia, thalamus, and brainstem reticular formation) that participate in feedback loops to assist with motor learning or coordination. While the movement is in progress, loops connecting the cerebellum and basal ganglia keep the movement smooth and well controlled by feeding information about how the task is proceeding back to the motor cortex.

The motor pathways from the cortex, whether directly from the cerebral cortex to the spinal cord, or indirectly from the cerebral cortex through the midbrain or reticular formation to the spinal cord, drive the motor nerve cells that make the muscles contract.

Eye movements

To effectively form a detailed visual picture requires that an image be held steady on the fovea of the retina, a region that is only a fraction of an inch across, for at least a tenth of a second. Even more demanding, depth perception requires both eyes to focus on an object simultaneously and when either or both the head and object are moving, the task of visual tracking becomes a prodigious challenge.

Voluntary movements of the eyes are commanded from a region in the frontal lobe called the frontal eye field. These commands are passed through the superior colliculus and special nerve cell groups in the brainstem reticular formation that coordinate eye movement in the horizontal plane (the paramedian pontine reticular formation—PPRF, otherwise known as the center for lateral gaze). The PPRF commands the motor nerve cells which drive the muscles that move the eyes in the level plane. Other nerve cell groups in the brainstem control vertical eye movements.

Eye movements coordinated with rotation of the head are commanded by circuits in the brainstem and cerebellum (see vestibulo-ocular reflexes, pp. 136–7), but tracking objects moving in space, while the head itself is still (optokinetic or smooth pursuit movements), requires a constant feedback between the visual cortex and the circuits that control eye movement. Optokinetic tracking starts with motion-sensitive areas of the visual association cortex that compute the rate of movement and command the frontal eye fields to move the eyes at the necessary rate to follow the object.

Changes in the distance of objects also require movements of the eyes: when an object approaches we need to turn the eyes inward to follow it. This convergence depends on areas of the visual cortex that judge visual depth and then pass commands to nerve cell groups in the reticular formation of the midbrain.

Reading the smile

Facial muscles can be under voluntary control by the cerebral cortex, or unconscious control by brainstem centers in the event of emotional responses. In other words, a smile can be warm and genuine, a courteous formality, or a calculating pretence. The sets of muscles used in a genuine smile are slightly different to those used in a deliberate smile. In particular, muscles around the eyes are more active during genuine smiles. When a person is using a smile to manipulate another, they often watch their subject's face intently to assess the effectiveness of their manipulation, so look for an intent look in the eye to judge if a smile is an authentic emotional response.

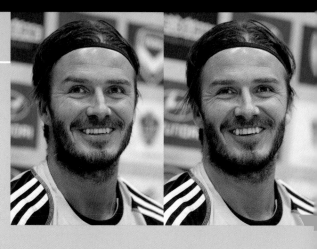

↑ **The involuntary smile on the right involves greater activation of the muscle that rings the eye (the orbicularis oculi) producing a slight lowering of the eyebrow and deeper "laughter lines" around the eyes. The angle of the mouth is also higher.**

Control of facial expression

Humans express their emotions through a rich range of facial expressions that mainly involve the lower two thirds of the face. Dozens of muscles around the lips, angles of the mouth, and around the eyes work in concert to produce a range of expressions from a smile to a frown.

Control of the facial muscles starts in the premotor cortex and the primary motor cortex, both located within the cerebral cortex. The primary motor cortex has a large area devoted to the face, indicating the behavioral importance of fine motor control of this region. The motor nerve cells that directly drive the facial muscles are located in the facial motor nucleus in the pons. The motor cortex sends messages to the facial nucleus via corticobulbar axons. These come from the opposite side of the cerebral cortex for motor cells driving muscles below the eye and from both sides for motor cells driving muscles in the upper third of the face.

Studies of people with brain injury show that more than one motor pathway may drive the facial muscles. For example, those with a stroke injury that causes paralysis of the entire side of the body and face, may nevertheless be able to smile on both sides of their face

in response to a joke. People with Parkinson's disease may have a masklike face under normal circumstances and have great difficulty in smiling voluntarily, but will produce a smile in response to spontaneous humor.

Pathways for skillful movement

The cerebral cortex has its own set of pathways that link directly to the brainstem and spinal cord motor nerve cells. These pathways are particularly important for fine, skillful movements of the face or fingers, but also contribute to movement of other muscle groups.

There are other, indirect, pathways to both the brainstem and spinal cord, incorporating intermediate connections in the midbrain and brainstem reticular formation. When the direct pathways from the cerebral cortex are damaged these indirect pathways can partially compensate. Nevertheless, the direct pathway from the cerebral cortex is crucial for skilled movements, like playing a musical instrument or fine needlework, that are a hallmark of human talents.

Routine motion

Many of our daily movements consist of patterns of motor activity that are routine and habitual. Walking swimming, running, swallowing, sucking, and yawning all consist of complex, but largely fixed, sequences of muscle activation at many different levels of the head, trunk, and limbs. It would be exhausting for our cerebral cortex to control every detail of those movements, so preset programs for the activation of muscles during routine movements are found within nerve cell networks in the reticular formation of the brainstem. The cerebral cortex simply needs to command the brainstem to activate one of these routines.

The cells of the reticular formation give rise to axons that run either to other parts of the brainstem to control swallowing, sucking, or yawning; or down to the spinal cord for regulation of walking, running, or swimming. In some animals there are also groups of nerve cells in the spinal cord that serve as central pattern generators, because they can produce rhythmic coordinated movements, even if isolated from the brainstem.

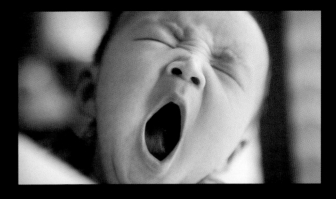

↑ **Yawning is an involuntary motor action controlled by nerve cell groups in the brainstem. Its causes remain uncertain.**

↓ **This complex motor task requires the activation of dozens of small muscles in rapid sequence. This is controlled by direct pathways from the cerebral cortex to the brainstem and spinal cord.**

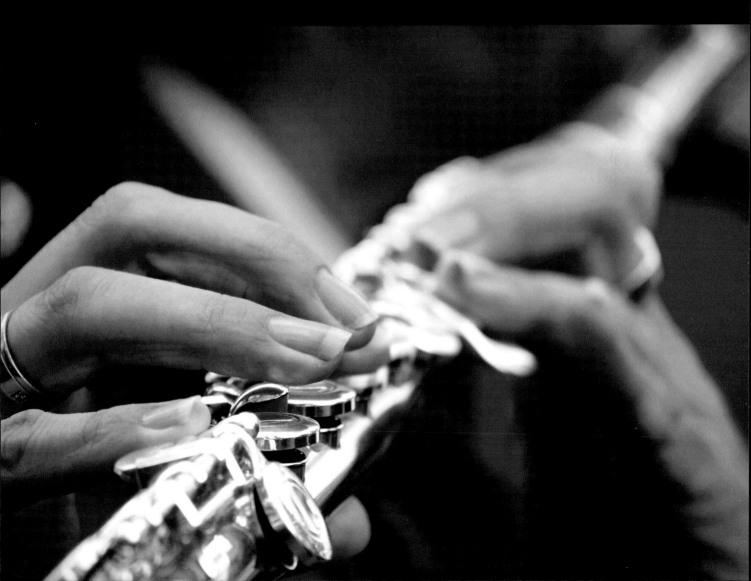

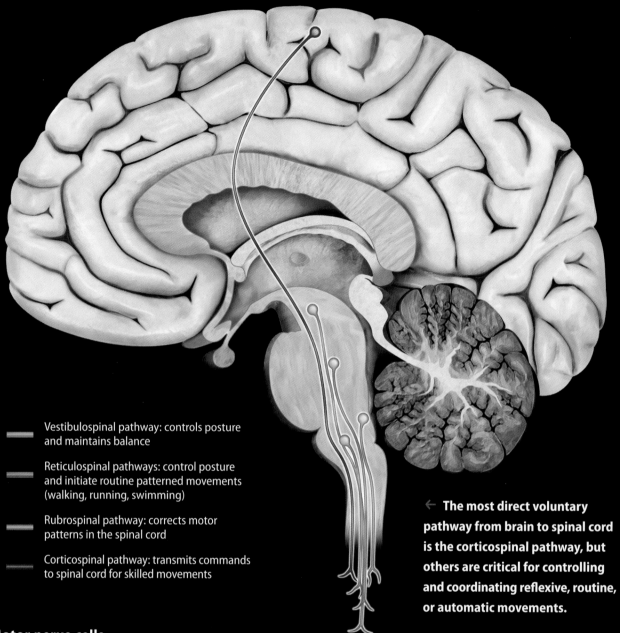

Vestibulospinal pathway: controls posture and maintains balance

Reticulospinal pathways: control posture and initiate routine patterned movements (walking, running, swimming)

Rubrospinal pathway: corrects motor patterns in the spinal cord

Corticospinal pathway: transmits commands to spinal cord for skilled movements

← **The most direct voluntary pathway from brain to spinal cord is the corticospinal pathway, but others are critical for controlling and coordinating reflexive, routine, or automatic movements.**

Motor nerve cells

Regardless of how motor commands are initiated in the cortex or brainstem, it is the motor nerve cells (often called lower motor neurons) that have the task of driving the muscles of our head, trunk, and limbs. Lower motor neurons for the muscles of the eyes, face, and neck are found in clusters within the brainstem (eye muscle nuclei, trigeminal motor nucleus, facial motor nucleus, nucleus ambiguus), and lower motor neurons for the muscles of the limbs and trunk are in the anterior (or ventral) horn of the spinal cord.

The phrenic nucleus in the neck part of the spinal cord is a relatively small group of motor nerve cells that drive the muscular diaphragm between the chest and abdominal cavity. If the phrenic nucleus is separated from the brainstem by a high spinal cord injury, breathing stops and the patient will die unless medical support is immediately available.

Some motor nerve cells are constantly active to maintain posture or keep sphincters closed. Others are only active in short bursts for specific actions. There are two general types of motor nerve cells: those that drive most of the muscle to produce obvious movements; and those that adjust the tension of small muscle fibers in the stretch sensory organs inside the muscle tissue.

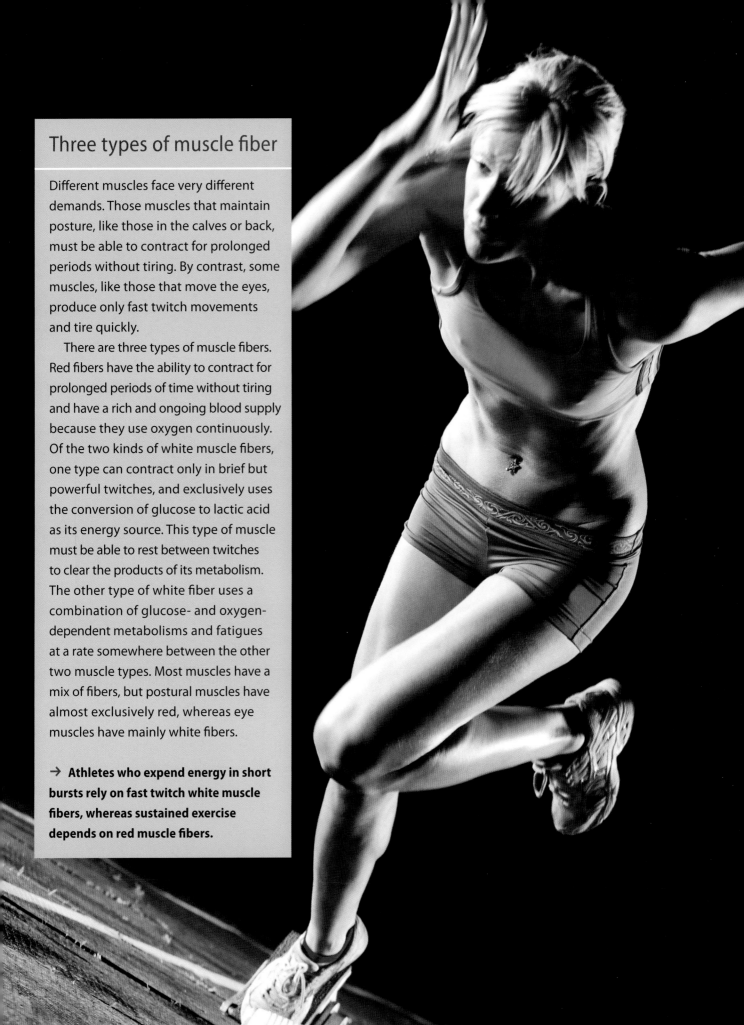

Three types of muscle fiber

Different muscles face very different demands. Those muscles that maintain posture, like those in the calves or back, must be able to contract for prolonged periods without tiring. By contrast, some muscles, like those that move the eyes, produce only fast twitch movements and tire quickly.

There are three types of muscle fibers. Red fibers have the ability to contract for prolonged periods of time without tiring and have a rich and ongoing blood supply because they use oxygen continuously. Of the two kinds of white muscle fibers, one type can contract only in brief but powerful twitches, and exclusively uses the conversion of glucose to lactic acid as its energy source. This type of muscle must be able to rest between twitches to clear the products of its metabolism. The other type of white fiber uses a combination of glucose- and oxygen-dependent metabolisms and fatigues at a rate somewhere between the other two muscle types. Most muscles have a mix of fibers, but postural muscles have almost exclusively red, whereas eye muscles have mainly white fibers.

→ **Athletes who expend energy in short bursts rely on fast twitch white muscle fibers, whereas sustained exercise depends on red muscle fibers.**

Coordination and reinforcement of movement

Producing a movement requires much more than simply making a decision in the cerebral cortex and instructing a muscle to contract. If we did not have systems for coordinating muscle activation, our movements would be uncontrolled, spasmodic, and exhausting.

Even the simplest task of reaching for a door handle involves the activation of dozens of muscles in the correct sequence, for the correct period of time, and with the correct amount of force. The slightest fault in that process can have disastrous effects. Looped circuits through the cerebellum ensure that our movements are controlled and coordinated. The basal ganglia play a slightly different, but no less important role: that of reinforcing desired motor behaviors and extinguishing unwanted motor behaviors.

Automatic eye movements

Some eye movement is controlled by conscious actions arising from the cerebral cortex, but much of the automatic movement of the eyes when we turn our head is coordinated by a small region on the underside of the cerebellum. This region (the vestibulocerebellum) has a rich input from the vestibular part of the inner ear, a sensory organ that detects rotation of the head in space. Rotation of the head stimulates sensory cells in the

→ **Automatic eye movements during head rotation rely on the semicircular ducts of the inner ear to sense rotation, along with vestibular nerve cells in the brainstem and the vestibulocerebellum (not illustrated) to coordinate eye movements.**

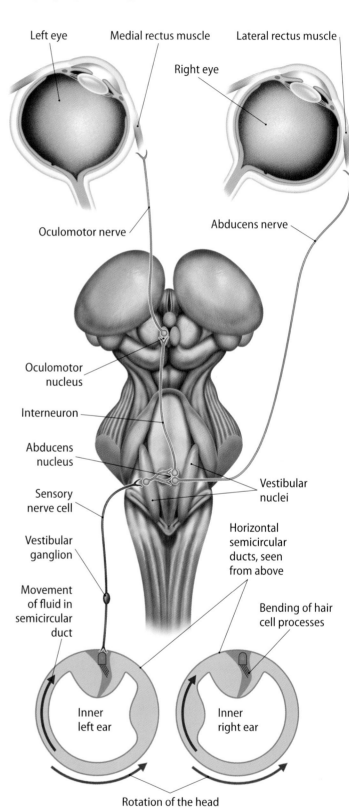

Left eye

Medial rectus muscle

Lateral rectus muscle

Right eye

Oculomotor nerve

Abducens nerve

Oculomotor nucleus

Interneuron

Abducens nucleus

Sensory nerve cell

Vestibular ganglion

Movement of fluid in semicircular duct

Vestibular nuclei

Horizontal semicircular ducts, seen from above

Bending of hair cell processes

Inner left ear

Inner right ear

Rotation of the head

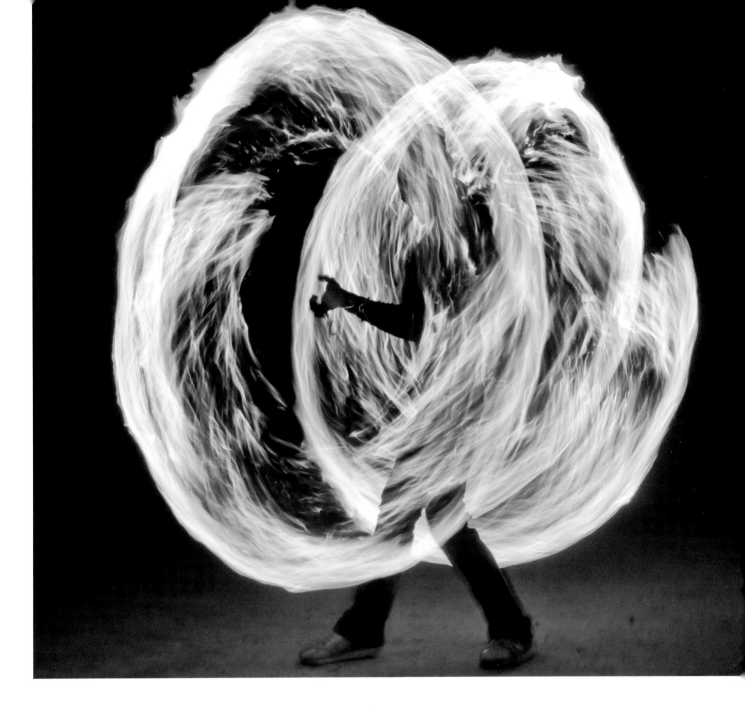

semicircular ducts of the inner ear and this information is conveyed to the brainstem or directly into the cerebellum. Other sources of information that are essential to coordinating eye movement include movements of the neck and the eyes themselves. Some Purkinje cells in the surface of the vestibulocerebellum receive information about all these movements and reach decisions about how to make eye movements to follow objects in the visual field.

Postural movements

The midline of the cerebellum, called the vermis, has a sensory map of the trunk of the body based on

↑ Rapid coordinated movement of the limbs requires constant feedback of information on joint position to the midline of the cerebellum to coordinate muscle groups quickly and precisely.

information from the spinocerebellar and cuneo-cerebellar tracts that connect with the spinal cord. The information comes from stretch receptors in the muscles and joints of the back and tells the cerebellum about deviations of the trunk to one side or the other. The vermis processes this information and makes decisions about which muscle groups to activate to

171

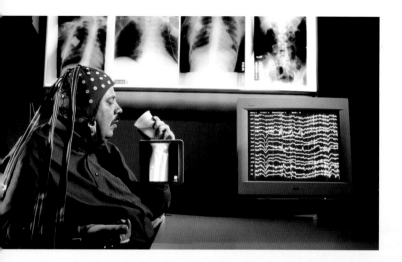

← **The brain can still issue motor commands when the body is disconnected. This quadriplegic is drinking with the aid of a sensor cap that detects his brain waves. These impulses are sent to electrodes implanted in his arm and finger muscles, allowing him to perform simple motor tasks.**

bring the trunk back to the upright position. The output from this part of the cerebellum is carried to nerve cell groups in the vestibular and reticular formation parts of the brainstem. Pathways from these nerve cell groups to the spinal cord regulate contraction of the muscles along the midline of the body.

This part of the cerebellum is also concerned with coordination of the habitual movements like walking and running that are driven by the reticular formation of the brainstem, particularly where those movements involve some swaying of the trunk from side to side.

Limb movements

The medial part of the hemisphere of the cerebellum (paravermal cortex) receives information from both the motor cortex and the spinal cord. This part of the cerebellum compares commands from the motor cortex with sensory information from the spinal cord about what is happening in the limbs as a result of those commands. This allows the cerebellum to check that movements are being performed correctly and to make small adjustments as needed. The outflow from this part of the cerebellum is back through the thalamus to the motor cerebral cortex to correct movements as they happen.

Circuits for skilled movement

The most lateral part of the cerebellum has a slightly different function from the paravermal cortex. Known as the cerebrocerebellum, it is part of an important loop circuit that allows us to plan movements (especially those of the limbs) and is active even before a movement begins. This loop circuit starts with the cerebral cortex, passes through the pontine nuclei of the brainstem, cortex and dentate nucleus of the cerebellum, and motor nuclei of the thalamus before returning to the motor and premotor cortex. The cerebrocerebellum is critically important for the acquisition of skilled movements, because the detailed motor routines for those must be imprinted in the cerebellum, before they can be successfully carried out.

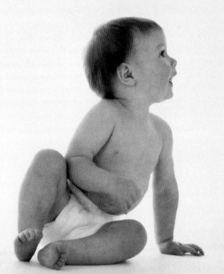

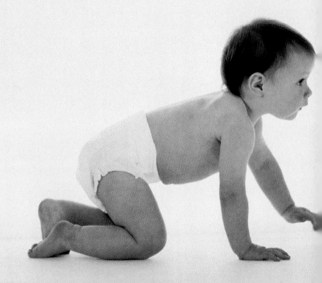

Basal ganglia circuits

The components of the basal ganglia form two looped circuits. One of these is known as the direct pathway and connects the cerebral cortex, striatum, internal part of the globus pallidus, and thalamus, and then runs back up to the cortex. The other loop is called the indirect pathway and connects the cerebral cortex, striatum, external part of the globus pallidus, subthalamic nucleus, the internal part of the globus pallidus, and thalamus before heading back to the cerebral cortex. The activity in these two loops regulates the level of movement of the whole motor system. Cortical activation of the direct pathway feeds back in a positive way to increase motor cortex activity. By contrast, cortical activation of the indirect pathway feeds back to reduce motor cortex activity.

Although the motor effects of disease and damage to the basal ganglia are well known, the precise role of the basal ganglia in its motor, emotional, and cognitive functions is still not well understood. Certainly, its role is much more complex than the simple muscle activity coordination performed by the cerebellar circuits.

One view of the overall role of the basal ganglia is that it selects and reinforces appropriate actions or behaviors, while extinguishing or inhibiting unwanted or inappropriate actions or behaviors. In the context of motor function, this means that the basal ganglia circuits strengthen complex patterns of motor actions that are behaviorally important and rewarding.

Diseases of the basal ganglia

Diseases that affect the basal ganglia result in either decreased or increased motor activity, depending on whether the direct or indirect pathway is damaged more. For example, damage to the subthalamic nucleus decreases activity of the indirect pathway to such an extent that the patient experiences violent flailing movements of the opposite side of the body. By contrast, damage to the dopamine-using nerve cells of the substantia nigra leads to increased activity in the indirect pathway and causes an overall reduction of motor activity so that the patient walks with small shuffling steps and has a masklike face.

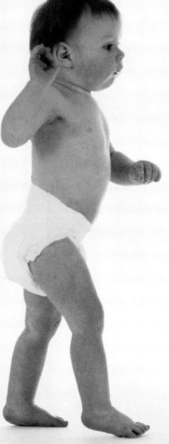

↓ **Developing motor skills during infancy requires the formation of complex circuitry in the forebrain and cerebellum and the myelination of axons in spinal cord motor pathways to allow those circuits to drive muscle nerve cells.**

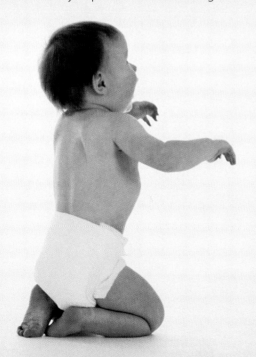

Head and neck reflexes

Reflex actions protect the body from damaging agents and actions and are hard-wired into the nervous system. Many are controlled from the spinal cord, but some that protect the airway and delicate sense organs of the face use direct pathways to the brainstem.

Many nerves in the head and neck can initiate reflexes that protect the delicate sensory cells of the eye and ear and prevent entry of foreign objects into the upper airway. Some of these reflex pathways are quite simple, while others are complex and circuitous.

Protecting the eye

Vision is the most important sense for humans, but the eyes are extremely vulnerable to damage. Two vital reflexes protect the eye from excessive light and injury.

When excessively bright light strikes the retina of one eye, the pupils of both eyes narrow to protect the retina from damage. This pupillary reflex is triggered when sufficient light strikes special retinal ganglion cells that send impulses to the brain along the optic nerve. These axons end in the pretectal region of the diencephalon, immediately in front of the midbrain. Pathways from

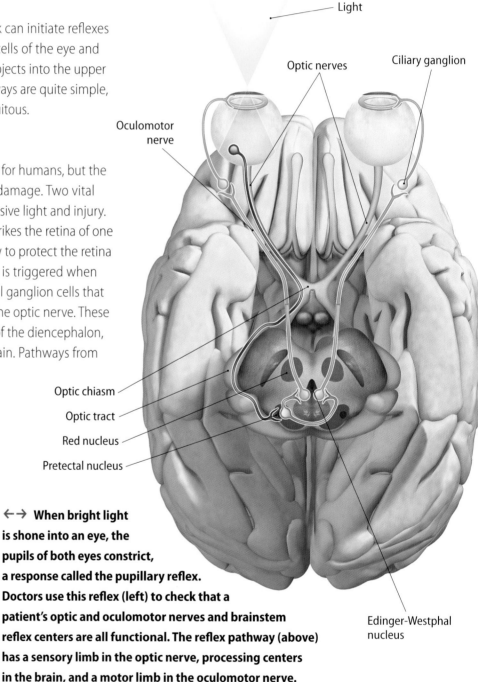

Light

Optic nerves

Ciliary ganglion

Oculomotor nerve

Optic chiasm

Optic tract

Red nucleus

Pretectal nucleus

Edinger-Westphal nucleus

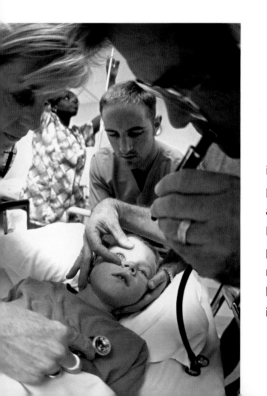

←→ **When bright light is shone into an eye, the pupils of both eyes constrict, a response called the pupillary reflex. Doctors use this reflex (left) to check that a patient's optic and oculomotor nerves and brainstem reflex centers are all functional. The reflex pathway (above) has a sensory limb in the optic nerve, processing centers in the brain, and a motor limb in the oculomotor nerve.**

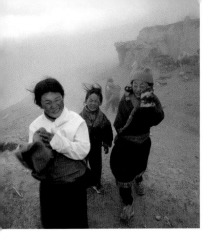

← **Wind-blown dust striking the cornea (as in these children in Tibet) induces the blink reflex to protect the eye from damage.**

here activate groups of parasympathetic nerve cells called the Edinger-Westphal nucleus on both sides of the midbrain. These nerve cells have axons extending out to the two eye sockets of the skull where a connection is made with parasympathetic nerve cells in the ciliary ganglion. Finally, axons from these nerves activate the smooth muscle in the eye that closes down the pupil and protects both eyes from the light.

The delicate surface of the cornea at the front of the eye is easily scratched and is protected by a blink reflex. When wind-blown dust or an eyelash touches the cornea, touch receptors are triggered and axons in the trigeminal nerve carry this information to the brainstem, where connections in the reticular formation activate muscle nerve cells in the facial nucleus. These nerve cells are connected to the muscle fibers encircling the eye and running across the eyelids (the orbicularis oculi muscle) and activate a brisk blink to clear the debris. A related reflex increases tear fluid secretion in response to corneal irritation.

Protecting the ear: the acoustic reflex

Loud noises can cause pressure waves in the inner ear that are strong enough to damage the delicate hair cells of the cochlea. When a loud noise enters one ear, a pathway from that ear to both sides of the brainstem is activated. The axons of this pathway trigger a tiny group of motor nerve cells that control the stapedius muscle in the middle ear. Contraction of the stapedius stiffens the chain of tiny ear bones (hammer, anvil, and stirrup) that carry sound waves to the inner ear, thereby dampening the transmission of sound vibrations to the fluids of the inner ear. The acoustic reflex also helps to block out low-frequency background noise during normal speech.

Protecting the airway: the gag reflex

When any object is introduced into the upper throat (pharynx) without having been chewed or in the absence of the voluntary activation of the complex swallowing maneuver, it evokes a strong contraction of the muscles of the interior of the throat. This reflex is designed to prevent the uncontrolled entry into the throat of foreign objects that might obstruct the airway. The sensation of an object touching the soft palate or side of the throat interior is detected and passed via the glossopharyngeal nerve to the brainstem, which activates the motor nerve cells that contract the throat muscles and close the pharynx entrance to expel the object. Vomiting may also occur in some people.

Ear protection

The acoustic reflex, in which loud noises cause middle ear muscles to contract, has its limitations. It is not fast enough to protect against gunshots, but shields to some extent against long-standing machinery noise. Nevertheless, the ears should always be protected against loud noise by earmuffs or plugs. Prolonged exposure to sound at a level above 100 decibels (the level of a loud orchestra) can be damaging to the hair cells of the organ of Corti in the inner ear.

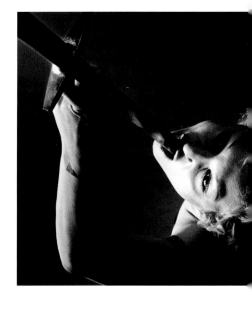

→ **The first obstacle in acquiring the skill of sword swallowing is overcoming the gag reflex. This can take months or even years to achieve.**

Spinal reflexes

The spinal cord is the simplest part of the central nervous system, but it contains vital reflexes for protecting the skin and tissue of the limbs during movement and interaction with the environment.

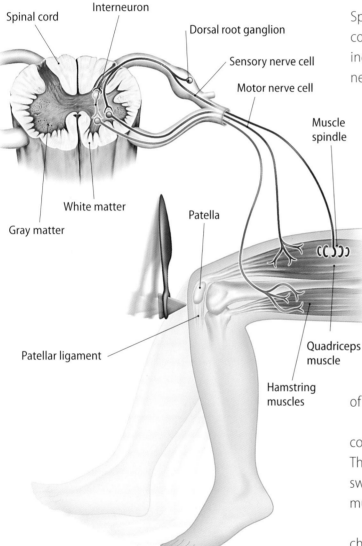

Spinal cord

Interneuron

Dorsal root ganglion

Sensory nerve cell

Motor nerve cell

Muscle spindle

White matter

Patella

Gray matter

Patellar ligament

Quadriceps muscle

Hamstring muscles

↑ **Tapping the tendon of a muscle causes a slight stretch that activates muscle spindle stretch receptors. When these sensory impulses in the sensory nerves (purple) reach the spinal cord, they activate motor nerve cells to reflexively contract the tapped muscle (red) or inhibit antagonistic muscles (blue).**

Spinal reflexes depend on the actions of interneurons contained within the spinal cord gray matter that link incoming sensory nerve cells with outgoing motor nerve cells. These bring about automated reflex actions that do not involve the brain.

The deep tendon reflex

All voluntary muscles contract in response to being stretched. This reflexive action is controlled by the simplest of all spinal cord reflexes, consisting of only two nerve cells and one synaptic contact.

Stretching a muscle puts tension on stretch receptors inside the belly of the muscle and sets up a train of impulses that pass along sensory nerves back to the spinal cord. This sensory axon enters the spinal cord and continues through the gray matter to the ventral horn where it contacts a motor nerve cell. The direct contact is excitatory so the stretch is immediately followed by a contraction of the same muscle.

During normal activity, stretch reflex circuits make constant automatic corrections during movement. They assist in maintaining an upright posture because swaying of the body to one side stretches and activates muscles to bring the body back to the upright.

In clinical practice, the stretch reflex is useful for checking that the sensory and motor nerves to a particular muscle are intact. Tapping the tendon of the muscle (hence the name for this reflex) with a tendon hammer briefly stretches the muscle, which in turn triggers a reflexive contraction that can be seen as a small jerk. A reduction of the deep tendon reflex activity may mean that sensory or motor nerve cells have been lost or damaged. The deep tendon reflexes

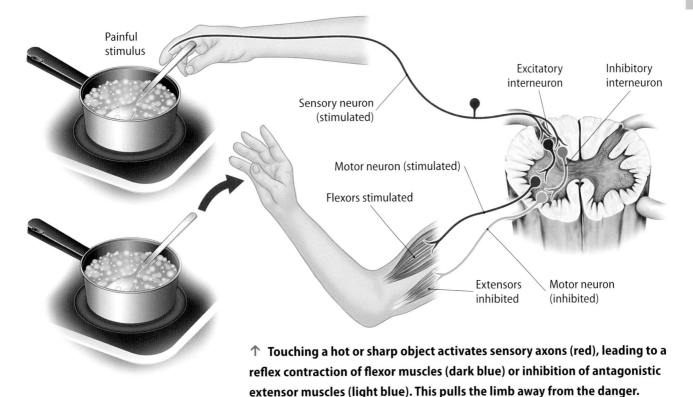

↑ **Touching a hot or sharp object activates sensory axons (red), leading to a reflex contraction of flexor muscles (dark blue) or inhibition of antagonistic extensor muscles (light blue). This pulls the limb away from the danger.**

are usually partially inhibited by motor pathways from the brainstem to the spinal cord, so damage to the spinal cord that interrupts the descending motor pathways causes increased activity of the deep tendon reflexes.

The flexion-withdrawal reflex

When a sharp or hot object comes into contact with an arm or leg, we withdraw the limb in a reflex action. This pathway involves many nerve cells in the spinal cord and spreads to several segmental levels. When it occurs to a leg while standing, this reflex activates not only a withdrawal response on the affected side, but also a pushing response in the opposite leg. This complex response withdraws the leg from potential injury while stimulating a stance response on the other side to support the body.

→ **Scratching the sole of the foot in a normal adult causes clawing of the toes downward. In cases of spinal injury, the same stimulus causes the toes to turn upward due to loss of brainstem control of the spinal reflex centers.**

The plantar reflex

In adults, touch stimulation to the sole of the foot induces a contraction of the muscles that bend the toes and ankle downward. This reflex facilitates standing by activating muscles that push against the ground when the sole of the foot is stimulated during weight-bearing. This automatic response ensures that the foot and calf muscles maintain a sustained contraction whenever the sole is compressed by standing.

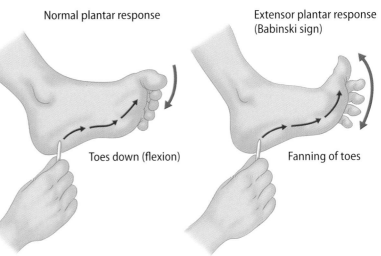

177

Abnormal movements

We perform complex movements involving dozens of muscles every second of our waking day. For most of our lives these movements are smooth and flawless and are carried out with very little conscious thought. It is only when the circuits that control our motor actions are damaged that abnormal movements emerge.

Abnormal movements are categorized according to motion, location, and pattern of occurrence. These observations can assist in identifying the underlying illness or nerve damage.

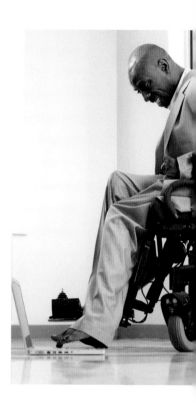

→ **Damage to the motor circuits can occur during development, after strokes, or from disease. Some limbs may be relatively unaffected.**

Tremor

The rhythmic shaking of a limb that we call tremor can be a sign of damage to one of the two major parts of the motor system, depending on whether the shaking is worst at rest or during an action.

A tremor that is worst at rest (resting tremor) is a characteristic sign of damage to, or degeneration of, one of the motor pathways of the basal ganglia. Parkinson's disease is a relatively common disease in which the dopamine-producing (dopaminergic) nerve cells of the substantia nigra in the midbrain degenerate. These nerve cells use dopamine as a neurotransmitter to activate target nerve cells in the striatum. The loss of

dopaminergic cells alters activity in the looped basal ganglia circuits and produces a tremor of the hand with an action like that of rolling putty into a ball (pill-rolling tremor). A resting tremor improves during voluntary movement, but gets worse during emotional stress.

A tremor that is only present during action, such as when reaching out to pick up a pen, is called an intention tremor. Intention tremor is characteristic of damage to the large, side parts of the cerebellum (the cerebrocerebellum) that coordinate fine movements of the hands. The damaged cerebellum is unable to smoothly activate the many muscles required for even the simplest action in the correct sequence and for the correct period of time. The result is a movement that wavers from side to side, and often over- or undershoots the target.

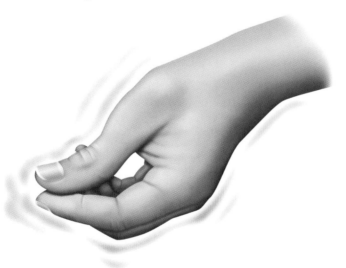

← **Damage to the dopamine-using nerve cells of the substantia nigra causes a pill-rolling tremor, as if the patient were rolling a ball of putty between fingers and thumb. A resting tremor (like the pill-rolling type) occurs when the muscles are relaxed. Pill-rolling is often seen in patients with Parkinson's disease.**

Drug-induced movements

Some drugs cause abnormal movements. Anti-psychotic drugs cause a type of movement called tardive dyskinesia, involving repetitive involuntary movements of the tongue and face (e.g., repetitive eye blinking, protruding the tongue, lip-smacking) and rapid movements of the limbs. These abnormal movements are thought to be due to the action of the drugs on the dopamine-containing nerve pathways in the brain.

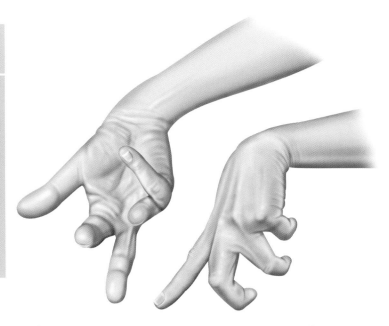

↑ **Slow, sinuous, twisting abnormal movements of the hands are called athetosis, a type of abnormal movement seen in some types of cerebral palsy.**

Slow, sinuous movements

Slow, writhing, aimless motor actions are called athetoid movements (a condition called athetosis, from the Greek for "without position"). These are seen at the ends of the limbs and usually result from damage to the striatum of the basal ganglia. Athetoid movements may be seen in cerebral palsy, a condition where the striatum is damaged around the time of birth.

Brisk, purposeless, dancing movements

Brisk or dancing movements of the limbs, face, and tongue that seem to be fragments of normal voluntary movements are called choreiform movements (a condition called chorea, from the Greek for "dance"). Chorea is seen in a serious genetic disease known as Huntington's chorea: a tragic, relentlessly progressive, degenerative disease of the caudate nucleus of the striatum and the cerebral cortex. People with this condition experience worsening abnormal movements, personality changes, and a loss of cognitive ability (dementia) resulting in death in as short a period as five years from diagnosis.

Violent, flailing movements

Wild, flailing movement of one side of the body is called hemiballismus (from the Greek for "half" and "jumping about"). It usually arises when the subthalamic nucleus is damaged by a stroke, resulting in bouts of violent movements on the side of the body opposite to the site of neural damage.

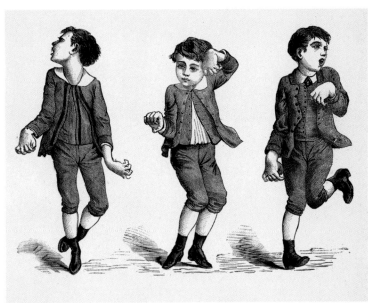

→ **Chorea in children is usually a delayed (and temporary) symptom of acute rheumatic fever. This French illustration of three boys with chorea dates from about 1880.**

Control without thought: the internal body systems

The maintenance of a constant internal environment is essential for survival, otherwise we would quickly die from catastrophic swings in blood pressure, blood gases, or temperature.

The nervous system (along with the endocrine system) controls the internal body environment, keeping conditions within a narrow range of acceptable levels in a process called homeostasis.

Controlling blood pressure

Changes in blood pressure stimulate nerve cells in the sensory nucleus of the solitary tract within the brainstem. These cells convey this information through a chain of nerve cells in the front and side of the medulla. One nerve cell group called the rostral ventrolateral medulla group (RVLM) links to the sympathetic nerve cells in the side of the spinal cord gray matter that control the smooth muscle in blood vessel walls and the force, rate, and speed of contraction of heart muscle. Damage to the RVLM or cutting of the pathway between it and the spinal cord causes a drop in blood pressure. People with damage to the nucleus of the solitary tract undergo a dangerous rise in blood pressure that may cause a stroke.

Responding to blood loss

Occasionally, there may be a sudden loss of blood volume due to internal or external hemorrhaging or through a break in the skin. This is a life-threatening situation because loss of blood flow to the heart or brain may cause death. The life-preserving response to blood loss involves a rise in heart rate, a restoration of blood pressure, a redirection of blood to vital organs, and reabsorption of as much water as possible from the urine to conserve circulatory fluid.

The pathways that bring about the changes in heart rate and blood flow are the same as those for controlling blood pressure, but an additional pathway controls the reabsorption of fluid and assists with blood pressure restoration. A sharp drop in blood pressure stimulates cells in the nucleus of the solitary tract, and an ascending pathway from the medulla (in the reticular formation of the brainstem) to the vasopressin-making nerve cells of the hypothalamus stimulates the release of vasopressin into the circulation. This hormone increases the reabsorption of water by the kidney and, in high concentrations, can raise the blood pressure by causing the smooth muscle in vessel walls to contract.

Controlling blood oxygen and carbon dioxide

It is essential that the concentrations of both oxygen and carbon dioxide in the blood are kept within narrow limits. Control of blood gas concentration is due to circuits that constantly measure the concentration of blood gases, nerve cells that analyze this information and make decisions about the rate and rhythm of breathing, and motor nerve cells that control the muscles that ventilate the lungs.

Information about the concentration of oxygen in the blood is gathered from a tiny structure called the carotid body, located alongside the beginning of the major artery to the brain, the internal carotid artery. This information is carried to the medulla along the glossopharyngeal nerve and enters the nucleus of the solitary tract. Cells that sense carbon dioxide also exist in the carotid body but most are located along the surface of the medulla itself.

Nerve cells in the medulla that drive the intake of breath are found in the upper medulla (the rostral

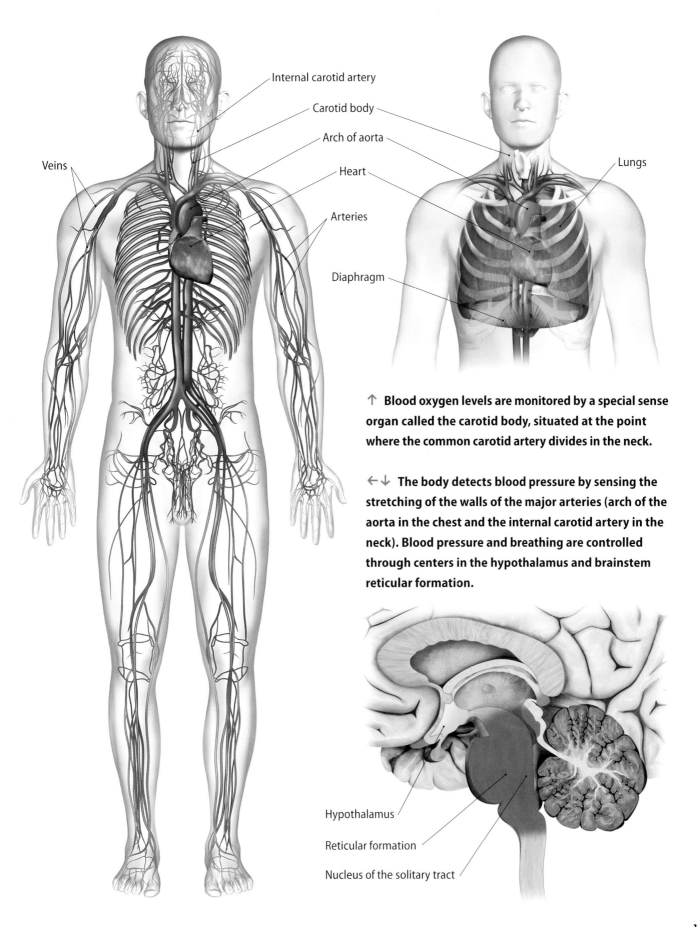

Internal carotid artery

Carotid body

Arch of aorta

Heart

Arteries

Diaphragm

Veins

Lungs

↑ **Blood oxygen levels are monitored by a special sense organ called the carotid body, situated at the point where the common carotid artery divides in the neck.**

←↓ **The body detects blood pressure by sensing the stretching of the walls of the major arteries (arch of the aorta in the chest and the internal carotid artery in the neck). Blood pressure and breathing are controlled through centers in the hypothalamus and brainstem reticular formation.**

Hypothalamus

Reticular formation

Nucleus of the solitary tract

Neurodegenerative disease

Many of the nerve cell groups that control the internal body systems are affected in degenerative disease of the nervous system. In a disease known as multiple system atrophy, several groups of nerve cells in the medulla that help regulate the internal organs begin to degenerate.

People with this disease are unable to keep a stable blood pressure when they rise from a prone position and are unable to alter their blood pressure in response to the needs of exercise. Loss of the serotonin-containing neurons in the midline of the medulla results in difficulty controlling body temperature. Degeneration of other nerve cell groups in the medulla and pons may also lead to abnormal control of the heart, gut, and the urinary bladder.

Those with Parkinson's disease also commonly experience problems with control of blood pressure and gut activity due to loss of nerve cells in the brainstem, but the effects are not as widespread as with multiple system atrophy.

ventral respiratory group or RVRG). Pacemaker cells (pre-Bötzinger cells) that set the rate and rhythm of breathing are located a little higher in the medulla, and other nerve cell groups in the pons oversee and regulate the pre-Bötzinger cells.

Pathways from the respiratory control centers in the brainstem to the spinal cord control the phrenic nerve cells of the upper spinal cord that drive the diaphragm, the main muscle for breathing in. Other pathways go further down the spinal cord to drive the nerve cells that control the muscles between the ribs for breathing in or out.

Breathing can be maintained in people who have damage to the brain at the midbrain level or above, provided that the pons and medulla of the brainstem are undamaged, indicating that the most important centers for breathing are in the lower brainstem.

Controlling body temperature

In response to cold, the hairs that hold air close to the skin become erect to provide insulation (goose bumps), blood is redirected from the skin to the body interior to reduce the loss of heat through the skin (vasoconstriction), and, when these measures are insufficient, groups of muscles vigorously and rhythmically contract to make heat (shivering). By contrast, when the environment is hot, we produce sweat to lose heat through evaporative cooling and shunt blood to the skin surface to lose heat by conduction (vasodilation). Nerve cell groups within the hypothalamus and brainstem control all of these actions.

Nerve cell groups in the hypothalamus detect the temperature of the blood and direct the actions of nerve cells in the midline raphe region (nucleus raphe magnus and raphe pallidus) of the brainstem that

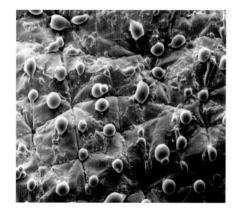
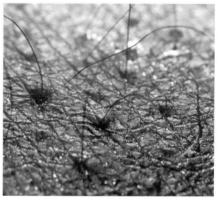

← **Body temperature may be lowered by increasing sweat secretion to enhance evaporative cooling (far left), or heat may be conserved by raising skin hairs to trap still air near the skin, improving insulation (left).**

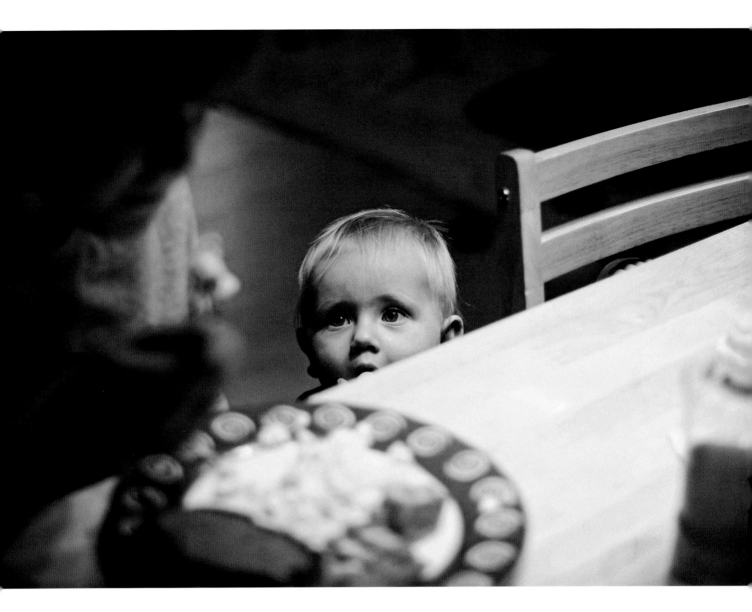

regulate the flow of blood to the skin surface. Some of these nerve cells may also control reserves of brown fat in the body that can be used to generate heat. Parts of the reticular formation on each side of the midline also contain nerve cells that are activated to generate heat through shivering. Finally, nerve cells in the reticular formation can activate sympathetic system nerve cells that increase sweating in response to heat or raise skin hairs in response to cold.

Controlling salivation

We all produce saliva in response to the sight, smell, or thought of food. The sensory act of experiencing or anticipating food arises in the cerebral cortex, but the

↑ The sight, smell, even the anticipation, of food stimulates activation of the parasympathetic parts of the autonomic nervous system that control the salivary glands, leading to watering of the mouth.

groups of nerve cells that control the production of saliva are in the brainstem. These nerve cells are found in two clusters, one that controls the parotid gland in front of the ear by pathways in the glossopharyngeal nerve, and the other that controls the sublingual and submandibular glands that lie below the tongue and jaw, respectively, and are controlled by pathways that run in the facial nerve.

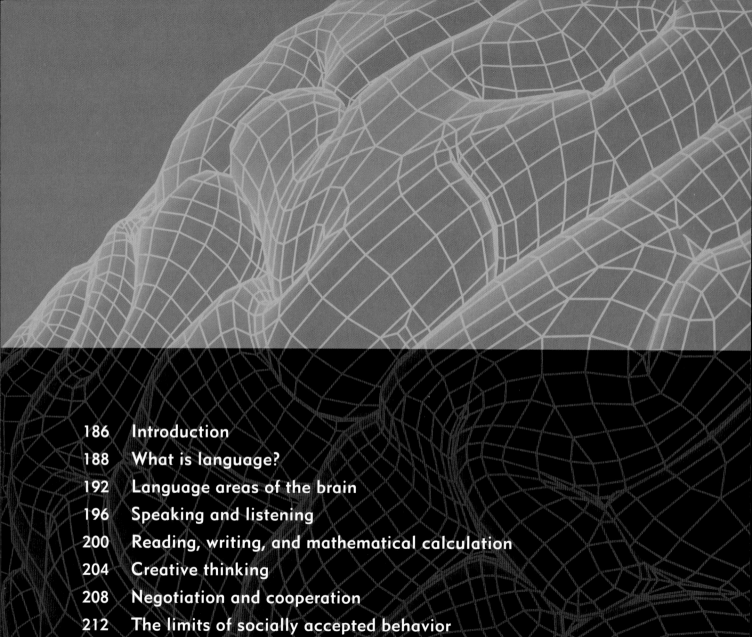

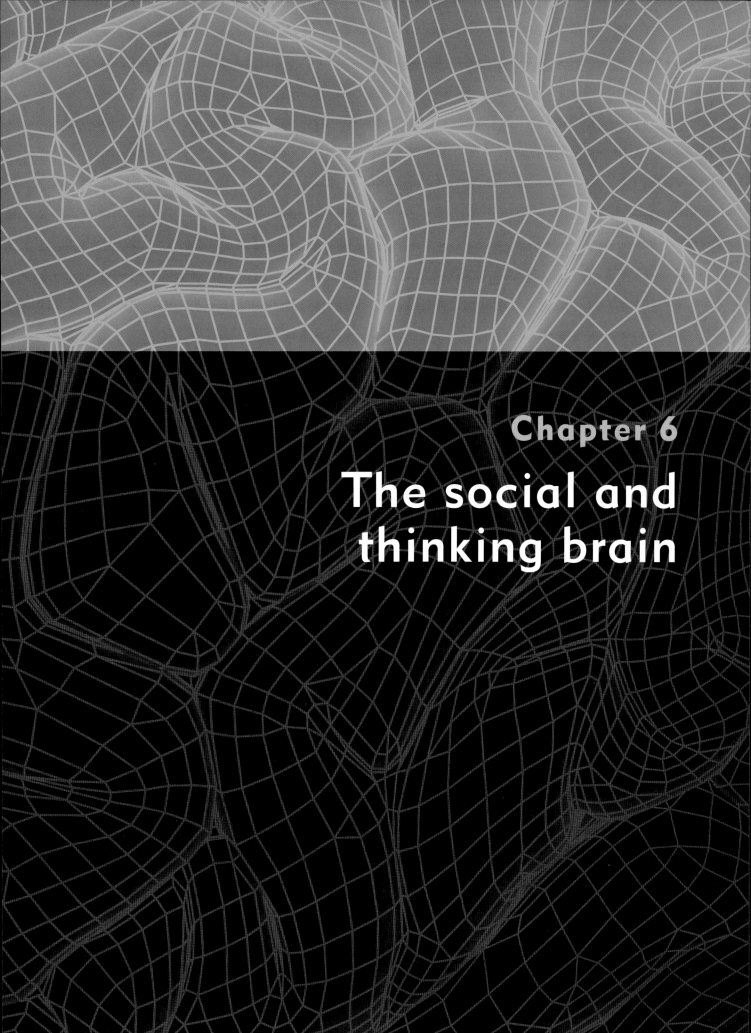

Chapter 6
The social and thinking brain

Introduction

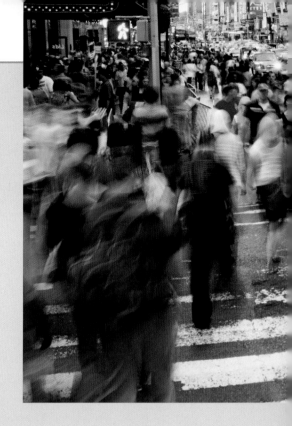

Our complex society requires us to cooperate without conflict, live together in close proximity, and make decisions together. This would not be possible unless we could understand the emotions of others, communicate effectively through spoken and written language, develop tolerance of the different viewpoints of others, and delay our own personal gratification in the interests of future benefits.

A theory of mind underlies all human social interactions. The theory of mind mechanism is believed to allow an individual to recognize that others have completely separate minds and to allow a person to form ideas about the beliefs of others. Understanding that another may have quite different beliefs and viewpoints from you is an important step during maturation of the human mind and occurs around the age of four years.

Spoken and written language and thought

All animals communicate to some extent, but humans have a far richer capacity to communicate complex ideas and feelings than other species. These abilities have arisen from a few key changes in the genes that control the development of the cerebral cortex. The human brain is also more lateralized than that of other species, with language abilities concentrated in the left hemisphere in most people. The ability to acquire spoken language appears to be innate, but written language requires years of training.

At least some of our daily thoughts are carried out through our language ability. Some neuroscientists argue that our unconscious thought processes are residues of a language not currently in use.

When did the modern social mind emerge?

Evolutionary psychologists suggest that humans have possessed a theory of mind for at least 40,000 years and that it underlies the explosion of art, culture, and technology that began at that time. Others argue that it may have arisen, alongside spoken language and advanced planning abilities, with the very first anatomically modern humans as long as 200,000 years ago.

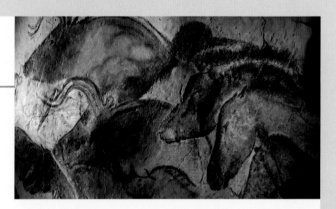

↑ **Prehistoric cave paintings may be evidence of our ancient ancestors' acquisition of a theory of mind.**

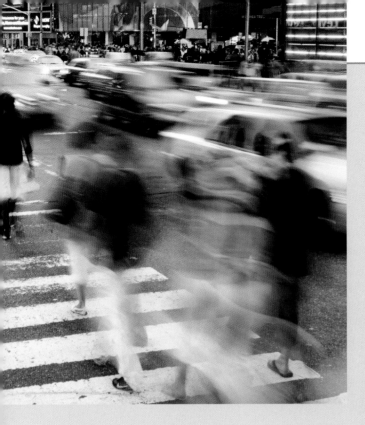

← We live in a complex, fast-moving, and crowded society that would collapse without cooperation, negotiation, and tolerance.

prefrontal cortex depends on an optimal level of input from dopamine-containing pathways from the brainstem. Impulsive and distractible behavior may result when that level of input deviates from the optimal level.

People who have a damaged prefrontal cortex appear to have lost the ability to apply those rules. They become stimulus-driven, engaging in activity simply in response to environmental cues, no matter how inappropriate that behavior is at the time.

Other individuals never develop a fully mature prefrontal cortex, and may exhibit antisocial personality traits and/or engage in criminal behavior. They may recognize that their lack of empathy and freedom from social rules liberates them to take advantage of the cooperative nature of most of the rest of the population.

The prefrontal cortex is also critically important for planning our goals and working toward them over periods of months to years. Patients with damage to their prefrontal cortex have profound deficits in the ability to pursue personal goals. They become aimless and undirected in their personal lives.

Why empathy is essential

Understanding and cooperating with another person requires empathy, the emotional identification with the feelings of another. Neuroscientist Vittorio Gallese has proposed that the emotions of others may be recognized and understood by a mirror neuron system in the cerebral cortex. Mirror neurons are nerve cells in the cortex that are active not only when performing a movement, but also when watching another person performing that same movement. These nerve cells were originally recognized for their role in learning by imitating, but some neuroscientists have argued that they also play a role in social cognition.

Other neuroscientists have questioned this, pointing out that simulating another's movements gives no information about that person's intentions. There may be another system of nerve cells, involving association areas in the upper temporal lobe, the amygdala, and the underside of the frontal lobe, for the cognitive aspects of understanding another's emotions.

The importance of the prefrontal cortex

We are all instilled with rules for appropriate social behavior during childhood. We internalize these rules in our prefrontal cortex, where we can access them to guide our adult social behavior. Maturation of the

↓ **The prefrontal cortex controls social and goal-directed behavior. Mature judgment is exercised here.**

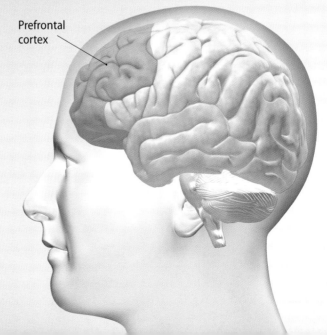

Prefrontal cortex

What is language?

Language is usually defined as a form of communication that uses words or symbols, according to agreed rules, to convey meaning to another person. It is important to remember that language may be verbal, written, or signed, because the brain pathways underlying each are not identical.

A wealth of evidence suggests that language (or more precisely speech) is genetically specified in the human brain. More accurately, it appears that children have a genetically determined ability to acquire spoken language provided they are exposed to speaking adults during the critical first five years of life. Children speak even if exposed to speaking adults and siblings for less than an hour a day, in contrast to apes who learn to sign only if rigorously trained in sign communication for more than half of their waking day. Furthermore, humans learn language even if the language they hear is fragmentary and full of false starts and interruptions. Even children who are otherwise intellectually disabled can learn language with informal and unstructured exposure.

↓ **Children have an innate ability to acquire the language they hear spoken by adults around them. They do so with no formal training in grammar and minimal correction of pronunciation.**

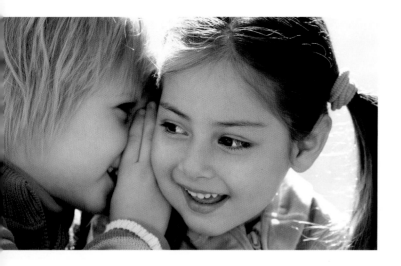

The diversity of human language

The first human language or languages have evolved into a rich family tree of around 6,500 living languages, some of which have sounds and grammatical structures that would seem strange to us. Nevertheless, all of these

The history of human language

It is generally accepted that all humans trace their ancestry to Africa, but when did the first language arise? Language does not fossilize, so our inferences on this question must be indirect. We know that many modern human populations (like the indigenous Australians) reached their modern distribution at least 40,000 and perhaps as long as 60,000 years ago. These modern hunter-gatherers have been relatively isolated from the rest of humanity and yet they have languages as rich and complex as that seen among hunter-gatherers elsewhere in the world. This suggests that language has a history at least 40,000 years old, and may even date back to the origins of the first anatomically modern humans more than 100,000 years ago. Geneticists have suggested that human language arose with the emergence of a distinctly human variant of a gene called *FOXP2*. Members of families with a mutation in this gene have specific language impairments including problems acquiring grammar rules, such as the formation of plurals or verb tense.

languages have the important attribute that they have the flexibility to express abstract and even mystical concepts and go beyond the mere utilitarian goals of day-to-day survival.

The click languages of southwestern Africa (e.g., the Nama or Khoekhoe language of Namibia) use clicking sounds in the back of the throat to modify the meaning of spoken words. In some of these there are as many as 48 different click sounds and native speakers can convey subtle differences in meaning that would be undetectable to a nonspeaker. At the level of the brain, this implies that the expressive language areas of the speaker must carry distinct motor programs for each click and that the auditory association cortex and receptive language areas

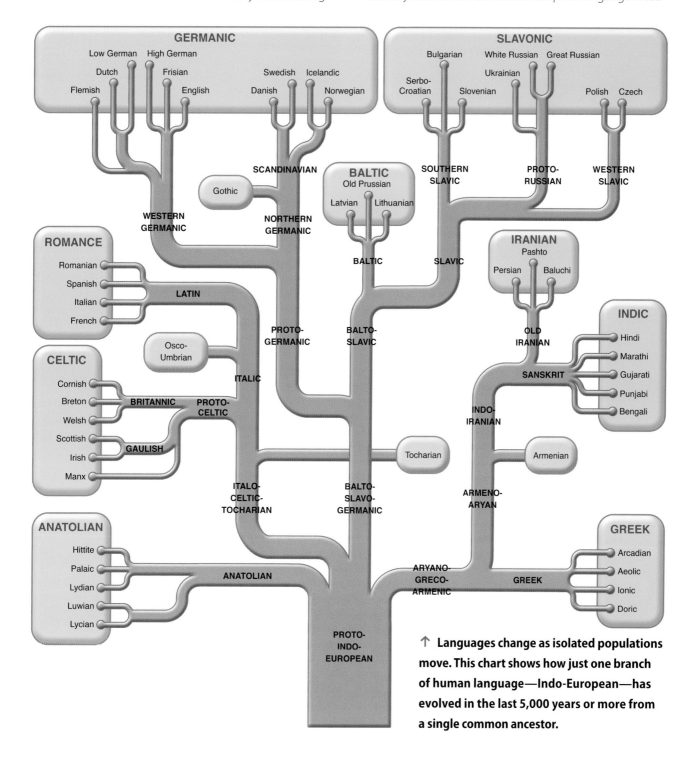

↑ **Languages change as isolated populations move. This chart shows how just one branch of human language—Indo-European—has evolved in the last 5,000 years or more from a single common ancestor.**

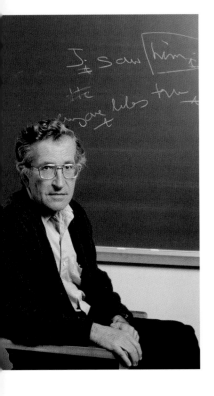

← Noam Chomsky is the most influential linguist of recent times. He proposed that the ability to learn grammar and use language with flexibility is innate to the developing human brain.

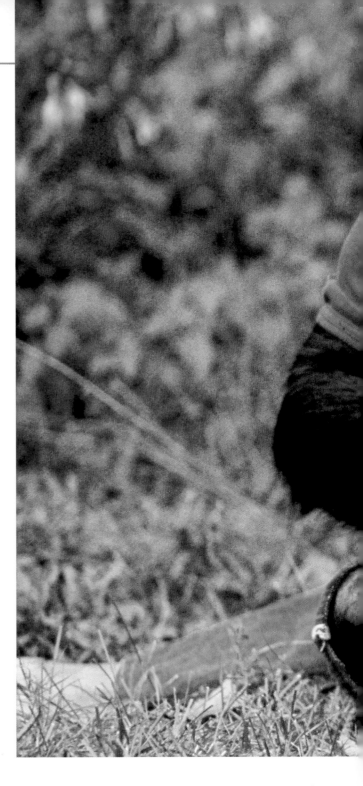

→ "Nim Chimpsky" (a pun on Noam Chomsky) learned approximately 125 signs and was able to communicate simple messages relating to his immediate context. But he did not learn language as most linguists define it.

of the listener must be able to distinguish very subtle differences between click sounds. The production of such a diversity of clicks also demands very precise control of the muscles of the throat, suggesting rigorous training of the cerebellum and brainstem circuitry that controls the relevant muscles.

Other languages use more familiar sounds, but have grammatical structure, inflections, and tones that would seem unusual to us. For example the Jingulu language spoken by the Jingili people of northern Australia has only three verbs: go, do, and come. These must be paired with different nouns to convey the actions that would be described by stand-alone verbs in other languages. Some languages combine all the concepts of a sentence into a single word. Yet other languages from eastern and southeastern Asia, as well as many parts of Africa, use pitch to modify the fundamental meaning of a word. The most familiar of these are Mandarin and Cantonese, which respectively have four and six distinct tones that can profoundly alter the meaning of spoken words.

Can we talk to the animals?

Innate animal communication is relatively simple and direct: a dog wags her tail when happy; she scratches the door when she wants to go out. But can an animal be taught to communicate as we do? Attempts to get apes to use human sign language have been moderately successful. Apes can master the use of dozens or even hundreds of words and can sequence them to convey simple messages. However, most linguists argue this achievement is not true language.

The linguist Charles Hockett argued that nonhuman communication differs from that of humans in at least

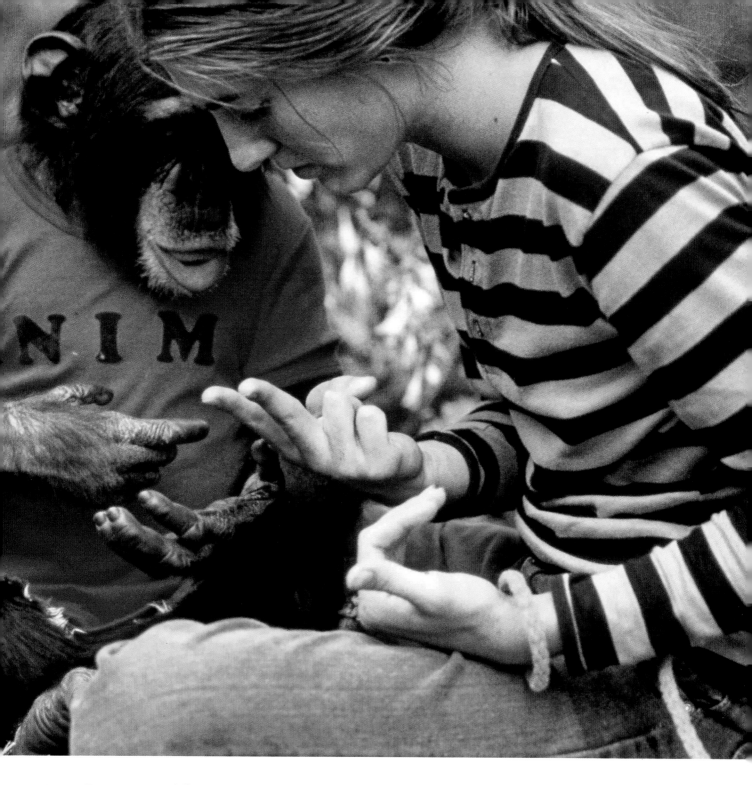

13 ways. Two important differences are displacement and productivity. Displacement means the ability to discuss objects and concepts that are not in the immediate environment of context or urgency. For example, humans can discuss at length the strange object they saw in the sky last night, whereas an ape would never do this. Apes can remember promises made hours earlier, but their overriding concerns are with meeting immediate needs. Productivity means the ability to use the simple building blocks of language in many different combinations, rather than confining communication to dealing with the quest for food or immediate pleasures. Children seem to innately grasp the flexibility of human language and will try to combine words in novel combinations to convey new meaning. The use of these novel language constructions can be reinforced or discontinued depending on the responses of adults and older children.

Language areas of the brain

In most individuals, the primary areas for spoken language production and comprehension are found within the left hemisphere of the cerebral cortex. However, the right hemisphere has an important part to play as do structures deeper within the brain.

Our knowledge of the relation between language and the brain traditionally rests on two types of evidence: damage to the brain with consequent disruption of language production and comprehension, and electrical stimulation of the surface of the cortex that produces similar, though temporary, effects. In the last decade functional imaging techniques have added a third and very powerful approach.

Language areas in the cerebral cortex

Two key areas have been traditionally recognized as critically important for spoken language: Broca's area (Brodmann areas 44 and 45) in the triangular and opercular parts of the inferior frontal gyrus; and Wernicke's area (Brodmann areas 39 and 40) in the angular and supramarginal gyri of the inferior parietal lobule and extending onto the upper surface of the superior temporal gyrus. Landmark studies by Paul Broca and Carl Wernicke of patients with strokes affecting those brain regions led to these discoveries during the 19th century, but we now appreciate that language function is much more complex and widely distributed.

Loss of speech due to brain disease or injury is known as aphasia and may involve language comprehension, expression, or a combination of both. Patients with damage to Broca's area have a major disturbance of speech production. Their spoken language is typically sparse and halting. Words are often poorly articulated, and key function words are frequently missing. These changes are consistent with a role for Broca's area in speech planning and production.

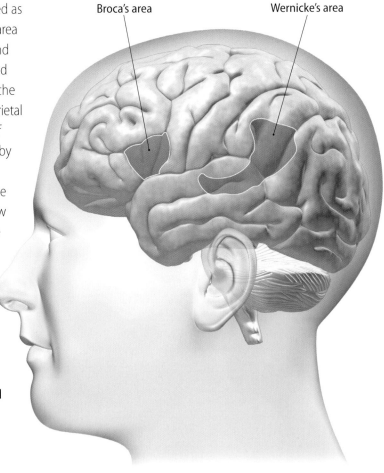

Broca's area   Wernicke's area

→ **Two key language regions of the cerebral cortex are Broca's and Wernicke's areas, named after the 19th-century doctors who linked particular language deficits with damage to specific parts of the brain.**

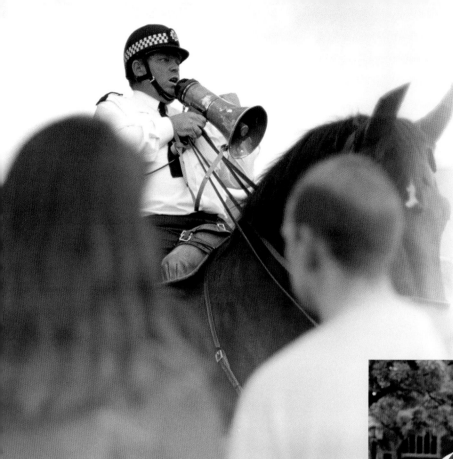

The tone, pacing, and inflection that a police officer uses to address an unruly crowd is completely different from that he would use to comfort a lost child. The non-literal aspects of language are known as prosody. Some instances of localized brain damage can leave people with aprosodia—an inability to convey or interpret prosody.

By contrast, patients with damage to Wernicke's area have a major disturbance of speech comprehension. Their speech may be fluent, but with disturbances of the sounds and grammatical structures of words. They are poor at repeating speech and naming objects. These changes are consistent with a role for Wernicke's area in holding permanent representations of the sound structures of words.

Broca's and Wernicke's areas are connected by a fiber bundle known as the arcuate fasciculus, which allows information transfer between the two. In particular, effective speech depends on the constant feeding of information from Wernicke's area, where word meaning is stored, to Broca's area, where words are constructed from motor programs for the component sounds.

Lateralization of language function

Most processing of language proceeds in one half of the brain, the dominant hemisphere. Almost all right-handed individuals (about 98 percent) have their language areas in the left hemisphere and about 60 to 65 percent of left-handed people also have language areas in the left hemisphere. The tendency for language function to be represented in the left hemisphere is matched by an asymmetry of the brain; in other words the left side of

the brain is shaped slightly differently from the right. The upper surface of the left temporal lobe is slightly larger than the right and includes a region called the planum temporale that is part of Wernicke's area.

Although most language processing occurs in the left hemisphere, the right hemisphere does retain some ability to understand concrete nouns. More significantly, the right hemisphere is important for interpreting prosody—the non-literal aspects of language, such as the tone of the conversation (for example whether it is humorous or serious); the emotional state of the speaker; irony and sarcasm; and distinguishing commands, statements, and questions.

Beyond Broca's and Wernicke's areas

Functional imaging has shown that spoken language processing is primarily carried out in the cortical areas of Broca and Wernicke, but other areas are also important for communication, particularly when we move away from spoken language. As a general principle, written language involves parts of the cerebral cortex closer to the visual cortex. Similarly, sign language involves brain areas closer to the motor areas involved in control of the hands, rather than the face and throat. Functional studies also indicate that an area in the lower front temporal lobe is involved in representing the meaning of words, and the frontal lobe just in front of Broca's area is also activated in tasks concerning word meaning.

Other parts of the cerebral cortex may be important for initiating language function and for maintaining the arousal and attention that is crucial for effective communication. Damage to the supplementary motor cortex on the inner or medial surface of the frontal lobe can lead to problems in the initiation of language, suggesting that this region acts as an activator of the language-processing systems. The cingulate gyrus on the medial surface of the hemisphere is important for focusing attention on language tasks and maintaining arousal during communication.

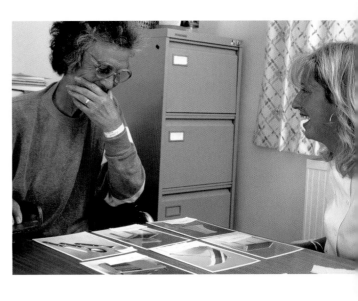

↑ **Stroke victims may lose the ability to use one or more aspects of language. Speech therapists must train them to use remaining brain areas so they may regain language.**

Language function beyond the cortex

Although the cerebral cortex is vitally important in comprehending and formulating language, deeper brain structures also play key roles.

Patients with strokes in the basal ganglia (caudate and putamen) and parts of the thalamus may also suffer language problems. This would be consistent with a role for the basal ganglia in laying down motor or behavioral rules for language, such as the regular aspects of word formation. The thalamus may also play a role in processing the meaning of words.

↓ **Making and interpreting sign language uses not only parts of the cerebral cortex known to be important for language, but also regions concerned with the motor control of the hands and visual analysis.**

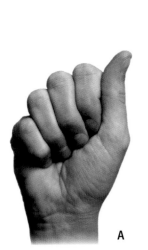

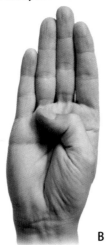

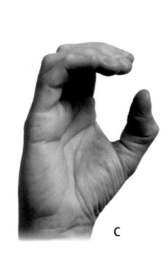

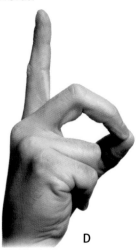

A · B · C · D

→ **What qualities make the best public speakers so effective? Clear ideas and well-constructed sentences are a start, but expert control over tone, rhythm, and intonation can give speech the power of great music and art.**

Functional studies have also suggested that the cerebellum is important in language. This may be through its role in motor coordination, because speech involves precisely timed control of muscle groups, but other scientists have suggested that it has a direct role in language and other cognitive functions.

Finally, articulating speech relies on motor nerve cells in the brainstem. Some of these control the breathing muscles of the trunk, and others exercise fine control over the many delicate muscles of the throat, tongue, mouth, and face that allow us to produce the range of vowels, clicks, and consonants that make up the wide range of human speech. Speech can only be produced during the expiration, or breathing out, phase of lung ventilation. This is because the sound of our voice must be produced by the forced passage of air between vocal folds that have been brought close together. Forcing air through this narrow gap produces the vibrations in the larynx at the front of the throat that can then be modified to produce the sounds of language. Without slow and controlled expiration it would be impossible to finish a phrase.

Lightning-speed listening

Experimental studies have shown that word recognition occurs in as little as one eighth of a second from the word starting, even while the word is still being said. How does the brain achieve this? Not only must the language components of the cortex work quickly, they probably achieve this high speed by processing information about different aspects of the word (e.g., individual sounds or phonemes, emotional content, or inflection) in parallel. In other words, the information conveyed in the word is broken down into its individual components and these are processed simultaneously before being brought back together for a consensus. It should also be noted that this process is largely unconscious, in that we can extract meaning from another person's words without being consciously aware of the fine details of the sounds of the words or the sentence structure.

Speaking and listening

Speech depends not just on language areas in the cerebral cortex, but on a complex set of circuitry running through the basal ganglia and cerebellum. The uniqueness of human speech is as much the product of our precise motor control of the muscles of our chest, upper airway, mouth, and face as it is of our language cortex.

Spoken words are composed of phonemes, the single distinct sounds that contrast with one another and allow different words to be distinguished (e.g., "pat" versus "bat"). The major distinction between different phonemes depends on vowels and consonants. Channeling the vibrations of the larynx through a relatively open upper airway produces vowels, whereas partial or complete constriction of the vocal tract during vibration of the air column produces consonants. American English has 25 consonant and 17 vowel phenomes, and coordinating the change in airway shape to produce them in a rapid sequence is a complex process.

Words and sentences

Words are constructed from phonemes and may designate actual objects, abstract concepts, actions, properties of objects, and logical connections between ideas. The information content of a word may go far beyond its concrete meaning and include unobserved properties that become associated with words through our experiences. For example, "dog" is the label for a particular animal, but when we think "dog" we bring to mind all our experience and knowledge of the animal such as barking or tail wagging. Words are often joined together to form other words, allowing an extra level of complexity and the communication of finer nuances of meaning; e.g., warthog means something quite different from the words "wart" and "hog," taken individually.

Words can be combined into sentences according to syntactic rules. The sentence level of language structure allows a richer expression of meaning than words alone, because a given word may have a number of different meanings depending on its position in a sentence or its modulation according to grammatical rules.

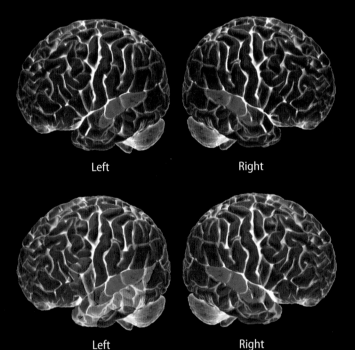

Left   Right

Left   Right

← **These colored PET scans show brain activity due to hearing an unknown language (top pair) and a known language (bottom pair). In the top pair, only the areas concerned with hearing are activated. In the bottom pair the red and green areas are for hearing. The yellow area deals with known words. The pink area is Broca's area, responsible for the production of speech.**

Beyond words

Understanding speech is a complex skill that combines information from many sources: the words and sentences themselves; the prosody (musical content) of the words; gestures; and linguistic context. We tend to look more closely and for a longer period of time at faces showing emotional expressions that match the emotional content of the speech we hear, suggesting that facial expressions are used as important additional clues to the meaning of spoken language.

Functional imaging studies of subjects given language tasks that demand the integration of auditory, visual, and linguistic information have shown that there are several key brain regions that deal with the convergence of this information. These are the posterior part of the superior temporal gyrus (on the upper surface of the temporal lobe), as well as a region called the fusiform gyrus (on the underside of the occipital lobe below the primary visual cortex).

Sentences are critically important for human thought and memory, because they encode facts or assertions about the world that can be incorporated into an individual's knowledge of the world and that may profoundly influence future opinions and behavior, e.g., "the price of freedom is eternal vigilance." Sentences serve to add information to semantic memory and help plan future actions. They may even underlie some types of critical thought.

Understanding speech

When we listen to spoken language, meaning must be extracted from at least three levels of information content: phonemes (the individual sounds); the words themselves (built from the individual phonemes); and syntax (the grammatical relationships between the words). The region known as Wernicke's area in the upper part of the temporal lobe is thought to play a central role in converting acoustic

information in language into phoneme representations. The information encoded in phonemes is then directed a little further forward in the upper temporal lobe, to a site on the left anterior superior temporal gyrus, where word meaning is extracted.

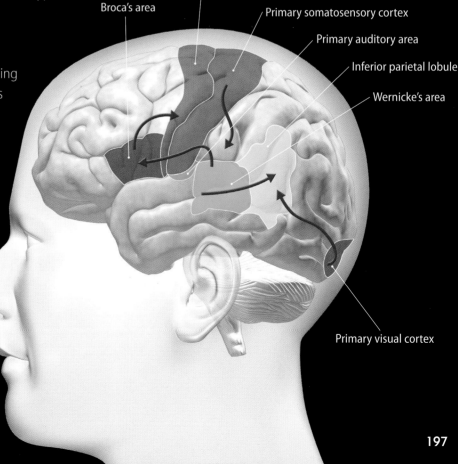

→ **Hearing, reading, and repeating language elicits a complex flow of information between the sensory, language, and motor areas of the cerebral cortex.**

Broca's area

Primary motor cortex

Primary somatosensory cortex

Primary auditory area

Inferior parietal lobule

Wernicke's area

Primary visual cortex

Problems with processing the information of phonemes tend to follow damage to the lower part of the parietal lobe, adjacent upper part of the temporal lobe, and sometimes Broca's area. Understanding word meaning is most affected by damage to the temporal lobe, but may also involve areas of the frontal lobe near Broca's area. Syntactic analysis appears to involve different parts of the cortical language areas in different people, suggesting that we each acquire slightly different ways of dealing with syntax during childhood.

Studies in patients with damage to the left hemisphere have shown that there are two key pathways involved in the analysis of the syntax of language. One of these is the arcuate fasciculus that runs in a curved course to connect language areas in the left temporal and frontal lobes. The other is a pathway that also joins the language areas, but does so by running a more direct course beneath the insular cortex, a region situated deep inside the lateral fissure of the left side of the brain.

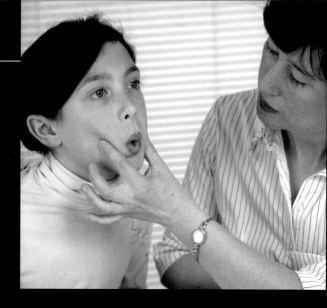

↑ **Most children master the demands of articulating their native language without formal instruction. However, in some cases speech therapy may be required when problems with the brain or airway passages prevent clear articulation.**

Equipped for speech

Many animals produce sounds to communicate, but only humans produce complex chains of sounds according to precise rules to encode detailed ideas. Is this distinction just about language areas in the cerebral cortex, or does it involve other parts of our anatomy? An important difference between the ape and adult human throat is that the larynx sits quite low in the mature human throat, providing a long column of air above the larynx for the production of a wide range of phonemes. By contrast, the entrance to the ape larynx sits so high that its upper tip is in contact with the soft palate. The high larynx of apes and infant humans reduces the risk of choking during swallowing, but greatly limits the range of articulate sounds that can be produced.

Speech depends on a combination of good control of expired breath to be able to articulate a full phrase, a full repertoire of motor programs in motor centers to form phonemes, and the skilled coordination of scores of tiny muscles in the throat, tongue, soft palate, mouth, and face to articulate the sounds of language. So the evolution of speech required much more than formation of language areas in the cerebral cortex. There must also have been major changes in the motor circuitry of the brainstem, cerebellum, and spinal cord.

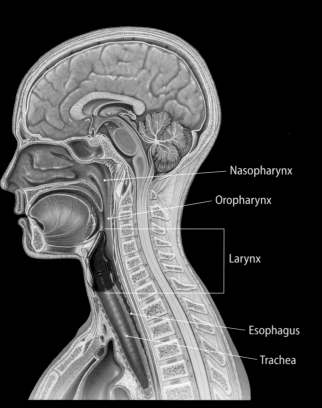

Nasopharynx

Oropharynx

Larynx

Esophagus

Trachea

↑ **The larynx, or voice box, sits quite low in older children and adults, allowing a rich repertoire of vowels, clicks, and consonants to be produced by changing the shape of the airway above it.**

Speech versus song

We take for granted the ability to distinguish between speech and song, yet the two forms of language are actually very similar acoustically. Functional imaging studies of people who hear words either spoken or sung have shown that distinguishing between speech and song depends on a network of eight brain regions in the temporal lobe. Most of these are on the upper surface of the temporal lobe in front of the primary auditory cortex or further back along the upper surface of the temporal lobe, particularly on the right side of the brain. This latter region is also associated with the comprehension of prosody, the rhythmic and musical aspects of language. This network of areas overlaps with brain regions concerned with the extraction of information about pitch from heard sounds, as well as the production of song.

↓ **Singing is a language function, but it also relies on areas in the right temporal lobe to blend words with melody and rhythm.**

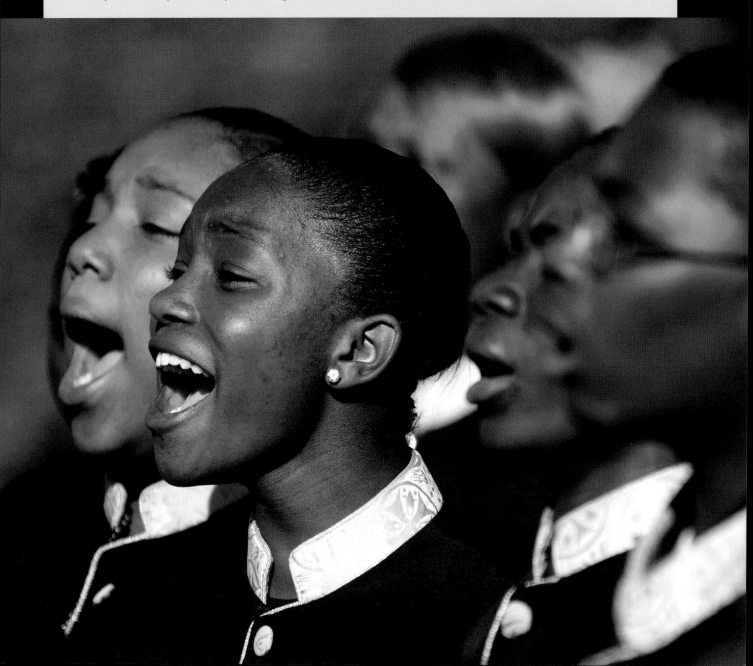

Reading, writing, and mathematical calculation

Spoken language has been an essential part of what it is to be a human for 60,000 years or more. Reading, writing, and mathematical calculation are much more recent developments. Although they are not talents that are hardwired in our brains, they have been instrumental in the story of civilization.

Whereas the ability to acquire spoken language may be innate, written language is far more difficult to obtain. Most of us spend more than a decade receiving close training from dedicated teachers to develop the skills to understand and express ourselves in written form. Skillful mathematical calculation and reasoning are even more difficult to acquire.

The reading challenge

Recognizing and interpreting written language depends on a complex sequence of processing events. The pattern of lines and dots must be interpreted as letters, then matched as a letter sequence to an internalized lexicon, before being converted to word meaning, and finally interpreted in the context of word order (syntax).

When we read we fixate on a point in the line for about one quarter of a second, before the gaze is moved on to the next point. There is a tendency to fixate on long content words, like nouns and major verbs, rather than smaller words like prepositions or pronouns. When we temporarily fixate during reading we can take in chains of words (about four words to the left and 15 words to the right of the fixation point in native English speakers).

The stream of visual processing concerned with form and object recognition (the "what" visual stream, see p. 156) involves pathways running from the primary visual cortex in the back of the occipital lobe down into the temporal lobe. It recognizes the shape of letters and the conformation of words based on a visual lexicon.

↓ **Reading is a complex process that requires the visual recognition of symbols and the conversion of their spatial sequence into meaning.**

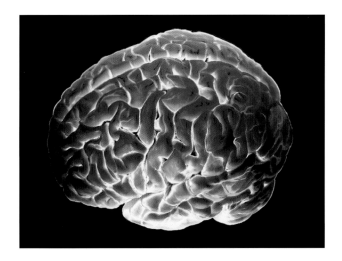

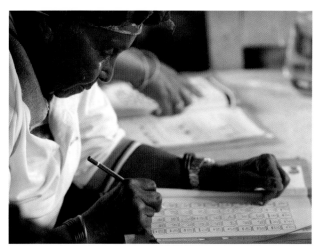

↑ **This MRI scan shows brain activity (red) while words are being read. The visual cortex (far right) is active, as well as an area of the temporal lobe (lower right), which is associated with comprehension of written words.**

↑ **Unlike spoken language, there is no critical period for mastering literacy. Learning to read is challenging at any age, but can be mastered with perseverance even in old age.**

This information is then passed up to Wernicke's area for the final comprehension of meaning based on word sequence. Damage to Wernicke's area may cause alexia, the inability to read.

Functional PET studies have shown activation of the primary visual cortex and a visuolexic area at the junction of the parietal and temporal lobes when the subject is viewing words and interpreting their meaning. Activity also extends up to the back part of Wernicke's area.

Writing

Writing requires the conversion of grammatical rules and word meaning into motor commands for the dominant hand. In many respects, written language requires a more precise following of language rules because written language crystallizes spelling, word order, and grammar.

Usually the same hemisphere that contains the language areas (the left) drives the motor dominant hand (the right), but in many left-handed individuals the language areas of the left hemisphere must channel commands through the corpus callosum to motor areas of the right hemisphere for control of the left hand. However, this does not seem to adversely affect the writing process.

The process of writing depends on Wernicke's area, where word meaning and grammatical rules are stored, as well as activation of the supplementary motor area, a region that is probably responsible for initiation of language expression. Information on word or character sequence and grammar (depending on the language) is

Pure alexia

Damage to the white matter connecting regions of the cerebral cortex can have profound effects even if the overlying gray matter is undamaged. In pure alexia, the person can write, but not read, not even his or her own writing. This is called "alexia without agraphia" and can happen after damage to the white matter beneath the primary visual cortex in the left hemisphere, provided the damage also involves those fibers at the back of the corpus callosum that allow the left hemisphere to get visual information from the right visual cortex. This type of damage disconnects the language areas of the left hemisphere from all their visual input, causing an inability to read.

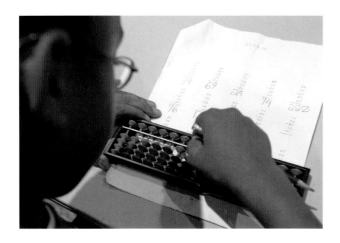

↑ **Before electronic calculators, tools like the abacus made performing arithmetic tasks easier by providing an external "working memory" during calculations.**

Mathematics also has some similarities to written language in that it depends on the manipulation of written symbols and the following of very precise rules, but the process of mathematical reasoning is always a conscious one and usually dominates our cognitive function while it is being performed. Most of us must pay close attention to the precise details of digits and symbols to effectively perform mathematical calculations. Some of this is due to the nature of numbers, where the position of a comma or decimal point can have profound significance, but most is due to the simple fact that mathematical calculation is not an innate ability with an inborn circuitry. Mathematical skills must be acquired by diligent training of brain circuitry that has been designed during evolution for other functions, such as spatial perception and language comprehension.

channeled forward from Wernicke's area to the cortex around Broca's area for choice of appropriate motor programs for letter construction, and from there to the part of the motor cortex where the upper limb is controlled. The level of motor coordination required for writing is prodigious and depends on precise motor routines learned over many years, so even the simple action of writing a shopping list involves activation of the looped circuits through the basal ganglia and cerebrocerebellum.

Damage to the expressive language area of the cortex (Broca's area) often causes agraphia (the inability to write) as well as aphasia, indicating that the final common pathway for both written and spoken language passes through the language areas of the left hemisphere. Agraphia may also result from damage to the lower parietal lobe near its junction with the temporal lobe (see box at right), a region that is within Wernicke's area in most people.

Mathematical reasoning

An important difference between spoken language and mathematical reasoning is that spoken language may be carried out without a fully conscious awareness of the details of sounds, whereas mathematics demands full conscious awareness of the symbols being used.

Gerstmann's syndrome

Damage to the parietal lobe where it meets the temporal lobe (usually on the left side) gives rise to a strange group of symptoms that are collectively called Gerstmann's syndrome. Patients often have problems recognizing or distinguishing fingers (finger agnosia), a confusion of left and right sides, an inability to write (agraphia), sometimes an inability to read (alexia), and a reduced ability to perform simple calculations (dyscalculia). The problem with calculation particularly involves a difficulty with distinguishing categories of numbers, e.g., tens, hundreds, thousands. This suggests that assigning the position of mathematical spacers or groupers, like decimal points and commas, depends on the same brain circuits that judge and assign the position of objects in space.

The nerve circuits responsible for mathematical calculation are poorly understood. Recognition of digits and mathematical symbols depends on the primary visual cortex and pathways through the upper temporal lobe that are concerned with the recognition of objects in the visual world. The precise rules governing mental arithmetic and the manipulation of mathematical symbols and digits are probably stored in the lower part of the parietal lobe, mainly on the left side of the brain, suggesting links between the rules for mathematical reasoning and grammatical rules for language.

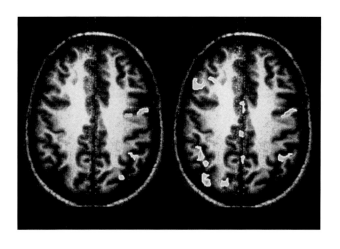

↑ **These images show EEG activity (yellow) during mathematical problem-solving superimposed on horizontal brain scans. At left, the subject is reciting multiplication tables, at right, the subject is performing repeated subtractions.**

↓ **Advanced mathematics requires the manipulation of symbols according to precise rules, much like the grammatical conventions for written language.**

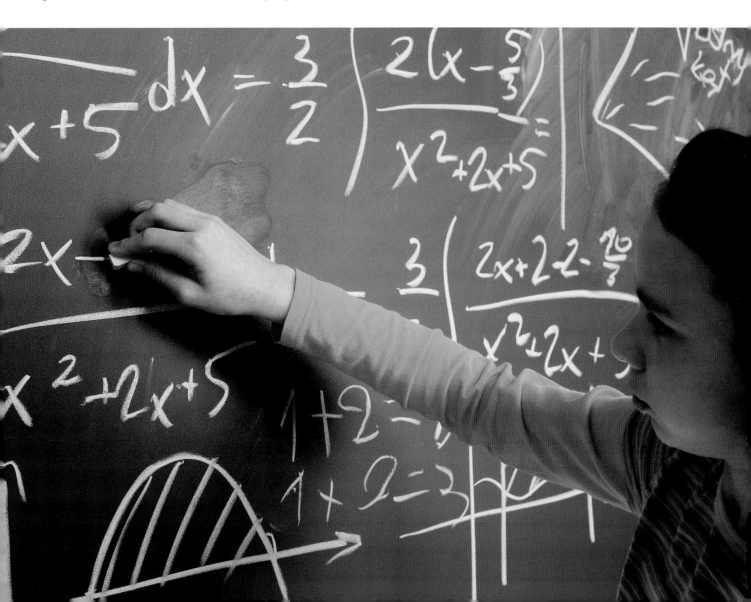

Creative thinking

The human mind has the ability to imagine novel objects and ideas and ponder difficult questions. What is the neurological root of our creative capacity? We often think that human capacity is limited to what an individual brain can achieve, but minds acting collectively have abilities that transcend the talents of the individual.

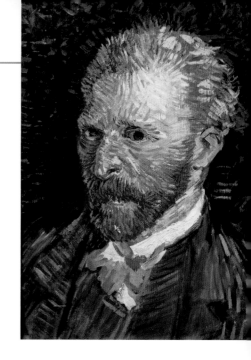

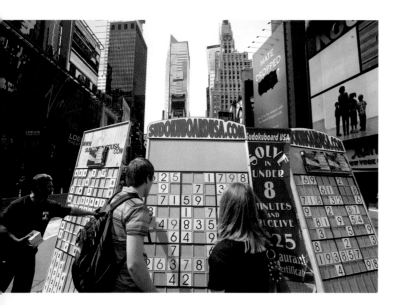

↗ **Recent studies suggest a possible link between damage to the temporal lobe and enhanced artistic creativity. It seems likely that the Dutch painter Vincent van Gogh experienced temporal lobe epilepsy caused by a brain lesion in that location.**

← **Problem solving involves the ability to create and test hypotheses about possible solutions. Imagination and testing against reality are key elements.**

Creativity is the ability to generate ideas, concepts, objects, or images that have never existed before. It is the cornerstone of what makes us human and yet it is a poorly understood function of our brains, mainly because creativity is often difficult to define and test in neuroscience experiments. Creativity is often divided into three types: divergent thinking, the ability to think in novel ways about problems; artistic performance, the ability to translate intellectual questions and ideas into novel forms of artistic expression; and insight, the ability to ponder the underlying causes of events and phenomena and to deduce connections between cause and effect, whether in human behavior or the physical and biological world.

Investigating creativity

Studies of creativity using modern imaging techniques (functional MRI and PET scanning) have shown that imagination and inventiveness are not critically dependent on any single mental process or particular brain region, although some brain areas do appear to be more active than others. Divergent thinking, in particular, appears to involve activation of diverse areas of the cerebral cortex, but with the medial prefrontal cortex and inferior frontal gyrus most consistently active. Artistic performance also involves widespread areas of cerebral cortex, but with particular activation of motor areas and the association cortex at the junction of the temporal and parietal lobes. Finally, insight appears to be the most consistent type of creativity with respect to regional brain activation, in that insight most actively involves the anterior (front) part of the cingulate gyrus (a part of the limbic system), as well as the prefrontal cortex.

The daydreaming mind

Goal-directed thinking has received most attention in neuroscience research, because it is easier to analyze, but much of our thinking is not directed toward a specific task. Daydreaming can not only be a pleasant way to pass the time, but may bring insights and ideas that goal-directed thinking does not. Daydreaming is a type of thinking that is not directly related to the current demands of the external environment. It requires two processes: the ability to disengage attention from current perception (perceptual decoupling); and the ability to draw information from the current contents of consciousness (meta-awareness). Thinking that occurs without any relation to events in the external environment can often interfere with the immediate processing of sensory information,

giving rise to inattentiveness and absent-mindedness. On the other hand, decoupling thought processes from the external world allows the mind to focus in detail on an internal train of thought and permits one to ponder problems and goals other than those of immediate concern.

Brain imaging studies suggest that perceptual decoupling involves activity in the anterior cingulate gyrus, the dorsolateral prefrontal cortex, and a region of cortex known as the precuneus, on the midline cortex between the somatosensory cortex and visual association cortex. Meta-awareness appears to primarily activate brain regions in the anterior cingulate gyrus, and the insular cortex deep inside the lateral fissure on the side of the cerebral hemisphere.

Is creativity a right hemisphere function?

Popular literature often ascribes creativity to the right cerebral hemisphere, but the scientific evidence for this is weak and often contradictory. Although there is some evidence that the right medial prefrontal cortex plays a critical role in networks that underlie creativity, this may be due to the fact that, unlike the left prefrontal cortex, it is not dominated by the demands of speech.

More recent studies of human creativity indicate that although the right hemisphere is more active than the left during creative tasks, interaction of many brain regions on both sides is critically important for creativity. This makes intuitive sense, because creativity requires the integration of many separate cognitive abilities that cannot all be in the same part, or even the same side, of the brain. If this view is correct, then people with the

→ **Artistic creativity is a uniquely human feature that has been around for at least 20,000 years, as shown by the Upper Paleolithic cave paintings of southern France and Spain.**

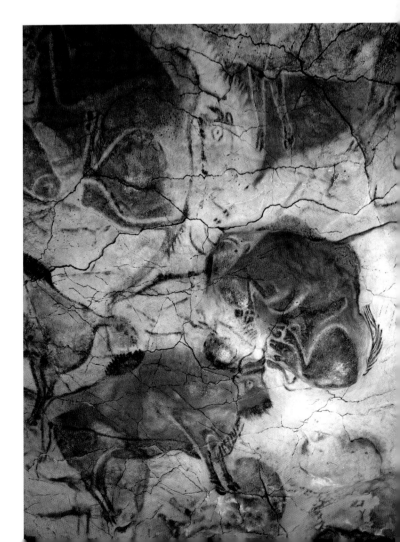

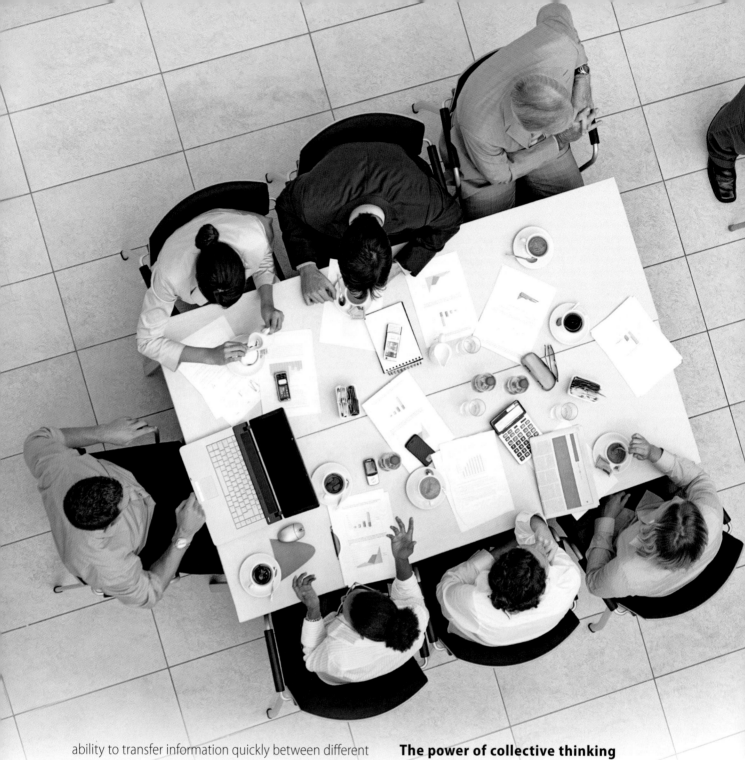

ability to transfer information quickly between different parts of the same hemisphere and between the two hemispheres (through the corpus callosum) should have the highest creativity.

It is often argued that the concentration of language abilities in the left hemisphere (lateralization) is a key feature for the advanced abilities of the human brain, but if creativity is most dependent on rapid transfer of information between hemispheres, then less lateralization may actually help creativity. In other words, lateral thinkers may not always be laterally minded.

The power of collective thinking

Although we value our own opinions and thoughts, democratic society is based on the aggregation of opinions from a wide range of minds. Whether it is guessing the number of jelly beans in a jar or deciding social policy, minds acting as a group are far more accurate and effective than the individual. In fact, the great social, economic, and military catastrophes of the 20th century can be seen as the result of the subjugation of the wisdom of the collective human mind to the extreme mindsets of a dominant few.

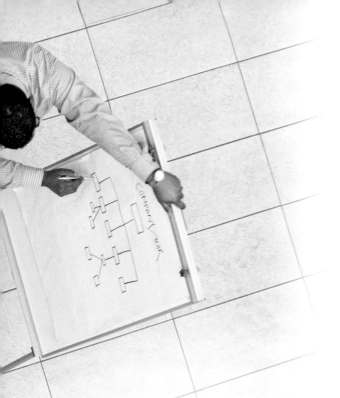

← **Collective intelligence in a small group amplifies the cognitive abilities of the group's individual members, provided they cooperate and have good rapport.**

How does this collective wisdom arise? Different sensory viewpoints appear to play an important role. Although individuals share similar anatomy and physiology, different experiences during life result in different neural mechanisms that process sensory information from the same sensory stimulus in unique ways. Collecting together and weighing up all these differing viewpoints ensures that none of the key elements of a sensory experience are missed.

When many minds work on the same problem or question simultaneously, effective solutions and answers can be arrived at quickly; much like the way parallel processing of sensory information speeds up the progression of perception in a single brain.

The reduction of "noise", which in the context of decision-making means the elimination of random or extreme viewpoints, is another benefit of collective decision-making.

→ **Market pricing, whether it be the value of a stock or the odds on a horse, is the product of many minds working in parallel on the same questions.**

Brain damage and insights into artistic creativity

Although much of human creativity appears to involve the prefrontal cortex, studies of patients with degenerative brain disease hint at important roles for other brain regions. Patients with focal degeneration in the left anterior temporal lobe have impaired language ability, but may experience enhanced artistic creativity. Furthermore, patients with progressive aphasia—a neurodegenerative condition that causes a gradual loss of speech, grammar, articulation, and syntax resulting from degeneration of the left inferior frontal gyrus—have increased visual and artistic creativity. It is as if articulate language impedes artistic expression and when language is lost, the potential of other cortical areas is realized (e.g., the right medial prefrontal cortex or posterior parts of the right hemisphere) such that artistic ability flourishes.

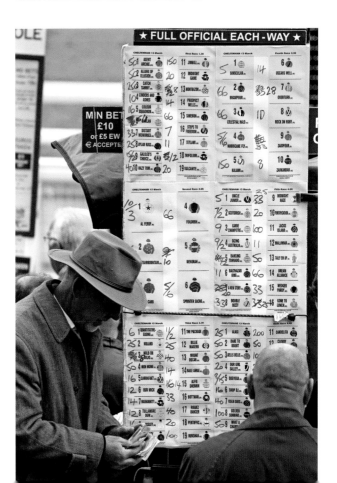

Negotiation and cooperation

Negotiating with other people is an important social skill for achieving mutual goals. Cooperation is a key component of human social structure and allows us to work collectively toward agreed objectives.

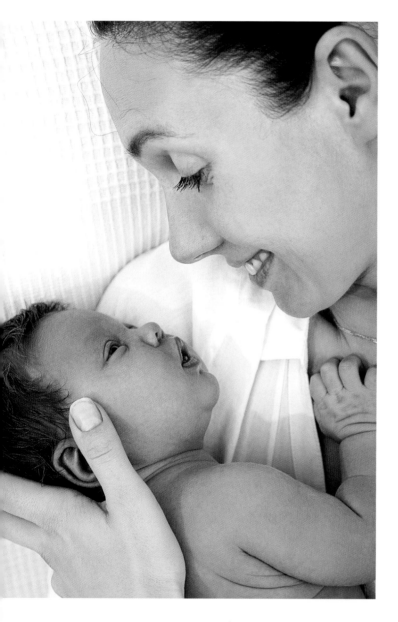

↑ **Making eye contact is the most powerful way of establishing an emotional link. During the first year of life, infants learn rapidly that the gaze of others conveys significant information.**

Both negotiation and cooperation require the ability to recognize that others have a different point of view, and to recognize and understand emotions in others. They also require that we are prepared to give up the short-term gratification of our own personal desires, so that longer-term goals of mutual benefit can be achieved. Of course, a keen understanding of the emotions and drives of others, without a sincere desire to cooperate, allows liars and schemers to gain personal advantage at the expense of others and the common good.

Psychologists have identified seven key behavioral elements involved in negotiation and cooperation:

- Recognizing others as separate minds.
- Understanding and/or sharing the emotions of others.
- Understanding the viewpoints and goals of others.
- Effectively communicating personal goals.
- Conceiving and planning long-term, large-scale projects.
- Being able to trade short-term personal goals for long-term mutual benefits.
- Being able to offer benefits to others in return for concessions.

How we read others' minds

The first step in negotiating with another person is to recognize that they have a different point of view from us and to deduce the differences between their point of view and ours. The theory of mind mechanism that allows this type of "mind-reading" is acquired around the age of four years, when children begin to recognize that others may have beliefs or points of view different from their own. Psychologist Simon Baron-Cohen has suggested that there are four components to this

→ **In this test for theory of mind, a child sees Anne moving Sally's ball. The child is asked: "Where will Sally look for her ball?" If they have theory of mind, they will know that Sally will think her ball is still in the basket. A child without theory of mind will think that Sally knows what they know—that the ball has been moved.**

For the greater good

Negotiating an agreement with another person, or society as a whole, depends on the ability to put off our own immediate short-term satisfaction, with the expectation that cooperation will bring greater long-term benefits. Planning for long-term benefit is probably a function of the prefrontal cortex, although such long-term planning (years to decades) has rarely been the subject of neuroscience research. Many projects require the concerted actions of thousands or millions of prefrontal cortices acting in unison, with each subordinating its personal goals to those of a greater good.

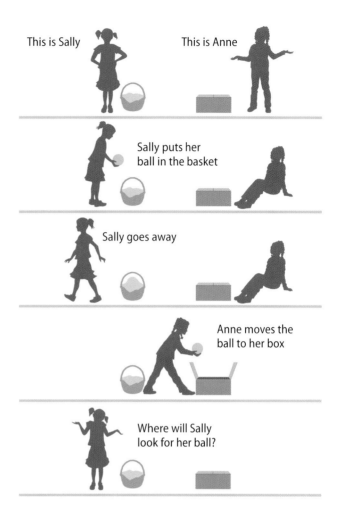

This is Sally   This is Anne

Sally puts her ball in the basket

Sally goes away

Anne moves the ball to her box

Where will Sally look for her ball?

"mind-reading" ability: an intentionality detector, an eye-direction detector, a shared attention mechanism, and a theory of mind mechanism.

A person's intentionality detector decides if an object has been moved because of an intention or by chance. The observer must decide if an observed event was because of the action of another mind or simply a random occurrence.

The eye-direction detector detects the direction of gaze of another person and infers what that person is seeing. The observer notes the point in space that another is watching and deduces the point of view that they will have.

→ **The underside of the frontal lobe (the orbitofrontal cortex) plays a vital role in recognizing the emotions of others and is key to social cooperation and empathy.**

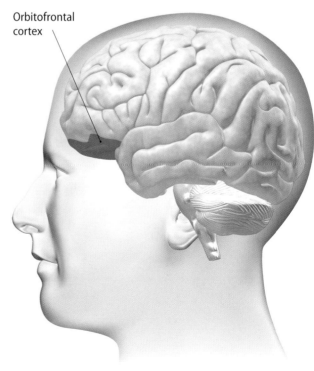

Orbitofrontal cortex

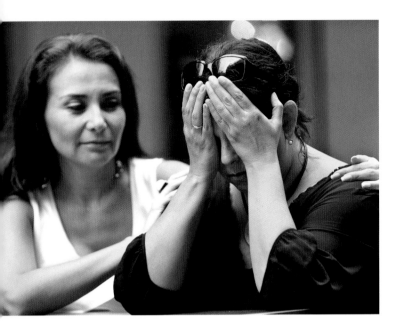

← Sharing the emotional state of another person (empathy) and understanding their emotional perspective is an important attribute of caring people.

Sharing emotions

Empathy is an emotional state caused by sharing the emotional and sensory state of another person. It should be distinguished from sympathy, which is an expression of concern or compassion for another. It should also be distinguished from the understanding of another person's beliefs, intentions, or desires, which is really a function of reason or cognition. In other words, understanding another person's emotions is very different from sharing them.

Both sharing another person's emotional state and understanding that state intellectually are important in human society. We are often motivated to help another when we share their emotions, such as assisting a mother who has lost a child in a crowded supermarket. Intellectually understanding someone's emotional state, even if we do not share the actual emotion, is also important in human relations, as when a health worker treats a patient's emotional distress with medications while maintaining a professional clinical detachment. Understanding what motivates another mind is also essential to effective negotiation, because you cannot

The shared attention mechanism decides if the self and the other person are looking at the same object or event. The observer must match up what they see with what they deduce another person would be seeing.

Finally, the theory of mind mechanism enables the self to form a mental model of what the other person is experiencing. The observer reaches a conclusion about the visual experience that another person will have and forms an image in their own mind of what that experience would be. This can then be used to predict the other's thoughts and actions.

What neuroscience cannot explain

Understanding the nervous system mechanisms that underlie human social function is a difficult area of research because society depends on a complex pattern of behaviors by large groups of people. We can get some insight into mechanisms at the core of empathy and planning, but what is the neural basis of democracy, nationalism, and patriotism? How can we explain the complex interactions between millions of citizens in modern democracies on the basis of drives and ambitions generated in nerve cell networks? Why are humans willing to give their lives for an ideology or nation state? And perhaps most importantly, how can dictators hold millions of otherwise rational human minds in thrall with a few stirring speeches?

← Dictators like Hitler entrance millions of rational minds with their rhetoric.

offer concessions to another, in return for your own benefit, unless you can model their goals and desires.

The prefrontal cortex plays a key role in recognizing emotions in others. The subdivision that is particularly important is the underside of the frontal lobe—the orbitofrontal cortex. A more intellectual understanding of the emotions and feelings of others probably involves other parts of the prefrontal cortex or the facial recognition areas on the underside of the temporal lobe. Some neuroscientists believe that empathy depends on the activation of mirror neurons in those very same brain regions that would be activated when the observer experiences the emotion, but other neuroscientists have argued that this activation does not necessarily carry the same emotional experience.

Lies and liars

All people lie, sometimes to ease social interaction (e.g., the polite excuse to avoid an unwanted social engagement), sometimes to avoid punishment, and sometimes to gain advantage. Clearly the effective function of human society requires the effects of lies to be kept to a minimum, but how do we detect and deal with liars?

Often lies go undetected because we do not attempt to detect them, a phenomenon dubbed the "ostrich effect" by psychologist Aldert Vrij. It may reflect the emotional cost of recognizing and dealing with lies—

in other words, people do not always want to hear the truth. Claims that lying can be detectd by EEG or functional MRI scanning have been disputed and the field remains a contentious part of neuroscience.

When psychopaths prosper

Psychopathy, or sociopathy, is a personality disorder characterized by a pattern of disregard for the rights of others. These individuals are often emotionally cold and callous and may manipulate others through lies and deceit to achieve their personal goals. Psychiatrists have traditionally seen psychopathy as an impairment or defect, but evolutionary psychologists argue that psychopathy may be an adaptive strategy that improves the psychopath's chances of surviving and prospering.

Provided the bulk of the population is trusting and cooperative, psychopaths can take advantage of the trusting natures of others to gain personal benefit. You would expect psychopaths to be able to understand the feelings and thoughts of others intellectually, because that allows them to better manipulate others, but research indicates they do not experience empathy.

Psychopaths can prosper only if there is a significant cost in time or resources for the rest of the population to check on the veracity of the psychopath's stories. Psychopaths often have to move on frequently to avoid their deceits being discovered.

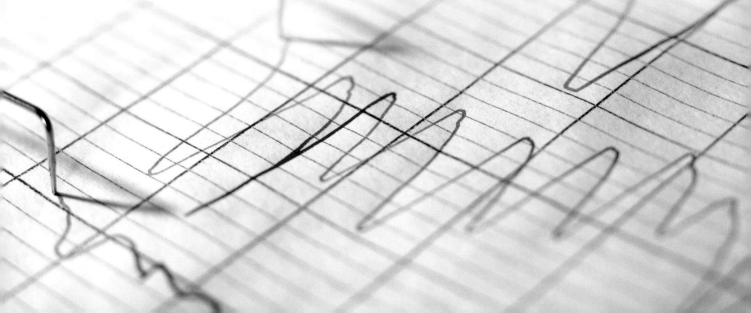

↓ **This polygraph (lie detector) readout records pulse, blood pressure, respiration, and other physiological processes while the subject answers questions. Proponents of this technique claim that false answers result in detectable physiological reactions.**

The limits of socially accepted behavior

Every day we interact with our fellow humans in ways that ensure that we all achieve our daily goals. Without the niceties and courtesies of social interaction, our society would collapse into chaos. How does the brain control this delicate social interaction? Why does it sometimes fail?

The prefrontal cortex is a large region at the front of the brain that is proportionally larger in humans than other primates. It performs an executive function, making complex decisions about social and planned behavior on the basis of sensory information about the world, our past emotional experiences, and our long-standing goals and plans. Neuroscientists recognize four main regions: the middorsal, dorsolateral, ventrolateral, and orbitofrontal cortical areas. The dorsolateral and ventrolateral regions are most closely associated with sensory areas of the cortex and probably receive information from the visual, auditory, and somato-sensory areas that is used to make social and planning decisions; the dorsolateral region also has close connections with motor areas of the cortex and is probably most involved in putting socially relevant decisions into action; and the orbitofrontal cortex is closely linked with the limbic system and is concerned with recognizing emotions in others. The orbitofrontal cortex allows us to decide how others are feeling and make socially appropriate decisions on that basis. Finally, all areas of the prefrontal cortex are interlinked to allow exchange of information.

Brains without inhibitions or empathy

Studies of people with brain injuries provide clues to the functions of specific areas. We know that damage to the prefrontal cortex during surgery results in a pattern of behavior known as the "dysexecutive syndrome." One of the most striking features of these patients is their lack of inhibition and behavioral control in social settings. Often quick to become angry, they are also impulsive and prone to making rude or childish comments.

Patients with prefrontal cortex damage are often said to be stimulus-bound, meaning that when exposed to a stimulus they react automatically without any thought as to whether the action is socially appropriate. As an extreme example of this, a doctor once placed a urinal on his desk before an interview with a patient whose prefrontal cortex had been damaged. On seeing the

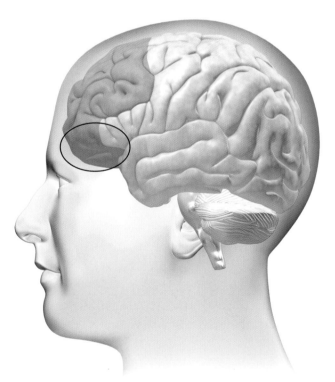

↑ **The orbitofrontal part of the prefrontal cortex (circled) is important for controlling socially accepted behavior, making considered decisions, and empathy.**

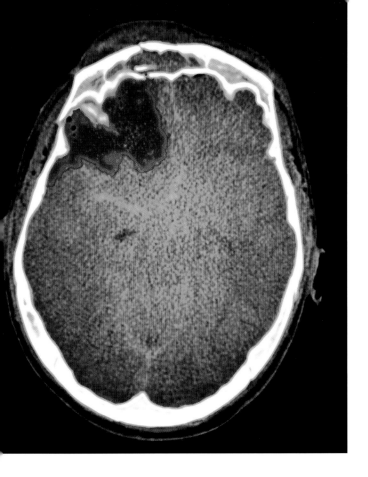

urinal, the patient proceeded to relieve himself into it, apparently oblivious to the inappropriateness of the act. Patients with prefrontal cortex lesions often behave impulsively, engaging in sex or getting married with no consideration of the consequences.

Patients with prefrontal cortex damage are also indifferent to their situation and the needs of others around them. They may laugh at the sight of someone crying and their sense of humor is often childish, compulsive, and facetious. Their actions indicate a general lack of empathy.

← **A CT scan shows hemorrhage into the prefrontal cortex, a lesion that would lead to the "dysexecutive syndrome," which is characterized by impulsive, uninhibited behavior.**

The strange case of Phineas Gage

In 1848, an American railway construction foreman named Phineas Gage suffered a horrific accident. While tamping a blasting powder charge into a drill hole, Gage struck the 3½-foot (1-m) iron tamping rod against the side of the drill hole, generating a spark that ignited the charge. Unfortunately, he was leaning over the hole at the time so the rod was propelled through his left cheek and on through his left orbit and frontal lobe. Miraculously, Gage survived the blast and avoided infection, but his behavior was altered forever. Prior to the accident he had been an efficient and capable foreman, but after recovery he was disrespectful and blasphemous, rude to his co-workers, and unable to organize or plan the workload. He soon lost his job and spent much of his remaining life exhibiting himself in a traveling sideshow. He was last heard of working on a stagecoach in South America. Gage's case advanced our understanding of the brain, providing evidence that the frontal lobes are closely involved in personality.

→ **An 1850 illustration of Phineas Gage's head injury involving a tamping rod.**

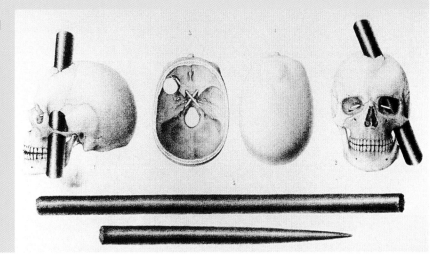

Planning and forethought

Planning for future goals is not a uniquely human attribute, but it does reach a high level of sophistication in our species, allowing us to individually and collectively plan years ahead to reach mutually desirable goals.

Simple forms of short-duration motor planning rely on working memory circuitry in the lower frontal cortex, but more complex planning over years is performed in a series of areas over the upper surface and underside of the frontal lobe.

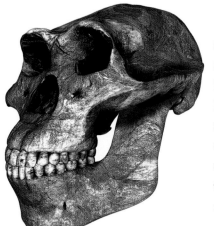

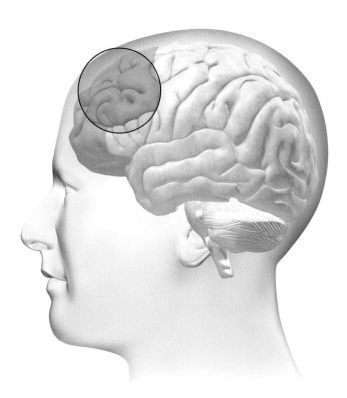

← ↓ **Early human ancestors like the australopithecines had a prefrontal cortex like that of modern apes. The expansion of the prefrontal cortex accompanied the emergence of modern humans.**

↑ **Planning ahead over months and even years is a human ability that relies on the upper and lateral parts of the prefrontal cortex (circled).**

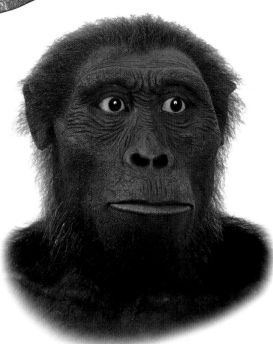

The prefrontal cortex and evolution

The human brain has increased in size about three-fold over the last two million years. The prefrontal cortex has undergone the greatest enlargement over that period. In fact, the prefrontal cortex of the modern human brain is more than 200 percent the size you would expect if our brain were simply a scaled-up chimpanzee brain. This expansion of the prefrontal cortex appears to have accompanied an increasing complexity of human social life, as shown by technology and art. An enlarged prefrontal cortex allows us to judge the emotions of other people and model their point of view, as well as planning ahead, from months to years. It is also critical for negotiation, cooperation, manipulating the behavior of others, and detecting deception.

Working memory and the ability to plan long term are both important in the evolution of a complex human society. Even for hunter-gatherers, working memory is critically important for the step-by-step processes involved in manufacturing tools. The more complex the tool, the greater the number of steps, so tool complexity would be expected to go hand in hand with the expansion of the prefrontal cortex. Long-term planning is also essential for organizing a hunt or a day's gathering of seeds, tubers, or fruits. In both these activities particular procedures or actions must be carried out in the correct sequence for success. This organized behavior requires motivation, the mental rehearsal of actions, and the ability to interact productively with other members of the group.

Working memory

Performing motor tasks with multiple steps requires that we hold information in mind for a few minutes—working memory. This is the sort of memory we use when reading and remembering a phone number before dialing. Working memory is held in mind for only a few minutes and is then forgotten as soon as it is no longer relevant.

Studies in monkeys have shown that working memory depends on a region of the prefrontal cortex on the side of the frontal lobe. Monkeys with damage in this area have problems performing tasks that require them to hold some type of information in their mind for a few seconds to minutes (called spatial delayed response tasks). These sorts of tasks might require them to remember the location of a stimulus, or the sort of behavior that will get them a reward, over a brief delay of several seconds.

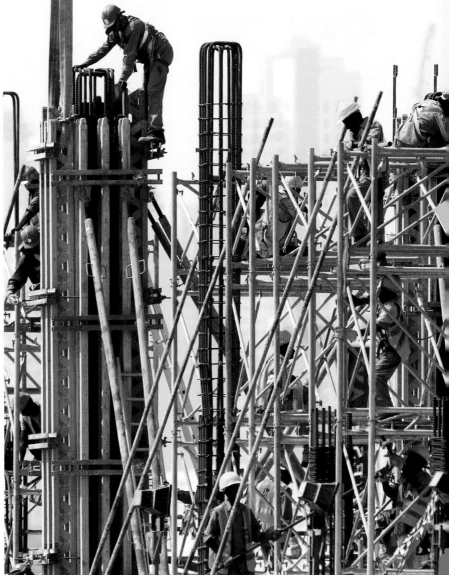

↑ **Building a skyscraper depends on long-term planning and a complex set of learned skills, with each worker carrying out a specific job in a sequence that is coordinated to produce the desired result.**

Initial studies testing the ability of humans with prefrontal cortex damage to hold information over a few seconds' delay did not demonstrate the same deficit, because humans could use their speech to help their memory. But when the test used abstract patterns that could not be verbally described, humans with prefrontal damage showed similar problems to the monkeys.

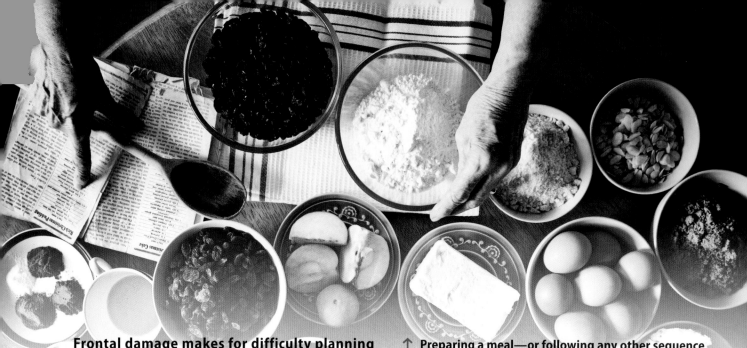

Frontal damage makes for difficulty planning

People with damage to the prefrontal cortex have difficulty planning and organizing their lives. They are unable to correctly order the sequence of motor tasks that must be performed to achieve a goal—following the many steps of a recipe to produce a cooked meal, for example. If patients are placed in a setting where they must work through a series of errands, such as shopping at the mall, they take much longer to perform the task than normal people. They tend to go into shops that are irrelevant to their task and are repeatedly distracted from working toward their main goal.

People with prefrontal cortex damage are also poor at assessing the consequences of their actions. This is

↑ **Preparing a meal—or following any other sequence of motor tasks in a certain order to achieve a goal—depends on the prefrontal cortex.**

tested in the clinical setting by gambling tasks that are designed to give the patient an early winning streak. Patients are given an initial stake of chips and work through a pre-programmed sequence of cards. High-scoring cards give the patient a win, low-value cards cost the patient some chips. Normal people stop playing when the losing streak begins, but patients with damage to the prefrontal cortex will continue to play until all their stake is lost.

The Tower of London Test

Neuroscientists use the Tower of London Test to examine a patient's planning ability. The test requires patients to think several moves in advance. A patient and an examiner both have a structure with three vertical posts; colored balls can be placed on the posts in various configurations and the three posts are of different lengths so they can hold between one and three balls. The examiner asks the patient to move the balls so that they match the arrangement of balls on his or her tower. There are rules: patients can only move one ball at a time, and they must hold the sequence of moves

in their head while they work through the task. Patients with damage to the prefrontal cortex have greatly impaired performance on this task, demonstrating the importance of this area for planning.

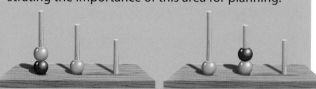

↑ **Move the balls from a start position (left) to match a goal position (right), by moving one ball at a time, and holding the sequence of moves in your head.**

Attention deficit hyperactivity disorder

Attention deficit hyperactivity disorder (ADHD) has symptoms that cluster in two principal areas: symptoms of inattention, and symptoms of hyperactivity and/or impulsivity. Patients may either have a combined type of ADHD or a version that has a predominance of inattention or hyperactivity.

Structural and functional imaging studies of the brains of patients with ADHD have found changes in the prefrontal cortex–striatum–cerebellum circuit. Analysis of the volume of brain regions has revealed a reduced volume of the right-sided prefrontal cortex, consistent with the greater role of the right side in attention to tasks. Reduction in the size of the striatum and the midline of the cerebellum has also been found in these patients.

ADHD is at least partially inherited. Particular genes concerned with dopamine transportation and receptors may increase the susceptibility of the prefrontal cortex to environmental damage. Some types of infection may produce antibodies that damage the circuits between the prefrontal cortex and the striatum.

Drugs that alleviate the symptoms of ADHD include stimulants like Ritalin (methylphenidate) and Adderall (a mixture of amphetamines). These

drugs may increase the release of dopamine and noradrenaline (norepinephrine) in the prefrontal cortex, optimizing levels of these neurotransmitters to reduce impulsivity and improve attention.

ADHD can be a controversial diagnosis and many child psychiatrists argue that it tends to be overdiagnosed, with potentially hazardous effects for the inappropriately medicated children.

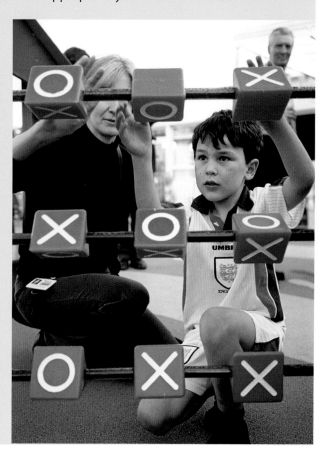

→ **A psychologist uses play activities to assess the attention span of a boy who may have ADHD.**

Functional subdivision in the prefrontal cortex

The prefrontal cortex is composed of several subregions, but the details of how these work together are still poorly understood. There is a major practical problem in dissecting out the functions of the prefrontal cortex because it is very difficult to subdivide the cognitive processes that make up planning.

Some researchers have suggested that the prefrontal cortex is organized according to function; i.e., specific

areas have specific functions. The underside of the frontal cortex is called the orbitofrontal cortex and is believed to be involved in emotional modeling and in the inhibition of behavior. The lower part of the side of the frontal lobe (ventrolateral prefrontal cortex) is thought to keep information in mind during working memory, whereas the upper part of the side of the frontal lobe (dorsolateral prefrontal cortex) is responsible for the manipulation of that information.

Music and the brain

Music of one kind or another is found in all societies: it is one of the defining characteristics of humanity. The appreciation and expression of music are complex abilities of the cerebral cortex that require many higher functional areas.

Music is similar to verbal language in some respects, because they both involve sequences of sounds, but the brain deals with music quite differently from language. The regions in the cerebral cortex for appreciating different aspects of music are not tightly grouped and may even be on opposite sides of the brain.

The human affinity for music
Music is a human invention that may be less than 60,000 years old. The earliest musical instrument ever found (a flute) is associated with the remains of the Neanderthals, but music does not appear to have become common until the emergence of fully modern humans. If music did not exist before humans invented it, why do we have brain circuits that allow us to enjoy it? It may be that brain circuits in the temporal lobe that allow us to interpret and recognize complex patterns of behaviorally significant sound in the natural world, such as bird song or the calls of prey animals, have been taken over for our musical appreciation. In non-musicians these appear to be mainly in the auditory association cortex of the right hemisphere and not directly associated with the language areas of the left hemisphere.

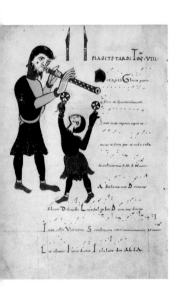

↑ **Making music has been part of human life from the late Stone Age. This 11th-century manuscript portrays a musician playing an oboe-like instrument.**

Amusia: musical blindness

The lack of musical appreciation skills is known as amusia. It mainly involves a problem in assessing pitch, but also includes musical memory and recognition of music. Some people (4 percent of the population) have a congenital form of the disorder and have a deficit in the fine-scale discrimination of pitch. The ability to appreciate music may also be damaged following strokes that involve the temporal lobe. Studies with patients suffering dementia have also indicated that the very front of the temporal lobe is important in the recognition of famous musical pieces. Although amusia may accompany problems with language (aphasia), these two conditions may also occur in isolation, supporting functional MRI studies that have suggested that language and music are mainly processed in quite different parts of the cerebral cortex.

The musical mind
Musicians and non-musicians process musical information differently. In people who have not had extensive formal training in music, the right hemisphere appears to be more important than the left in the perception of a complex series of sounds like a melody. By contrast, trained musicians show higher activity in the left hemisphere when listening to a melody. In fact, for trained musicians musical ability appears to involve the language-dominant left hemisphere more than in

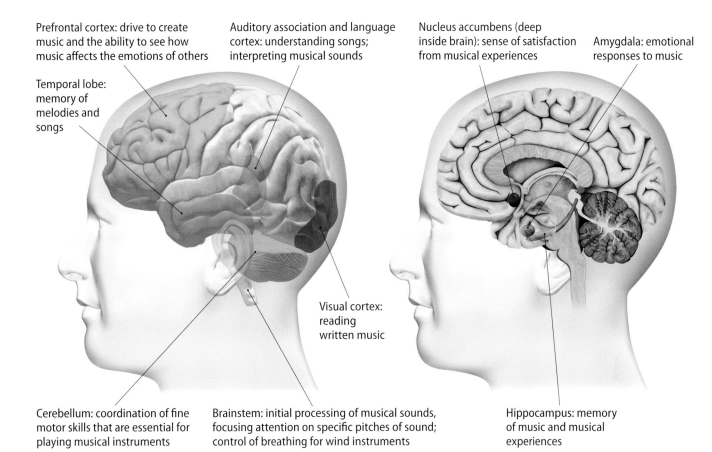

Prefrontal cortex: drive to create music and the ability to see how music affects the emotions of others

Temporal lobe: memory of melodies and songs

Auditory association and language cortex: understanding songs; interpreting musical sounds

Nucleus accumbens (deep inside brain): sense of satisfaction from musical experiences

Amygdala: emotional responses to music

Visual cortex: reading written music

Cerebellum: coordination of fine motor skills that are essential for playing musical instruments

Brainstem: initial processing of musical sounds, focusing attention on specific pitches of sound; control of breathing for wind instruments

Hippocampus: memory of music and musical experiences

↑ **The many facets of music-making and musical appreciation involve diverse areas of the cerebral cortex, cerebellum, and brainstem (left), as well as deeper brain structures (right).**

other individuals, suggesting that language areas can take up the detailed analysis of sequences of musical sounds, if they are trained to do so. The greater involvement of the right hemisphere in the appreciation of the emotional aspects of music is consistent with the role of that side of the brain in prosody, the perception of emotional content in language.

On the other hand, when it comes to simpler aspects of music, such as rhythm, the left hemisphere is more active in both trained musicians and non-musicians. The left hemisphere is also more active when a listener is paying close attention to the music, rather than listening to the music in the

background. Transfer of information between the motor areas of the two hemispheres is also better developed in trained musicians, as suggested by a slightly larger front part of the corpus callosum, the fiber bundle between the two hemispheres, in trained musicians.

Imagining a familiar tune activates the auditory association cortex around the right auditory cortex and the frontal cortex on both sides. Imagining playing music triggers the brain's supplementary motor area, which is important for rehearsing rhythmic actions in a precise sequence.

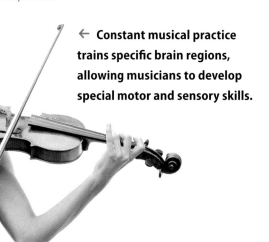

← **Constant musical practice trains specific brain regions, allowing musicians to develop special motor and sensory skills.**

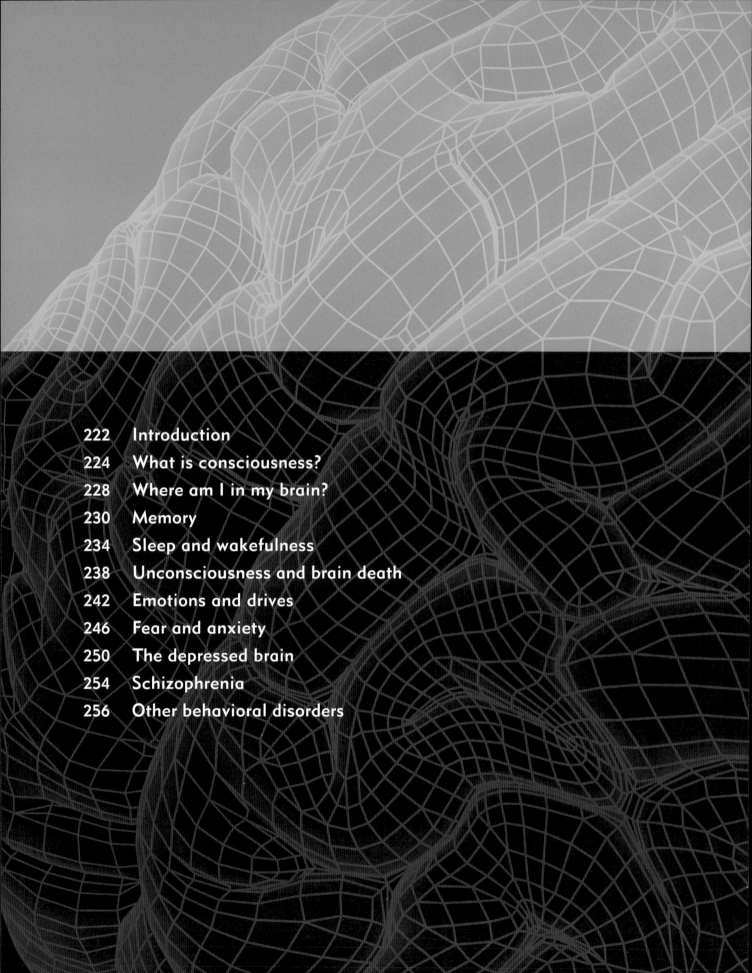

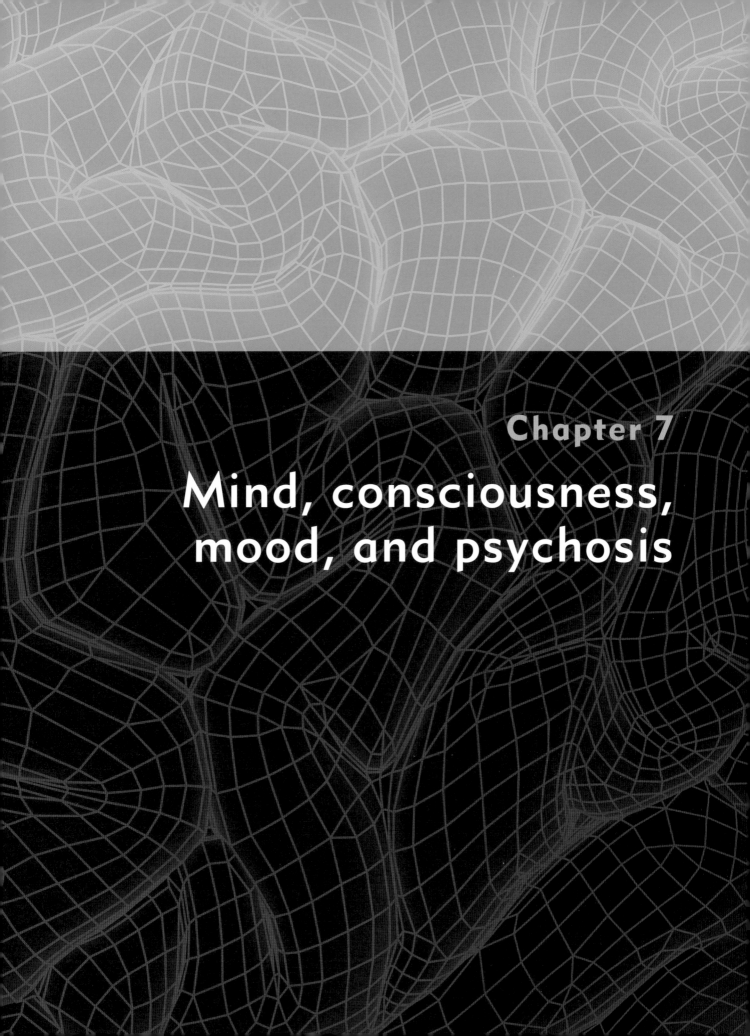

Chapter 7

Mind, consciousness, mood, and psychosis

Introduction

What is the mind? What is consciousness? And how are these produced and maintained by the brain? Although we experience "mind" and "consciousness" every day of our waking lives, details of how the internal activity of our brain produces our conscious experiences are still poorly understood.

Consciousness arises from the relationship between the mind and the world. But consciousness is not a continuous process; our sensory attention is discontinuous in both time and space and is directed at will depending on which aspect of our perceptions are most relevant to our behavior at any given time.

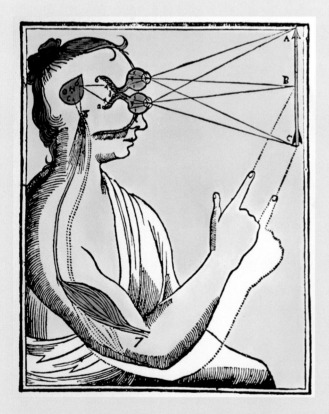

↑ **Descartes suggested that the material world and the realm of thought interacted in the pineal gland, the purple structure in this 1660s illustration.**

A philosophical conundrum

In the 17th century, philosopher and mathematician René Descartes argued that consciousness is lodged inside an immaterial domain that he called the realm of thought, as opposed to the domain of material things, which he called the realm of extension. He suggested (incorrectly) that the interaction between these two domains lay in a small structure between the cerebral hemispheres called the pineal gland. This distinction between the material and immaterial is called a dualist approach and is to be contrasted with monist approaches, which argue that there is only one realm of being and that consciousness and matter are both aspects of this.

Naturally, modern-day neuroscientists (such as Gerald Edelman and Antonio Damasio) seek to explain consciousness on the basis of events within the material brain, and this is the approach taken in this book. Nevertheless, the scientific study of consciousness is fraught with problems, not least of which is the difficulty of establishing an agreed scientific definition of the mind and consciousness. Our contemporary conception of consciousness and the mind is that they arise as an emergent property from activity in circuits and networks of the (very material) cerebral cortex, thalamus, striatum, and brainstem.

Memory and mood

Memory is essential not only for a reflective and contemplative experience of life, but also for carrying out even the simplest daily tasks. Neuroscientists recognize many different types of memory, from a short-term working memory that allows us to remember a phone number through to long-term declarative memory that lets us recall events from childhood. Much of our procedural memory does not even reach conscious awareness, but works in the background to reinforce skills when we train or practice. Our emotional memory is extremely important for shaping future behavior, but it can be tormenting when emotionally overwhelming events are recalled in flashbacks.

↓ Memory can be of many kinds, including emotive recollections of childhood, facts and figures, as well as learned motor skills.

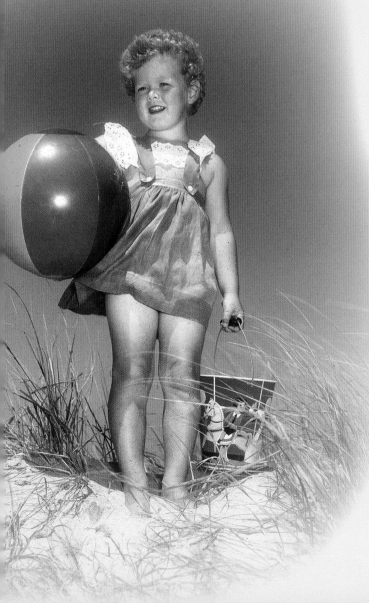

Altered states of consciousness

Philosophers may argue endlessly about what our consciousness is, but there are clinically important aspects of brain function surrounding our conscious experience. Sleep is essential for health but is still poorly understood. It probably serves to keep animals inactive when they are at a behavioral disadvantage and to catalog and store sensory experiences for future reference. Sleep disturbances are an important cause of disability and even fatalities in the community.

Questions of what controls different levels of consciousness are also clinically important. Many brain-injured patients spend prolonged periods of time in a vegetative state, in which brainstem reflexes are present but higher cortical function is essentially absent. The issue of how brain death is defined is of great practical significance in neurology and transplantation medicine.

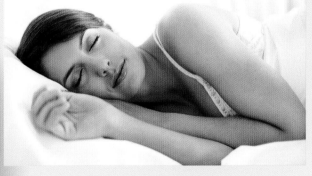

Disorders of mood are a major cause of disability and death worldwide, and depression is found in every human culture. For most of us, sadness is a passing experience when we suffer setbacks or loss in our daily lives, but for some people depression becomes a dark beast that haunts their every waking moment. Some form of depression is common in Western society, affecting between 20 and 30 percent of the population at some stage in their lives. For about 2 percent of the population depression becomes a psychosis, meaning that the feelings of sadness have a nature and intensity far beyond the normal range of human experience.

What is consciousness?

Everyone thinks they know what consciousness is, but it is an extremely difficult concept to define and even harder to pinpoint in the brain.

Philosophers and scientists alike have long speculated about the nature of consciousness. The contemporary US philosopher John Searle has defined consciousness as the "inner qualitative, subjective states and processes of sentience or awareness." We recognize that we come to consciousness when we wake up in the morning and give up consciousness when we go to sleep, lapse into a coma, or die.

Consciousness: a matter of unity and content

An important feature of consciousness is that we perceive ourselves as whole and are aware of the boundary between the external world and us. In terms of the brain's function, this means that all the different types of information (touch, vision, taste, and so on) that our brain deals with are incorporated into a single or unitary model of our self. Brain injury patients lose this sense of self when their right parietal lobe is damaged.

Another important aspect of consciousness is content. We cannot separate our awareness from our subjective sensations, inner imagery, motives, moods, and thoughts. However, only an already conscious brain can experience

Know thyself: what sensory neglect syndrome tells us about consciousness

Damage to the back part of the parietal cortex in monkeys causes a syndrome of neglect of the opposite side of the body, even though the sense of touch from the affected region is unaffected. Damage to the right lower parietal cortex in humans causes a similar effect on the left side of the body. These patients ignore the left halves both of external objects and their own body. The patients may not be aware that anything is wrong and may even claim that the left side of their body belongs to someone else. They also have a general problem with spatial orientation and are unable to use maps or judge distances in the visual world. Patients with this syndrome have a deficit in the unity aspect of consciousness, because they no longer recognize all of their body as belonging to them.

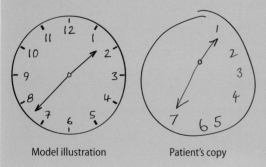

Model illustration   Patient's copy

← **A patient is asked to copy a drawing of a clock. Those suffering from sensory neglect syndrome ignore the left side, as shown in the patient's copy.**

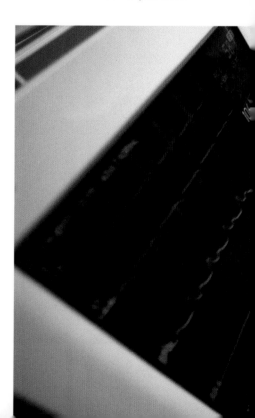

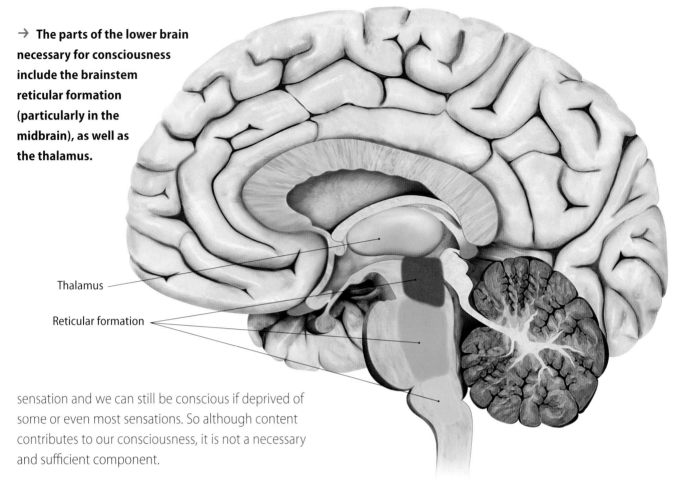

→ **The parts of the lower brain necessary for consciousness include the brainstem reticular formation (particularly in the midbrain), as well as the thalamus.**

Thalamus

Reticular formation

sensation and we can still be conscious if deprived of some or even most sensations. So although content contributes to our consciousness, it is not a necessary and sufficient component.

Our consciousness is not continuous

We like to think that when we are awake we are continuously aware of the world around us, but this

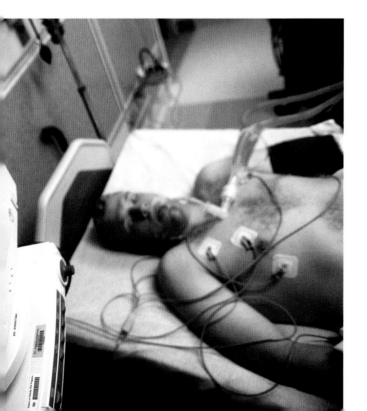

is far from the truth. Stage magicians know that visual attention is discontinuous or even sporadic and exploit this in their sleight of hand. Although we think we are aware of everything that happens throughout our range of vision, our awareness of the visual world is actually concentrated on just a few degrees of central vision. Our eyes constantly flick from one object of interest to another and our visual cortex forms our visual perception on the basis of one tenth of a second grabs of visual information. If we are concentrating on a particular feature in the visual world it is easy to ignore important events in the periphery.

We should also remember that not all our mental processes occur under conscious awareness. In some

← **Consciousness depends on the coordinated activity of the brainstem, thalamus, and cerebral cortex. Any medical condition that interferes with the function of those regions can cause unconsciousness.**

↓ **Focusing on counting basketball passes, many of those who watched the video of this test of inattentional blindness did not see the "gorilla."**

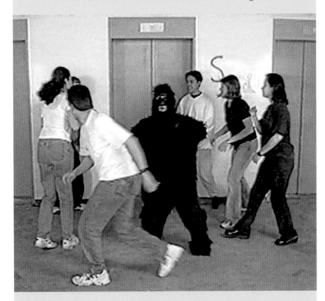

Gorillas in their midst

In 1999, two American psychologists, Daniel J. Simons and Christopher F. Chabris, conducted a test that demonstrates inattentional blindness. They used a video of two groups of people, wearing black or white T-shirts, passing a basket-ball between them. Subjects were asked to count the number of passes made by one of the teams, while a woman walked through the midst of the basketball players in the video either carrying an umbrella or wearing a gorilla suit. In most groups studied, 50 percent of the subjects failed to notice the "gorilla" or the woman carrying the umbrella. This simple experiment demonstrates that our perception of what is happening in our field of vision is determined more by our focus of attention than we realize.

→ **Infants certainly appear to be conscious, but we cannot accurately assess how they perceive themselves and the world until language emerges.**

respects, consciousness is like a searchlight that can be turned to objects or situations of particular behavioral importance. Much of our day-to-day activity actually goes on outside that spotlight. We have all had the experience of thinking about a problem while walking, only to realize at the end of our walk that we have no recollection of any of the scenery on the way.

How is consciousness produced?

Consciousness is an emergent property of the brain; in other words, it is the product of activity in nerve cell networks, but if we move beyond this simple statement we come up against a philosophical problem. The scientific approach to brain function is inherently reductionist—neuroscientists study the constituent parts of the brain to dissect and understand distinct aspects of brain function—but consciousness is inherently unitary. Put simply, the production of consciousness is more than the sum of the functions of the brain parts.

This means that there is no such thing as a locus of consciousness: consciousness must be a distributed function of widespread areas of the brain (but mainly the cerebral cortex). Although our conscious state depends on normal function of the reticular formation of the midbrain, this is not to say that the midbrain is the center of consciousness, any more than the power supply to a computer is the seat of its information processing capacity.

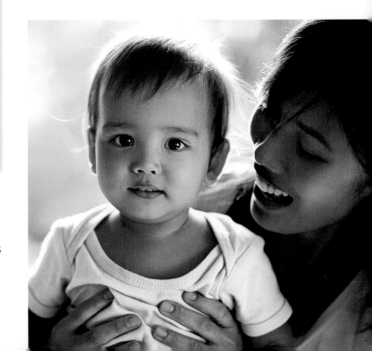

→ **States of consciousness can be detected by an EEG trace. The frequency and shapes of these brain waves change with different states of arousal and attention.**

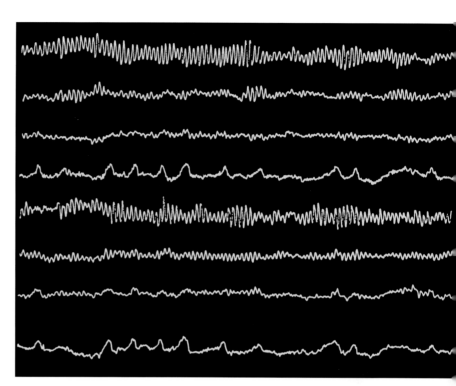

The cerebral cortex is clearly essential for our higher mental functions, but consciousness probably depends on coordinated activity between the cerebral cortex, thalamus, striatum, and brainstem. That is to say, consciousness is more about active circuits than brain regions.

Unified field consciousness

One promising model of consciousness is the unified field consciousness hypothesis. This model emphasizes synchronized activity that functionally binds together nerve cells in diverse regions of the brain. A particular network that may be central to our experience of consciousness is the frontoparietal network that links regions in the prefrontal cortex concerned with planning and social behavior, with regions in the parietal lobe that integrate sensory information from vision, touch, and hearing. Support for this conception comes from observations that conditions that reduce the level of consciousness, such as coma, general anesthesia, deep or slow-wave sleep, and the vegetative state, all involve some reduction of activity in the frontoparietal network.

How do we study consciousness?

Neuroscientists use functional imaging techniques (e.g., functional MRI or PET scanning) and EEG to study the activity of the conscious brain. EEG involves using electrodes fitted to the scalp to measure the brain's electrical activity—effectively, the firing of nerve cells. One type of electrical activity detected by EEG is called an alpha wave. When the brain is at rest with the eyes closed, the EEG shows alpha wave activity across the cortex. These are relatively slow (8 to 12 cycles per second) and of high amplitude, and indicate a state of the cortex known as synchronization, in which nerve cells fire in unison. When the eyes are opened, the EEG immediately changes to alpha waves of lower amplitude and higher frequency, a pattern called desynchronization that is found during thinking tasks such as calculation. Synchronization between different brain regions is associated with conscious awareness and probably indicates ongoing transfer of information between the synchronized regions of the cortex. In experiments, subjects are asked to view images that may be either meaningless or represent a face; evidence of synchronization between diverse regions in the cortex is seen only when the image has meaning.

Focusing our sensory attention

How do we direct our attention at will and avoid distraction by irrelevant sensory information? The reticular formation of the brainstem is key to focusing attention on one sensory stimulus at the expense of another. Descending pathways from the raphe nuclei of the brainstem to the spinal cord can suppress the transmission of pain information through the spinal cord. Similarly, the reticular formation controls the transmission of visual, auditory, and other sensory impulses higher up in the brain.

Where am I in my brain?

The mind/body problem—the question of where the person resides in their body—is one that has challenged philosophers for centuries. Even today, with our vastly increased knowledge of neural processes, many questions remain.

Somewhere inside the brain is our mind. We know this because modern medicine can transplant many of our bodily organs without making any change to the personality or behavior of the recipient. But where exactly in the brain does the mind reside, or does this question even have a meaningful answer?

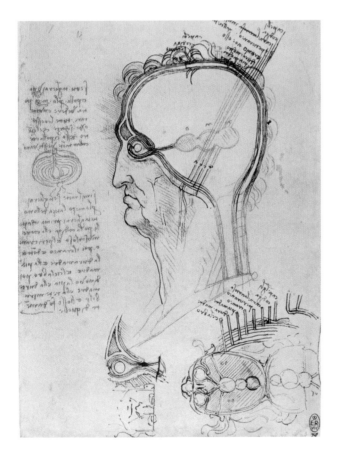

↑ **For da Vinci, the fluid-filled cavities called ventricles played major roles in the mind's workings. He believed that the first ventricle gathered data, the middle one processed data, and the third one stored memories.**

Insights from brain disease and injury

We can begin to approach the problem by considering what various brain diseases tell us about the seat of the mind. Some diseases clearly produce profound alterations to the personality and behavior of patients, whereas others do not. If we can determine which regional damage produces what behavioral effects, we can get an idea as to which brain parts are most important for the entity we call our mind. The problem with this approach is that the patient with the damaged brain may not be aware that their personality has changed, so the assessment of changes to the mind can only be made by an external observer.

Damage to the spinal cord, cerebellum, and much of the brainstem does not produce major changes in personality, although it will have profound effects on motor function. Some damage to specific brainstem regions—e.g., the midbrain reticular formation—can profoundly affect the level of consciousness, but this may be more analogous to damaging an on/off switch rather than altering the mind. On the other hand, maintenance of mood and cognitive ability is critically dependent on pathways from the brainstem to the cerebral cortex that use the neurotransmitters serotonin and dopamine, so those aspects of the mind (as a neurophysiologist or psychologist would define it) rely on interactions between these brainstem systems and the cerebral cortex. Damage to the thalamus and hypothalamus can cause changes in quite complex patterns of behavior, including sexual function and appetite, but this also does not produce major effects on the individual's personality.

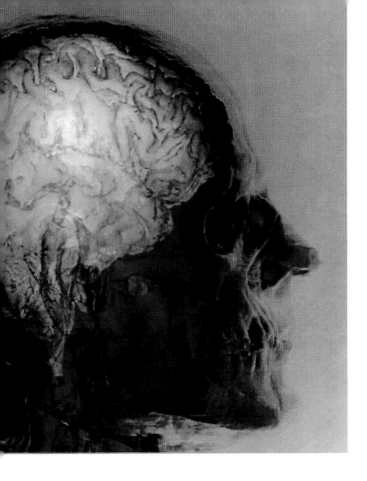

↑ **The cerebral cortex, seen in this CT scan, is critical to our conscious mind, but deeper brain structures, such as the thalamus and brainstem, play vital roles.**

It is when we move into the forebrain that we come closer to critical areas for those aspects of behavior we call the mind, but these should be seen more as key circuits rather than distinct brain regions. The circuit that is vital for social function and planning probably determines the bulk of what an external observer would consider the mind of a person. This circuit involves various regions in the prefrontal cortex, the striatum, pallidum, and thalamus. Our perception of our body's position in space and even awareness of the whole left half of our body is dependent on function in the right parietal lobe of the cerebral cortex. Our ability to store new memories depends on the hippocampus in the temporal lobe, although patients with amnesia from damage there usually have the same personality. Finally, our mind communicates through our language areas that are usually localized in Broca's and Wernicke's areas in the left cerebral hemisphere, so damage to those regions impairs our mind's ability to express itself.

The big question: what is the mind?

What exactly *is* the mind? Different scholars give different answers. A neurophysiologist would define the mind on the basis of information processing and motor activation, saying that the mind is the sum total of all the neural processes that receive, code, and interpret sensations, as well as recalling and correlating stored information and acting upon it. In Freudian psychiatry, the mind or psyche is often considered as a combination of the conscious, preconscious, and unconscious. A psychologist would define the mind on the basis of observed behaviors, saying that the mind consists of reasoning, intellectual, and understanding faculties taken together.

↓ **In Freud's iceberg model of the mind, only the small upper part is visible (the conscious); the rest (the preconscious and unconscious) is unseen.**

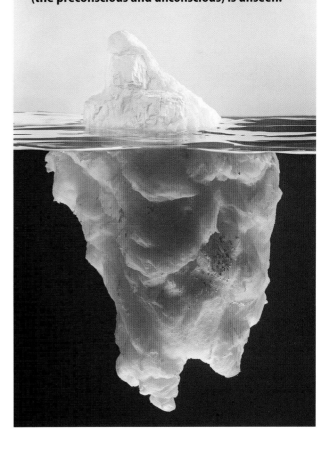

Memory

In our daily lives, we remember a huge number of things, from how to drive and where we live, to the names of our children and the sound of a friend's voice on the phone. We take memory for granted, but what exactly is it and how are memories formed and organized?

Memory is the ability to store and recall past events, information, and skills. There is no single universal mechanism for storing and retrieving information in the brain. Different memory systems use different mechanisms and any single memory system can use a variety of mechanisms at the cellular level. All these mechanisms have in common some temporary or semi-permanent change in the structure and function of nerve cells.

Types of memory

Memory is a complex process with many different types, some conscious and some unconscious. The tasks of our day-to-day life usually combine the many types of memory seamlessly to achieve our goals.

Declarative, or explicit, memory is the ability to remember items of information that are directly accessible to our conscious minds, such as knowing the meaning of a word (semantic memory) or recollecting events or facts (episodic memory). Declarative memory involves parts of the cerebral cortex in the inner part of the temporal lobe and the medial parts of the thalamus.

Some memories do not readily reach consciousness, but nevertheless profoundly influence our future behavior and physiology. Non-declarative, or implicit, memory includes a wide variety of skills and learned

→ **Long-term memory comes in many different forms, ranging from the emotional, through motor skills, to recollections and factual information.**

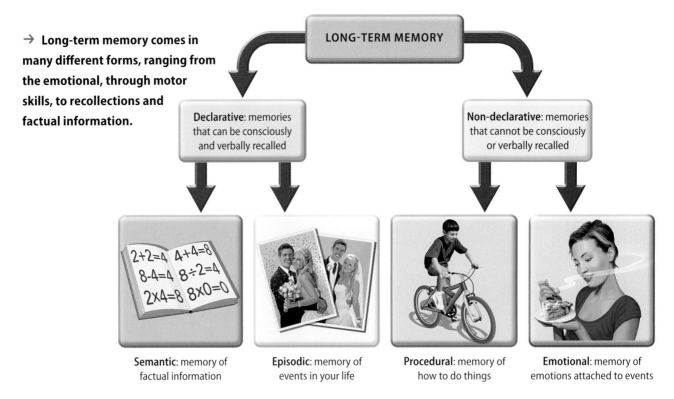

LONG-TERM MEMORY

Declarative: memories that can be consciously and verbally recalled

Non-declarative: memories that cannot be consciously or verbally recalled

Semantic: memory of factual information

Episodic: memory of events in your life

Procedural: memory of how to do things

Emotional: memory of emotions attached to events

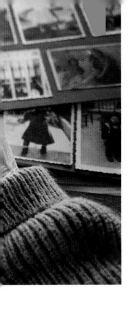

← **Many aspects of memory are linked to our visual experiences. Looking at old photographs may trigger a flood of memories.**

responses, from playing a difficult piece of music, to semi-automatic emotional responses to previously experienced situations and events, such as distress when remembering a past failure or humiliation. Non-declarative memory can be divided into two types: skills, habits, and conditioned motor routines (procedural memory); and emotional associations (emotional memory). Skills and habits are acquired with the aid of the looped circuits between the cerebral cortex, basal ganglia, thalamus, and cerebellum; whereas emotional associations between events and feelings depend on the amygdala.

How memories are made

We acquire memory in a step-by-step process. When we are exposed to novel information, the initial storage is by working memory, the storage of a small amount of information that we can keep in our minds for a few minutes, such as remembering a phone number for a few minutes while we enter the digits to make a phone call. Studies in monkeys have shown that damage to a specific region of the lateral prefrontal cortex (Brodmann area 46) causes a selective problem with spatial working memory (remembering the position of objects), whereas damage to other parts of the lateral prefrontal cortex causes problems with non-spatial (remembering a sequence of tasks) as well as spatial working memory.

Some working memory is worth retaining for the long term. This information undergoes a process of consolidation to become our long-term memories. Consolidation itself is a two-step process, requiring changes in synapses over a period of minutes or hours; and a reorganization of memories in different regions of the cerebral cortex over a period of days to months.

The role of the amygdala

Behaviorally important information often has an emotional component—we have all noticed that our recollection of emotionally charged events is much stronger than for emotionally bland events. The amygdala is an almond-shaped group of nerve cells in the front of the temporal lobe that plays a key role in linking the perception of objects and situations with their emotional significance. For example, the sight and smell of a particular type of food may become associated with feelings of comfort and love because that is what our mother cooked when we were young.

Pathways from the basolateral part of the amygdala to the hippocampus help to determine which particular events and experiences will be stored in long-term memory. Damage to the amygdala impairs a person's ability to learn the association between events and their pleasurable or painful outcomes.

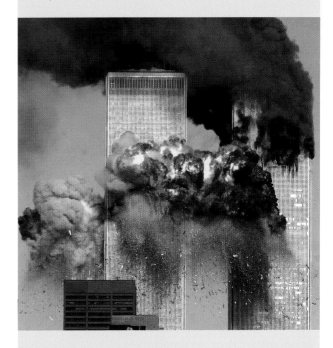

↑ **Memories are much more intense when they are linked with strong emotion. Events like 9/11 illuminate our memories like a camera's flash.**

Cellular changes that underlie memory

Nerve impulses (action potentials) are passed from one nerve cell to another through a junction called a synapse. Memory relies on adjustments in the strength of synaptic connections between nerve cells. The best studied examples are two processes that affect the activity of synapses: these are known as long-term potentiation and long-term depression.

Long-term potentiation (LTP) is the persistent increase in the strength of a synapse between two nerve cells, as measured by the electrical response of the downstream nerve cell, following a brief burst of nerve impulses in the stimulating nerve cell. LTP has been found in the hippocampus, cerebellum, cerebral cortex, amygdala, and peripheral nervous system. LTP allows nerve connections that are repeatedly activated to become more effective, reinforcing that pathway and influencing behavior. The induction of LTP involves several cellular mechanisms that produce increased concentrations of calcium ions in the downstream cell. Some involve different types of receptors in the nerve cell membrane that bind with the neurotransmitter glutamate.

Long-term depression is a reduction in the activity of a synapse in response to long-term activation of a nerve pathway. Believed to be important in learning involving the cerebellar circuits, it may also be important in reversing the effects of LTP in the hippocampus.

Long-term potentiation and depression can act in seconds to minutes to adjust the strength of synapses; both processes are suited to the changes associated with short-term memory. Long-term memory may use LTP, but also requires the manufacture of new protein to build new structures within nerve cells. This may involve changes in the architecture of dendrites (the branching projections of nerve cells) and their spiny protrusions.

Where is memory stored?

Memory is stored in different parts of the brain. Brain regions involved in declarative memory include several association cortex regions in the prefrontal, parietal, and temporal areas; some cortical areas around the hippocampus in the temporal lobe; and the hippocampus

Amnesia and the hippocampus

During the middle of the 20th century, neurosurgeons trying to treat brain disease found that when they removed the hippocampus on both sides a serious problem with memory resulted. Patients had normal working memory, but severe anterograde amnesia—they were unable to form new episodic or semantic memories, even though the acquisition of procedural memory (e.g., learning a jigsaw puzzle) was unaffected. There was also some loss of retrograde memory—events that occurred shortly before the surgery—that was worse for episodic than semantic memory. By contrast, memory of events months to years before the surgery was unaffected.

Fornix (fiber bundle)

Hippocampal commissure (fiber bundle)

Mammillary body (of hypothalamus)

Hippocampus

← **The hippocampus is vital for laying down new memories. Its major outflow pathway is the fornix, which carries information to the mammillary bodies. The hippocampal commissure connects the hippocampuses on each side.**

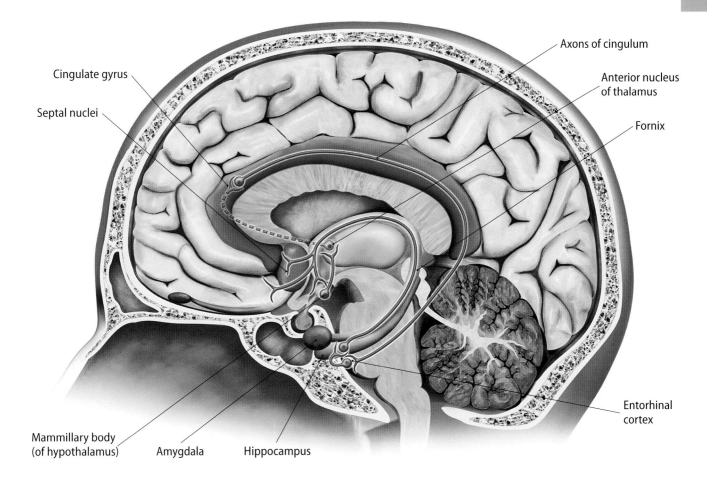

Cingulate gyrus

Septal nuclei

Axons of cingulum

Anterior nucleus
of thalamus

Fornix

Entorhinal
cortex

Mammillary body
(of hypothalamus)

Amygdala

Hippocampus

itself. Declarative memory requires the streaming of sensory information from the association cortex through the temporal lobe to the hippocampus, where long-term potentiation reinforces some conjunctions of information that are behaviorally important. The coded information is then streamed back to the association cerebral cortex for long-term storage, probably by a combination of LTP and structural changes in nerve cells.

Procedural memory is the learning of habits, skills, and sensory-motor adaptations that occur in the background whenever we train ourselves in new tasks. Procedural memory can be divided into the acquisition of skills and habits (e.g., playing the piano or learning to ski); or the learning of sensory-motor adaptations and adjustments of reflexes (e.g., adjusting the force that a muscle develops in response to a change in load or a new stimulus).

The learning of skills and habits depends on the looped circuit between the cerebral cortex, striatum, thalamus, and cerebral cortex. This type of learning involves not just the skills themselves, but also the

↑ **The Papez circuit, shown here in red, connects the hippocampus with other parts of the limbic system, and plays an important role in the formation and consolidation of new memories.**

unique elements of personal style that individuals bring to their performance of those skills. The circuits in this system mainly act to modify the motor routines stored in the cerebral cortex. Parkinson's disease patients, whose striatum does not receive the normal supply of dopamine from the substantia nigra in the midbrain, have great difficulty in learning new skills.

The learning of motor routines that ensure that actions are performed smoothly and effectively depends on the looped circuit from the cerebral cortex through the pontine nuclei, cerebrocerebellum (side parts of the cerebellum), thalamus, and cerebral cortex. Patients with damage to these parts of the cerebellum have great difficulty in adjusting the force and speed of contraction of muscles during new motor tasks.

Sleep and wakefulness

Throughout the animal kingdom, sleep and wakefulness alternate as part of a biological rhythm. Although still a poorly understood type of brain activity, sleep is vital; lack of sleep has a serious effect on the brain's ability to function. Sleep is certainly an essential function, but exactly why it is essential, and how its beneficial effects are mediated, remain a mystery.

Despite external appearances, sleep is an active process and is found in a wide variety of animals, from reptiles and amphibians to birds and mammals. It differs from coma in that we can be aroused from sleep, and sleep plays an important part in normal brain function, particularly in learning and memory.

Two types of sleep

We experience two distinct types of sleep, which alternate several times during the night. Non-rapid eye movement sleep (non-REM sleep) includes a number of stages during which the waves of brain activity on an electroencephalogram (EEG) become progressively slower. The eventual state of non-REM sleep is slow-wave sleep, when the EEG is dominated by slow waves of less than four cycles per second. Muscle tone and cerebral blood flow are reduced, parasympathetic activity is increased, and heart rate and breathing are slow and steady. Slow-wave sleep owes its electrical features to rhythmical activity of nerve cells in the thalamus that interact with the cortex to produce the slow rhythm. Dreams are very rare and vague in slow-wave sleep.

About every hour to 90 minutes, the average person changes to a period of desynchronized sleep. The EEG activity in this state looks rather like the waking state, with a great deal of high-frequency, low-amplitude activity, but the person is very difficult to rouse when in desynchronized sleep. Muscle tone is almost completely lost in the limbs and sensory transmission is greatly reduced. Regulation of body temperature is also temporarily impaired and breathing and heart rate become irregular. Probably the most striking external feature of desynchronized sleep are bursts of rapid eye movements, which give this state its other name—rapid eye movement, or REM, sleep.

Large sensory areas of the cerebral cortex and the limbic emotional system are active during REM sleep to produce dreams, but there is no external sensory input. The activity of executive parts of the cortex concerned with social conformity, planning, or spatial perception are also relatively reduced during REM sleep, so the internal cortical activity generates dreams that may be both behaviorally and spatially bizarre.

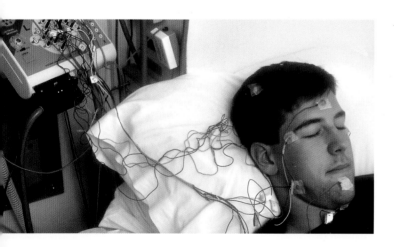

← **Changes in the electrical activity of the brain during sleep are usually detected with an EEG.**

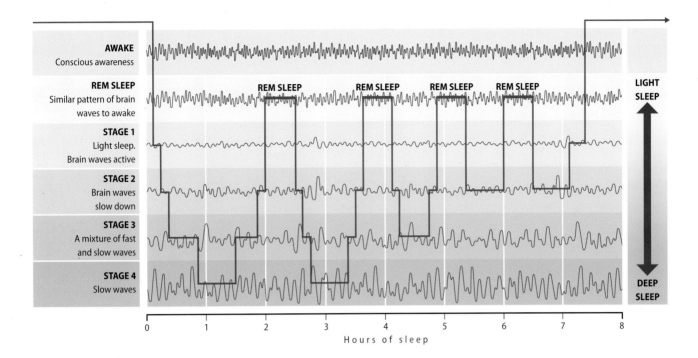

AWAKE
Conscious awareness

REM SLEEP
Similar pattern of brain
waves to awake

STAGE 1
Light sleep.
Brain waves active

STAGE 2
Brain waves
slow down

STAGE 3
A mixture of fast
and slow waves

STAGE 4
Slow waves

REM SLEEP   REM SLEEP   REM SLEEP   REM SLEEP

LIGHT
SLEEP

DEEP
SLEEP

0   1   2   3   4   5   6   7   8

Hours of sleep

↑ **During the night, we pass from a state of wakefulness (top trace) through four stages of sleep, occasionally returning to rapid eye movement (REM) sleep, in which we dream.**

What brain circuits control sleep?

The circuits for the control of switching between sleep and wakefulness are located in the brainstem and hypothalamus and have been best studied in animals. Damage to the reticular formation of the upper brainstem causes the subject to have a continuously synchronized EEG much like slow-wave sleep, in other words, they cannot attain full wakefulness. On the other hand, damage to the reticular formation of the lower brainstem causes the subject to show a state of continuous wakefulness and is unable to effectively sleep.

The hypothalamus and parts of the forebrain are also important in regulating sleep, and some circuits using particular chemicals play key roles. Nerve cells in the hypothalamus that use orexin as a neurotransmitter have excitatory connections—increasing activity—with the nerve networks that promote wakefulness. Nerve cells using histamine also contribute to arousal, which is why antihistamine drugs, which act against the release of histamine, cause drowsiness.

The brain circuits controlling REM sleep are more precisely localized than those for slow-wave sleep. When we have been in non-REM sleep for some time, nerve cells in the reticular formation of the pons (in the brainstem) become periodically active, causing nerve cells in other parts of the reticular formation (the locus coeruleus and the raphe nuclei) to stop firing and the acetylcholine-using nerve cells of the midbrain to fire faster. This latter change, in turn, causes the thalamus to

Changes in the sleep cycle during early life

Newborns have as much as eight hours of REM sleep each day, and their sleep rhythm consists of about 50 to 60 minutes of sleep usually starting with REM sleep. By the age of two, the amount of REM sleep has dropped to about three hours and the sleep cycle is much more like that in adults. REM sleep probably dominates sleep before birth and during infancy because it is essential for the development of nerve cell processes and the formation of connections in the cortex, especially in the prefrontal region.

→ **Sleep and wakefulness are regulated by several nerve pathways. One set uses the neurotransmitter orexin, which is produced in the lateral and posterior hypothalamus and streams to the cortex and brainstem.**

● Lateral and posterior hypothalamus
○ Mammillary nuclei of hypothalamus
● Ventral tegmental area
● Locus coeruleus
● Raphe nuclei
● Pontine reticular formation

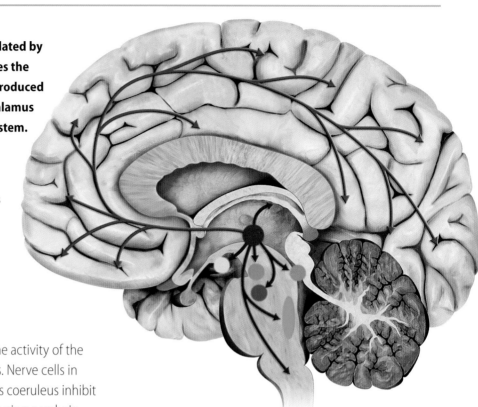

become more active and to begin the activity of the cortex that we experience as dreams. Nerve cells in the reticular formation near the locus coeruleus inhibit muscle activity during REM sleep, causing paralysis.

What do dreams mean?

Dreams may signify nothing more than the cerebral cortex exercising its ability to generate internal images, but dreams occupy such a central role in mythology, art, literature, and psychotherapy that their study remains a source of fascination. Psychoanalytic models of human behavior maintain that dreams relate in a disguised form to our inner conflicts and problems, in other words those memories and anxieties that continue to trouble us in our daily lives. In these ideas, dreams supposedly give us access to behavioral tensions that are not available to our conscious minds, and an experienced

↓ **Dreams may seem as vivid as reality, and it is tempting to assign special significance to them, but their purpose and meaning remain elusive.**

psychotherapist can use that access to begin a healing process. While these ideas are contentious, it is true that dreams may help a person develop coping strategies, particularly when those require the integration of new and old experiences, and may also ensure that inner conflicts do not impede learning and appropriate behavior. That is, dreams may allow a person to play out methods of dealing with stressors in a way that does not interfere with daily activity. Nevertheless, this line of research remains controversial.

Insomnia

Between 25 and 35 percent of people experience some difficulty sleeping each year, and the problem is more common with increasing age. Insomnia is usually associated with anxiety, and may enhance pain and suffering from other medical conditions. Patients with insomnia have at least one feature of disrupted sleep

Narcolepsy

Narcolepsy affects three million people world-wide, and is characterized by uncontrollable episodes of falling asleep at any place or time. People who suffer from narcolepsy also have cataplexy (a sudden loss of muscle tone), particularly during emotional situations. Night-time sleep may be interrupted by periods of wakefulness and terrifying dreams.

Studies using structural MRI have shown that people with narcolepsy have less gray matter in the lower temporal and lower frontal lobes, although it is uncertain whether this is the cause or the consequence of the sleep problem. Studies of the brains of narcoleptics have also found a reduction in the number of orexin nerve cells in the lateral or side parts of the hypothalamus. Orexin is an important excitatory chemical for maintaining arousal through its connections with the locus coeruleus nerve cells of the brainstem.

the primary goal of management of insomnia is to reduce the cause of the anxiety. Medication to increase sleep is of limited benefit unless the underlying cause of stress is addressed.

Regulating the sleep cycle

Most adults sleep for seven to eight hours each night, but we go to sleep earlier and for longer if we have lost sleep the night before. The cyclical nature of sleep and wakefulness is controlled by part of the hypothalamus called the suprachiasmatic nucleus—only 10,000 nerve cells on each side of the brain just above the crossing of the visual pathways. The suprachiasmatic nucleus receives input from the retina about light levels and has a natural cycle of activity of about 25 hours duration.

↓ **Our daily (circadian) body rhythms are controlled by a complex circuit that is reset by daily light exposure at the retina and involves our sympathetic nervous system and pineal body (gland).**

(problems with sleep onset, frequent awakenings, prolonged periods of awakening, or an early awake time) despite an adequate opportunity for sleep. As well, they experience fatigue, cognitive impairment, or emotional effects during the day.

The underlying cause of insomnia is usually anxiety, because anxiety leads to hyperarousal and a disruption of the normal sleep–wake cycle. In the natural world, anxiety is usually caused by danger (e.g., an attack by a predator), so the hyperarousal state and insomnia may be an adaption to increase vigilance until the danger is past. The hyperarousal may also activate aggression pathways involving the amygdala. Nevertheless, in the modern world this state of hypervigilance is most definitely not adaptive, and

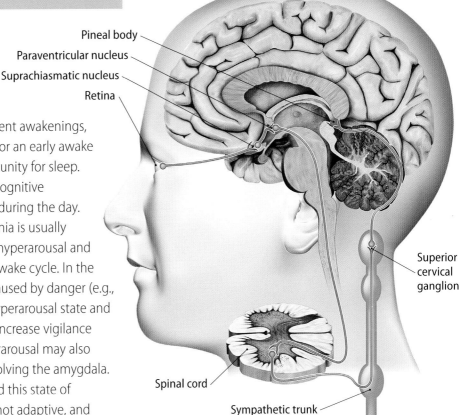

Pineal body
Paraventricular nucleus
Suprachiasmatic nucleus
Retina
Superior cervical ganglion
Spinal cord
Sympathetic trunk

Unconsciousness and brain death

Unconsciousness involves a complete or almost complete lack of awareness of surroundings and unresponsiveness to stimuli. Coma is the most extreme form of this condition, and brain death is the irreversible end of brain activity.

↓ **If a major artery to the brain is blocked (e.g., by a blood thrombus from a plaque in the common carotid artery), brain tissue may be deprived of blood, resulting in a period of unconsciousness.**

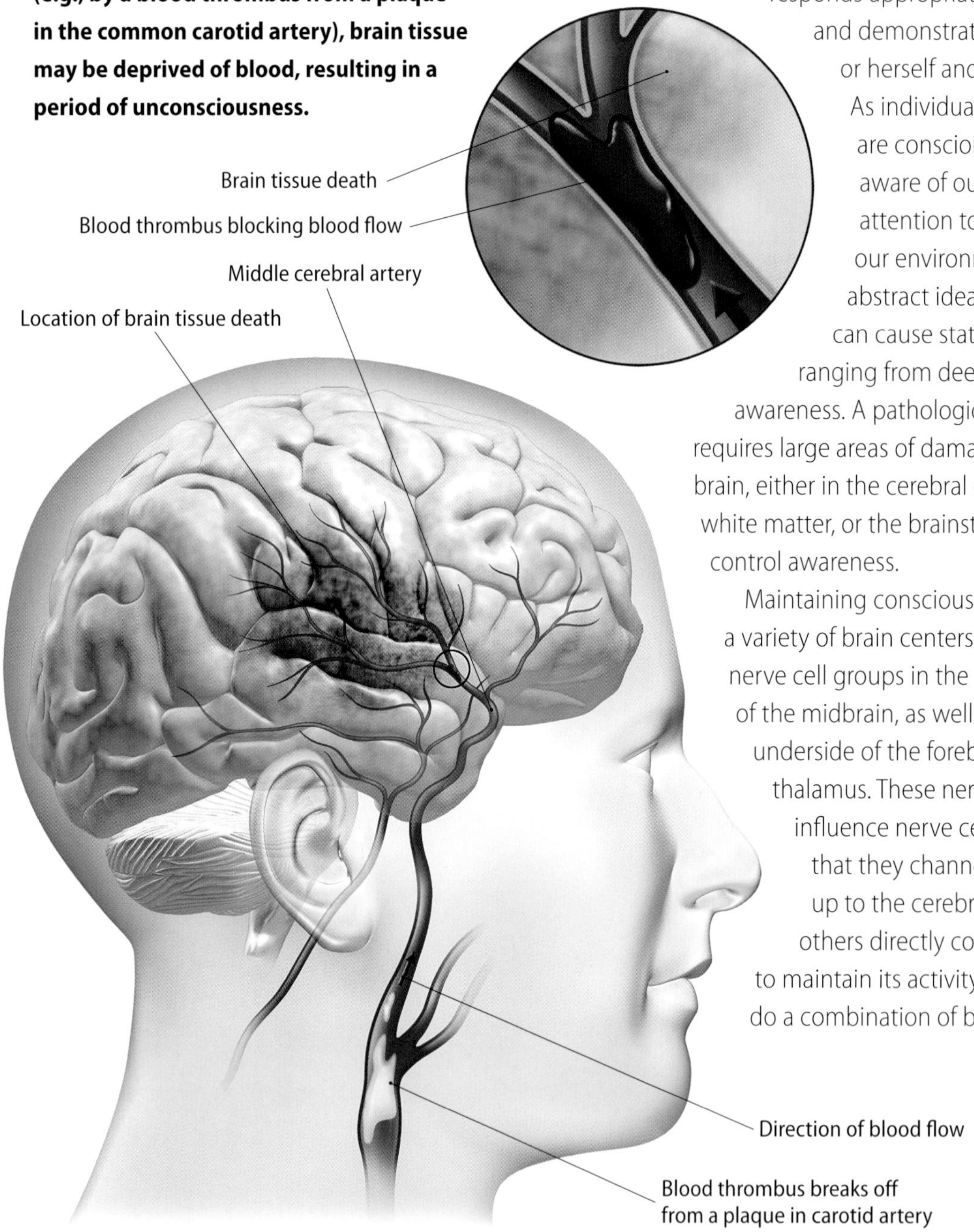

Brain tissue death

Blood thrombus blocking blood flow

Middle cerebral artery

Location of brain tissue death

Consciousness is a state in which a person responds appropriately to external stimuli, and demonstrates awareness of him- or herself and their surroundings. As individuals, we know that we are conscious because we are aware of ourselves, can direct our attention to important aspects of our environment, and contemplate abstract ideas. Damage to the brain can cause states of consciousness ranging from deep coma to almost full awareness. A pathological loss of consciousness requires large areas of damage to *both* sides of the brain, either in the cerebral cortex, its underlying white matter, or the brainstem networks that control awareness.

Maintaining consciousness requires activity in a variety of brain centers. These include certain nerve cell groups in the reticular formation of the midbrain, as well as nerve cells in the underside of the forebrain, and in the hypo-thalamus. These nerve cell groups may influence nerve cells in the thalamus so that they channel sensory information up to the cerebral cortex, whereas others directly connect with the cortex to maintain its activity, and yet other groups do a combination of both.

Direction of blood flow

Blood thrombus breaks off from a plaque in carotid artery

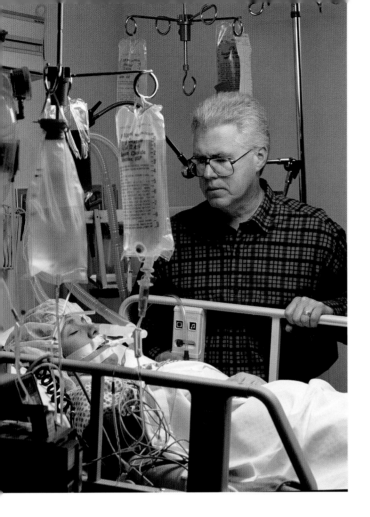

↑ **Unconscious patients require constant nursing to maintain body fluids and kidney function, sustain breathing and circulation, and prevent pressure sores.**

The Glasgow Coma Scale

Clinicians need a scale to reliably record the level of consciousness in head injury patients. This is important both for charting their patients' recovery from brain injury and for assessing the benefits of treatments. Graham Teasdale and Bryan Jennett, professors of neurosurgery at the University of Glasgow, developed the Glasgow Coma Scale (GCS) in 1974. The modified GCS scale rates patients on three tests (eye movements scored out of 4, verbal responses scored out of 5, and motor actions scored out of 6) that are added to arrive at a minimum score of 3 (coma or death) through to a maximum score of 15 (fully awake). Severe brain injury is a GCS score of 8 or less; moderate brain injury is a GCS score from 9 to 12, inclusive; whereas minor brain injury is a GCS score of 12 or better.

Eye response	Open spontaneously	4
	Open to verbal command	3
	Open to response to pain	2
	No response	1
Verbal response	Talking/Oriented	5
	Confused speech/ Disoriented	4
	Inappropriate words	3
	Incomprehensible words	2
	No response	1
Motor response	Obeys commands	6
	Localizes to pain	5
	Flexion/Withdrawal	4
	Abnormal flexion	3
	Extension	2
	No response	1
Maximum score		15

Coma and persistent vegetative state

Coma is a state of unconsciousness in which a patient appears to be sleeping, but cannot be aroused. Causes include a head injury, disease, liver or kidney failure, stroke, reaction to drugs and alcohol, or an epileptic seizure. The midbrain reticular formation is particularly important for maintaining consciousness, so a common cause of prolonged unconsciousness is temporary or permanent dysfunction of both sides of the midbrain. Coma may also be caused by damage to the thalamus and cortex on both sides. But coma does not arise if the damage is confined to one side of the brain.

Coma is a serious sign of brain dysfunction, but usually lasts only a week or two, after which time the patient's state may change into a slightly different condition known as persistent vegetative state. Patients in this condition may have functional brainstem reflexes, with some aspects of the sleep/wake cycle, but they show no sign of interaction with the environment. Vegetative patients may open their eyes in response to strong stimulation and may even briefly fix their gaze on objects or people, but they do not speak and show no

Causes of altered consciousness

Altered consciousness may result from any of a number of different causes, ranging from head injuries and epilepsy to brain tumors and intoxication.

Cause	Reason for loss of consciousness
Head injury	Twisting or tearing of nerve fibers or changes in the blood flow to the brainstem may be responsible. Serious head injury may also cause brain swelling or compression of the brainstem against the skull interior due to bleeding.
Epilepsy	Epilepsy is a recurrent abnormal electrical discharge in the brain that may be inherited or the result of other disease. Epileptic seizures often temporarily deactivate the brainstem centers that maintain consciousness.
Intoxication	Drugs (sedatives, alcohol, tranquillizers) and poisons (solvents) have a direct depressive effect on the brainstem and cerebral cortex.
Vessel disease	Loss of blood supply to the brainstem due to blockage of blood vessels or low blood pressure can disable the nerve networks that maintain awareness.
Infection	Infection of the membranes around the brain (meningitis) or of the brain tissue itself (encephalitis) raises the pressure inside the skull and compress the brainstem against the skull. The products of inflammation and fever may also impair the function of the brainstem.
Space-occupying lesions	Diseases that cause swelling inside the skull (e.g., growing brain tumors or bleeding into the confined space of the skull interior) may push the brainstem against the skull base, blocking the activity that keeps the cerebral cortex alert.
Metabolic problems	A variety of metabolic problems (low blood glucose, diabetic ketoacidosis, kidney and liver failure, low thyroid hormones) cause abnormal brainstem function and a loss of consciousness. These may act through starving the brainstem of nutrients or by their toxic effects on nerve cells.

awareness of their surroundings. Functional MRI studies of patients in the vegetative state have shown that they may have activity in some areas of the cortex when appropriately stimulated (e.g., when asked to imagine playing golf), even though they remain unconscious. They may also have activity in language areas when exposed to speech, but are unable to speak and do not show any responsiveness to language.

Some patients may pass from acute coma into a state known as chronic coma. This is a condition that differs from the persistent vegetative state, in that patients display only reflexive behavior without any sleep/wake cycles and do not direct their gaze to objects or people.

→ **Patients in a persistent vegetative state may have regained some brainstem reflexes but show no interaction with the environment.**

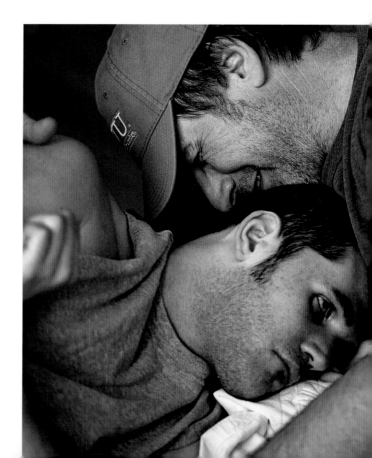

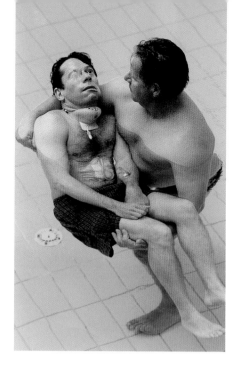

↑ **An actor plays Jean-Dominique Bauby in the film of his book, *The Diving Bell and the Butterfly*, which he dictated by blinking his left eye while a victim of locked-in syndrome.**

→ **This MRI scan of the brain of a comatose man shows damage to the temporal regions (upper center). The patient was declared brain dead.**

Locked-in syndrome

Sometimes a patient may appear unconscious, but be fully awake, a condition known as locked-in syndrome. This may happen when there is a stroke affecting the front of the brainstem that destroys the motor pathways to the brainstem and spinal cord, but leaves the sensory pathways and brainstem arousal systems undamaged. The patient is unable to move or talk, but is otherwise fully conscious and mentally alert.

Brain death

Brain death is an irreversible loss of all brain activity, including the automatic functions like breathing and control of the cardiovascular system. In most parts of the world, death of either the whole brain or the brainstem is the important indicator for death of the patient. The careful assessment of a patient for brain death is critically important, because it determines whether a patient's life support may be turned off and their organs removed for transplantation.

The criteria for brain death include: no spontaneous breathing; no response to pain; no eye movements in response to infusion of warm or cold water into the external ear; no constriction of the pupil in response to light; no blinking in response to touch on the cornea; and no "doll's eye" movements in response to turning of the head (oculocephalic reflex). The EEG must be flat on two occasions 24 hours apart, or a cerebral blood flow scan must show no flow of blood inside the skull.

It is also very important that the patient's body temperature is within normal limits and that they are free of consciousness-altering drugs when the assessment is made. Low body temperature, e.g., following immersion in very cold water, may reduce the EEG activity even though the patient is able to recover brain function when the body temperature returns to normal.

Emotions and drives

Emotions—such as happiness, sadness, and fear—interact
with drives—such as thirst and hunger—to influence the way
we react to and interpret the world we live in.

The anthropologist Paul Ekman identifies seven basic
emotions in humans: happiness, sadness, anger, fear,
disgust, surprise, and contempt. Our feelings are
ultimately designed to reinforce behaviors that promote
our survival and that of our species, but often the brain
pathways that control or express our emotions may be
affected as part of disease processes that cause suffering.

What are emotions made of?

There are three aspects to an emotion: the behavioral
(e.g., the facial expression), the physiological (e.g., the
changes in blood pressure or heart rate), and the verbal
or cognitive self-report (the distinctive subjective report
of the way the emotion feels). Each of these aspects
may serve a different function—communicating to
others, preparing the individual for action, or reinforcing
behavior, respectively. That means that even if they
occur at the same time, they are not always expressed
to the same degree.

This neat division into three components nevertheless
leaves us with the question of whether our experience
of emotions is the result of the physiological response
feeding back to our brain, or whether it is our subjective
experience that drives our physiological response.

Where emotions come together

Early conceptions of how the brain produced emotions
emphasized a ring of structures around the edge of the
forebrain. These were called the limbic system (from the
Latin *limbus* meaning "edge" or "border"). This original
conception included the cingulate gyrus and
septal nuclei near the midline, the amygdala and
hippocampus in the temporal lobe, and assorted
pathways and nerve cell groups in the thalamus
and hypothalamus.

Our modern conception of how the brain
processes emotions is much more complex than
the original limbic lobe model. Functional MRI
studies have shown that parts of the cerebral
cortex not originally included in the limbic
system are important in the processing of
emotions. In particular, the prefrontal cortex has
two regions (orbitofrontal and ventromedial cortex)

Reality testing and
error monitoring

Top-down guidance of
attention and thought

Inhibition of
inappropriate actions

Regulating
emotion

Striatum

Hypothalamus

Amygdala

← **The prefrontal cortex regulates our emotions and
drives through connections with other cortical areas,
as well as the striatum, hypothalamus, and amygdala.**

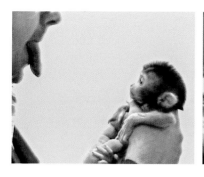
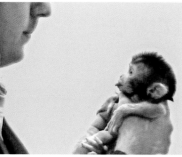

← **Monkey see, monkey do: nerve cells in some cortical regions are active both when performing an action (sticking the tongue out) and watching another make the same action. Some neuroscientists believe that these "mirror neurons" are important in modeling the minds of others.**

that are important for the behavioral flexibility that allows us to choose between emotionally conflicting behaviors (e.g., suppressing fear so that a task may be performed). The front part of the insula, a region of cortex deep inside the lateral fissure, may be important for emotions such as admiration and compassion.

Even within brain regions originally included in the limbic lobe, subregions serve different functions. The front of the cingulate gyrus is concerned with the regulation of mood, whereas the back part is more concerned with cognitive tasks.

Mirror neurons

Observing others experiencing an emotion (the third-person experience) activates the part of the brain concerned with that particular emotion just as much as if we experience the emotion ourselves (the first-person experience). This phenomenon is said to be due to "mirror neurons" that "reflect" the activity that would be occurring in the brain of another person. Functional MRI studies of the brains of subjects viewing others with facial expressions of disgust showed activation of the front of the insula, a region that lies deep inside the

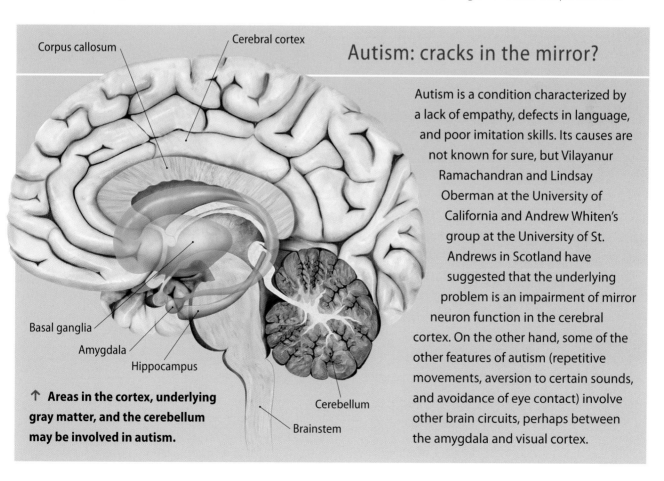

Corpus callosum
Cerebral cortex
Basal ganglia
Amygdala
Hippocampus
Cerebellum
Brainstem

↑ **Areas in the cortex, underlying gray matter, and the cerebellum may be involved in autism.**

Autism: cracks in the mirror?

Autism is a condition characterized by a lack of empathy, defects in language, and poor imitation skills. Its causes are not known for sure, but Vilayanur Ramachandran and Lindsay Oberman at the University of California and Andrew Whiten's group at the University of St. Andrews in Scotland have suggested that the underlying problem is an impairment of mirror neuron function in the cerebral cortex. On the other hand, some of the other features of autism (repetitive movements, aversion to certain sounds, and avoidance of eye contact) involve other brain circuits, perhaps between the amygdala and visual cortex.

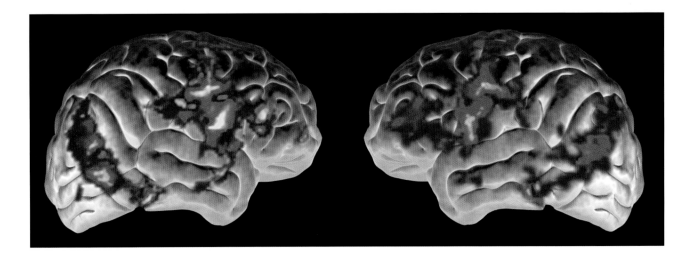

↑ **In this PET scan, the same sets of nerve cells in the cerebral cortex are activated when watching an action (left) as when performing it (right), evidence that mirror neurons are at work.**

lateral fissure. This is the same region of the cerebral cortex that is activated by subjects personally experiencing a disgusting stimulus, e.g., an unpleasant odor.

This common activation of emotionally significant parts of the cortex, whether the emotion is personal or a third-person observation, may be the anatomical basis for our ability to empathize with the experiences and emotions of others. Empathy is an important skill that underlies effective participation in human society.

The amygdala: linking senses and emotions

The most important task performed by the amygdala is to link sensory stimuli and emotional experience. This allows us to learn whether experiences are positive or negative and is profoundly important for regulating future behavior. The amygdala also lets us recognize anger and fear in the faces of others. Stimulation of the amygdala in humans produces a feeling of anxiety and the experience of déjà vu (the feeling of having experienced the same situation before). On the other hand, damage to the amygdala leaves patients unable to recognize emotions in others and causes a social disinhibition—a patient may urinate in public, for example, or expose themselves.

Through its connections with the hypothalamus, the amygdala also directs the physiological expression of emotions—changes in heart rate, blood pressure, and blood flow to the skin. Some patients who have had damage to the amygdala on both sides of the brain do not show the physiological effects of emotions even though they are subjectively experiencing great anxiety.

A drive to survive

Drives are directed to ensuring survival of the individual and the species. We are all subject to drives, some basic, such as seeking food or water; some complex, such as finding a sexual partner and having children; and some abnormal, such as seeking rewarding sensations from drugs of addiction or gambling.

Drives and their satisfaction depend on a complex interaction between the cerebral cortex for conscious plans and goals, reward systems in the brain that use dopamine as their signaling chemical and provide feelings of pleasure as a result of behavior, and nerve groups in the hypothalamus that control appetite and physiological responses.

Many of the more basic drives (feeding, drinking, and sexual activity) are controlled through the hypothalamus, a part of the brain that is generally concerned with maintaining a relatively constant internal environment (homeostasis).

A good deal of research has centered around our drive for food. Early studies suggested that the lateral hypothalamus induces feeding behavior, whereas the

How we hunger

The drive to satisfy hunger is a basic one, but the control of food intake and body weight is complex and still poorly understood. Clearly, though, understanding feeding behavior is very important in the management of people who are greatly overweight. Signals that tell the brain that there is an abundance of fat tissue (adiposity signals) from the mass of fat in the body feed back to the hypothalamus to inhibit nerve cells in the arcuate nucleus that make the neurotransmitter neuropeptide Y and stimulate nerve cells that make another chemical, proopiomelanocortin (POMC). These chemicals in turn influence the balance between catabolic (energy-expending) pathways through the paraventricular nucleus of the hypothalamus and anabolic (body-mass building) pathways through the lateral hypothalamus. The balance between these two pathways influences the centers in the brainstem that interpret signals from the liver and gut about stomach fullness and energy intake to determine when the individual feels satisfied during a meal.

medial hypothalamus reduces feeding, but more recent studies have shown that the control of feeding is far more complex. Food intake is normally regulated by feedback loops that ensure that food intake is kept within an optimal range for a desired weight. Signals from fatty tissue and internal organs feed back to the hypothalamus and nucleus of the solitary tract to reduce food intake. Psychological factors may perturb this balance, causing the body to drift away from its set-point weight, resulting in obesity.

↓ **Advertisers seeking to sell us products have long exploited our drives to gain social status and impress a potential sexual partner, as this jeans ad shows.**

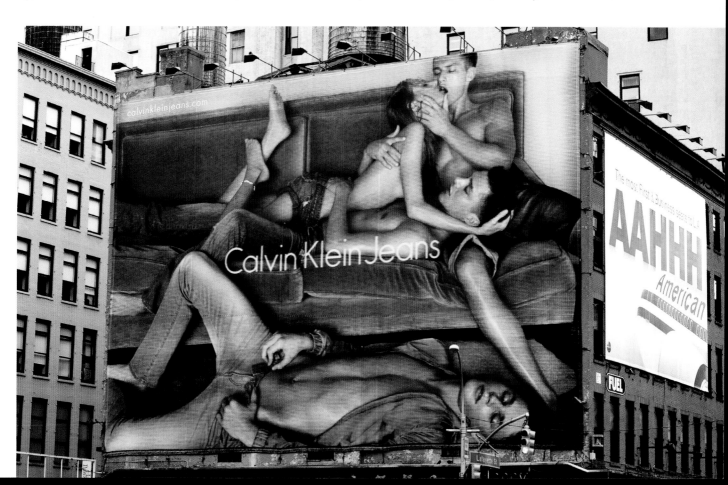

Fear and anxiety

The emotions of fear and anxiety have adaptive or beneficial roles when they warn us of dangerous situations and alert us to change our behavior, but when they come to dominate our lives they can paralyze us with distress and indecision.

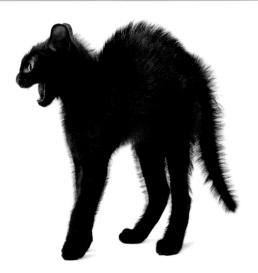

↑ **This kitten's fight-or-flight response includes physiological changes that increase the apparent body size. The equivalent human response can also manifest in aggressive, combative behavior.**

The terms "fear" and "anxiety" are often used as synonyms, but there is a real difference in meaning between the two. Fear is the acute emotion that is usually experienced when confronted with a dangerous or painful situation, whereas anxiety is the anticipation of painful or unpleasant experiences and may be felt over a much longer period of time.

Conditioned fear and the amygdala

Why do we feel fear in particular circumstances? Classical conditioning experiments in both animals and humans pair a sensory stimulus with an uncomfortable electrical shock. When lab rats are placed in a chamber and hear a tone immediately before a shock is administered to their feet, they come to associate the tone with the shock and begin to show autonomic responses (e.g., a rise in blood pressure and heart rate) and behavioral responses, such as

freezing of limb movement and emitting a high-pitched keening sound, even before the shock is felt. Even more significant, rats that have been exposed to this learning situation for several days come to associate the environment of the test chamber with the painful stimulus and will freeze as soon as they are placed in the chamber.

This conditioned fear response depends on the amygdala in the temporal lobe, because the amygdala links sensory stimuli in the environment (in the rats' case, a musical tone) with their negative consequences for the individual (an electrical shock). This process also happens in our day-to-day lives, when we link

Fears and phobias

All of us have fears of everyday objects, situations, or creatures, but some of these fears may be considered unreasonable and interfere with daily life, in which case they are called phobias. Phobic patients know that their fear is unreasonable and disproportionate to the situation, but are unable to apply the cognitive control that other people use to

regulate the fear. Here are some common causes of phobias, with the approximate percentage of the population affected:
- Potentially dangerous animals (e.g., spiders, mice, snakes, bats): 22 percent
- Heights: 18 percent
- Water: 12.5 percent
- Public transportation: 10.5 percent

→ **The physiological changes of the fight-or-flight response depend on nerve centers located in the amygdala, hypothalamus, and the three parts of the brainstem reticular formation.**

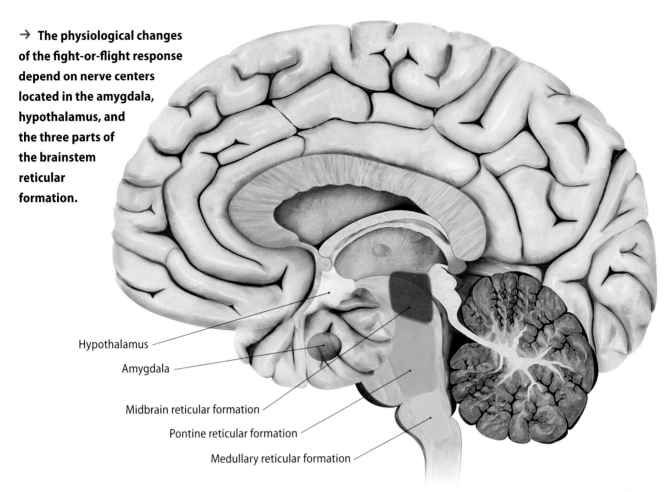

Hypothalamus

Amygdala

Midbrain reticular formation

Pontine reticular formation

Medullary reticular formation

situations and experiences with unpleasant consequences for us. Eventually, even imagining the situation may cause a rise in blood pressure and heart rate that we experience as anxiety.

Expressing fear

Fear conditioning has a host of effects on the body and behavior that are mediated by pathways through other regions of the brain. Some of these will release hormones to act on the body, whereas others will trigger the internal feeling of the emotion in the cerebral cortex.

The hypothalamus plays a key role in the regulation of the internal body environment, so most pathways for the behavioral expression of fear and anxiety pass from the amygdala through the hypothalamus. For

example, a pathway through the stria terminalis, a fiber bundle starting in the amygdala, and the hypothalamus causes the release of the stress hormone cortisol from the cortex of the adrenal gland on top of each kidney. Another pathway through the hypothalamus and the medulla activates the sympathetic nervous system to raise heart rate and blood pressure.

→ **Crises, such as being caught in a hurricane, activate sympathetic pathways that make energy stores in the liver available to deal with dangers.**

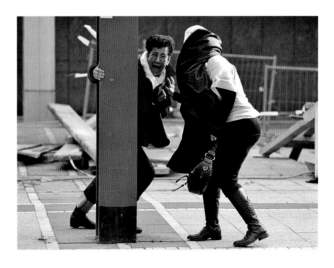

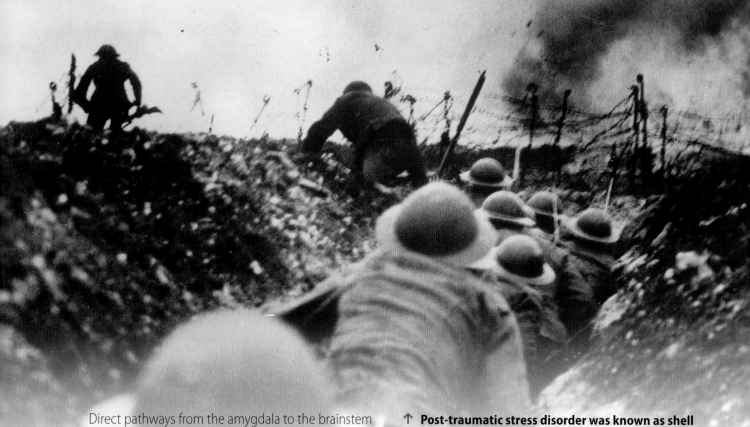

Direct pathways from the amygdala to the brainstem mediate other effects of stress and fear. A pathway to the gray matter of the midbrain leads to the emotional behavior of fear, while a pathway to the reticular formation of the pons increases the activity of muscle reflexes.

Finally, a pathway running from the amygdala to the acetylcholine-using nerve cells on the underside of the forebrain activates systems that increase the level of arousal of the cerebral cortex and focus sensory attention on stressful stimuli in the environment.

Stressful events and hormones

Memories of emotionally charged events are often more vivid than those of bland, unexciting events. Emotional arousal from fear-inducing situations increases our attention toward particular events. As the saying goes: there is nothing like being shot at to focus the mind. This has some benefits, in that we will learn to avoid dangerous situations in future. Emotionally charged events cause release of adrenaline (epinephrine) and cortisol from the adrenal gland, hormones that influence memory storage. Noradrenaline (norepinephrine), adrenaline, opioid peptides, and cortisol all act on the basolateral part of the amygdala to enhance memory storage in the cerebral cortex. Drugs like diazepam impair the memory of unpleasant events by acting on the basolateral amygdala.

↑ **Post-traumatic stress disorder was known as shell shock in World War I because it was thought to be caused by the shock waves of exploding shells.**

Post-traumatic stress disorder

Exposure to situations that cause extreme psychological trauma—perhaps involving the threat of one's own death or the death of a loved one, or the threat or experience of torture or sexual assault—may result in post-traumatic stress disorder (PTSD). Working in very dangerous situations—e.g., as an emergency service worker, or in the military during battle—may also cause this severe anxiety disorder. Children may also develop PTSD as a result of bullying or abuse. An extreme form of psychological stress, PTSD overwhelms the person's ability to cope and will lead to symptoms occurring many months to years after the event.

Symptoms of PTSD include reexperiencing the original trauma through flashbacks or nightmares, difficulty falling or staying asleep, anger, and hypervigilance. A formal diagnosis of the condition requires that the symptoms last for more than one month and cause a significant impairment of day-to-day functioning in the patient's social or working life. If symptoms last for fewer than 30 days, the condition is known as an acute stress disorder.

Dealing with stress

The most damaging aspects of psychological stress are due to a combination of factors, including loss of control over the stressful situation; unpredictability of the timing of the stress; absence of a physical outlet; and lack of social attachments. If a stressful situation cannot be avoided, doctors recommend recognizing individual limits and adjusting the circumstances so that the amount of stress involved in a situation will benefit, rather than hinder, an individual. Stress may also be relieved by getting plenty of regular exercise and maintaining an active and supportive social network.

Most patients diagnosed with PTSD have low secretion of cortisol from the adrenal cortex but high levels of adrenaline and noradrenaline in their urine. This is in contrast to the normal fight-or-flight response, where both cortisol and adrenaline are secreted in large quantities.

One theory of PTSD attributes the abnormalities to a hyperexcitable amygdala and an inability of the prefrontal cortex to extinguish the feelings of fear and intense anxiety. A genetic predisposition may also play a role.

Stress and disease

Stress is usually defined as something that is perceived by the individual as a threat to their ability to maintain their health and life. It can also describe the body's response to a threatening or dangerous situation, or to demands arising from a new or changing situation. Stress can be physical or psychological, but the reactions of any group of people to physical stressors are more similar to each than those to psychological stressors. In other words, some people show an extreme reaction to

psychological stressors. Constant exposure to stressful situations is likely to give rise to anxiety because the individual comes to anticipate pain or injury.

Our reactions to stress consist of autonomic, endocrine, and motor responses, with most of these orchestrated by the hypothalamus. The reaction to physical stress is usually adaptive, in that it maintains life and health. Psychological stress may also be beneficial when it prepares us for additional mental demands, such as during an examination or public performance. Measuring blood levels of two key hormones, adrenaline and cortisol, can be used to assess activation of the sympathetic nervous system and adrenal cortex, respectively.

Psychological stress lasting months or years may not only damage our psychological health, but also contribute to chronic physical disease through elevated blood pressure or excess cortisol secretion triggering the development of diabetes. Eliminating the causes of psychological stress in our environment is therefore very important for optimal health.

↓ **The responsibility for thousands of lives moving at high speed through complex airspace makes an air traffic controller's job a particularly stressful one.**

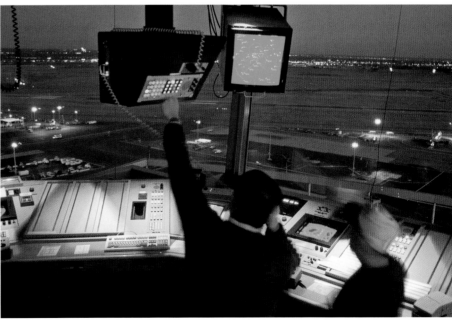

The depressed brain

In contrast to the normal emotional experiences of sadness, loss, or passing mood states, depression is persistent and can interfere significantly with an individual's ability to function. It is a medical disorder, like high blood pressure.

Depression is a serious mental illness affecting between 20 and 30 percent of the population at some stage of their life and is life-threatening when it leads to suicide. Most depression is unipolar, in that the person experiences only one abnormal state, that of depression and its associated symptoms. Unipolar depression may be reactive—a response to some painful event such as the loss of a loved one, redundancy at work, or personal failure—or it may arise from inside the person (endogenous depression), and have nothing to do with life events. Endogenous depression is usually more serious than reactive depression. Another type of depression is bipolar. It is characterized by episodes of mania followed by depression (see p. 252).

Major depressive disorder

A diagnosis of major depressive disorder is made if a person has five or more of the symptoms (see "Symptoms of depression," opposite) and impairment in usual functioning nearly every day during the same two-week period. Major depression often begins between ages 15 and 30, or even earlier, and episodes typically recur. An estimated 5 percent of adults aged 18 to 54 suffer from major depressive disorder in a given year. Unipolar major depression is the seventh-greatest cause of disease burden worldwide.

Other types of depression

Dysthymia is a chronic type of depression, where the symptoms last at least two years but are not as severe as major depression. At least two of the symptoms of depression persist and, while not as disabling as in major depression, dysthymia can keep a person from functioning well or feeling good. Researchers estimate that 1 percent of adults aged 18 to 54 have dysthymia in a given year. Many people with dysthymia also have major depressive episodes.

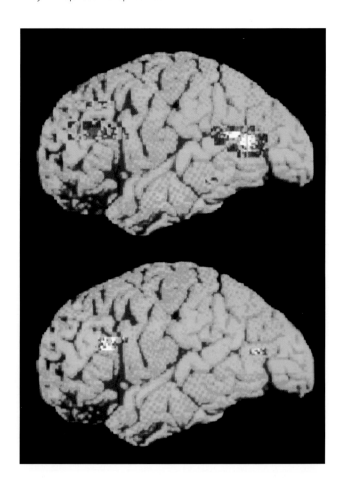

→ **The depressed brain (top) in these PET scans contains large areas of low activity (red and yellow areas) in the prefrontal (at left) and parieto-temporal (at right) cortex. The brain treated for depression (bottom) shows metabolic activity returning to normal.**

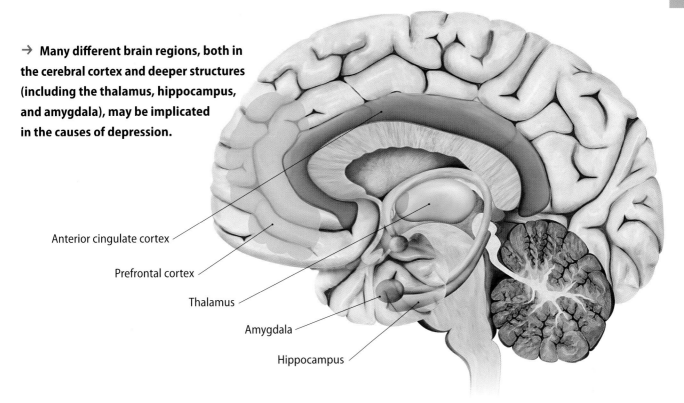

→ **Many different brain regions, both in the cerebral cortex and deeper structures (including the thalamus, hippocampus, and amygdala), may be implicated in the causes of depression.**

Anterior cingulate cortex

Prefrontal cortex

Thalamus

Amygdala

Hippocampus

Symptoms of depression

The major symptom is persistent sad, anxious, or empty feelings. A person suffering from depression may also experience a range of associated symptoms:

- Loss of pleasure in activities that were once enjoyable, including sex
- Frequently feeling guilty, worthless, hopeless, or helpless
- Persistent feelings of decreased energy, tiredness, or listlessness
- Difficulty thinking, concentrating, making decisions, or remembering
- Disturbed sleep—sleeping too much or too little; insomnia, waking too early, or oversleeping
- Appetite loss or overeating
- Frequent feelings of either restlessness and irritability or feeling slowed down
- Thoughts of suicide or wishing you were dead
- Persistent physical problems (such as pain, headaches, and stomach or bowel problems) that do not respond to treatment

Patients experiencing minor depression have fewer than five of the depression symptoms, have not had a major depressive episode, and their symptoms have not persisted for two years. Less common forms of depression include atypical depression (mood changes in response to actual life events), seasonal affective disorder (mainly experienced during the winter months), and postpartum dysphoric disorder (major depression experienced by women within four weeks of their giving birth).

What causes major depressive disorder?

Depression can be caused by some general medical conditions, including strokes, nutritional deficiencies, and infections. It may also be the result of alcohol or substance abuse (substance-induced mood disorder), in which case it is often associated with symptoms of withdrawal and intoxication. In many cases, though, it is due to neither medical conditions nor substance abuse, and in these circumstances there are underlying neurobiological causes. These causes include a genetic predisposition, pregnancy and delivery, changes to neuroanatomical structure, alterations in the balance of neurotransmitters in the brain, and changes in hormonal levels.

The mechanisms that control the secretion of the stress hormone cortisol from the adrenal cortex are abnormal in some patients with major depressive disorder. Severe depression is associated with increased levels of the hypothalamic messenger corticotropin releasing factor (CRF) in the fluid around the brain, and increased secretion of both the pituitary hormone adrenocorticotrophic hormone and the adrenal cortical hormone cortisol. These patients appear to have a chronic activation of the pathways that cause secretion of cortisol and a reduced sensitivity in the brain to the effects of cortisol in turning off the production of CRF. This chronic activation of the stress hormone pathways may be an underlying cause of the long-standing depression of mood.

People with major depression have also been found to have abnormalities in the neurotransmitters in the brain, in particular serotonin, dopamine, acetylcholine, noradrenaline, gamma aminobutyric acid, and endogenous opiates. Functional imaging studies of patients with major depression have shown that blood flow and use of glucose are higher than normal in some parts of the brain (e.g., the front of the cingulate cortex and the underside of the frontal lobe, the amygdala, thalamus, and lower parts of the striatum).

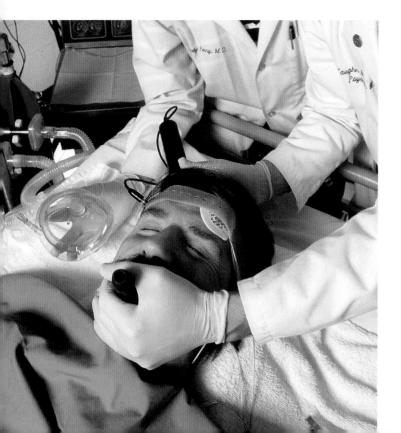

Bipolar disorder

Bipolar disorder, or bipolar mood disorder, used to be called manic depressive psychosis. It is a psychiatric illness characterized by extreme mood swings and usually starts in late adolescence or early adulthood. A person may feel euphoric and extremely energetic at one time (hypomania), only to drop into a period of paralyzing depression, in an ongoing cycle of elation and sadness. It is different from normal mood states of happiness and sadness, because the symptoms of bipolar disorder can be severe and life-threatening.

It is estimated that around one in 50 people in Western countries develops this illness, which affects men and women equally. Most of those affected are aged between 20 and 30 when first diagnosed. Patients with bipolar disorder are often intelligent and artistically creative.

What causes bipolar disorder?

Doctors do not yet fully understand the underlying mechanisms of bipolar disorder, and a number of environmental factors may be involved, although a genetic predisposition has been clearly established. The identical twin of a patient with bipolar disorder has a risk of developing the condition as high as 70 percent.

One theory is that the illness might be linked to particular neurotransmitters that help regulate mood. Experience with the effects of drugs and analysis of the brains of bipolar sufferers suggest that the neurotransmitter dopamine is of central importance in the disease, but it is likely that dopamine's role involves complex interactions with other neurotransmitter systems. Studies of patients with bipolar disorder have also discovered abnormalities in pathways in the brain that use the neurotransmitters serotonin, noradrenaline, and acetylcholine.

← **Electroconvulsive therapy (ECT), shown here, has a negative public image thanks to books and films such as *One Flew Over the Cuckoo's Nest*, but such treatment may be necessary—and effective—for some severely depressed people with suicidal thoughts.**

Symptoms and signs of bipolar disorder

Bipolar disorder is a type of psychosis, which means the patient's perception of reality is markedly altered. They may realize that others consider their actions irrational, but fail to understand it themselves. Typically, bipolar disorder involves alternating cycles of mania and depression—each lasting days, weeks, or months. Some people experience more highs than lows; others report more lows than highs. The severity of the mood swings and the symptoms also vary from person to person.

MANIA
- Feeling extremely euphoric or energetic
- Going without sleep
- Thinking and speaking quickly
- Delusions of self-importance
- Reckless behavior, such as overspending
- Extreme sexual behavior
- Aggression
- Irritability
- Grandiose, unrealistic plans

DEPRESSION
- Withdrawal from people and activities
- Overpowering feelings of sadness and hopelessness
- Lack of appetite and weight loss
- Feeling anxious or guilty without reason
- Difficulty concentrating
- Suicidal thoughts and behavior

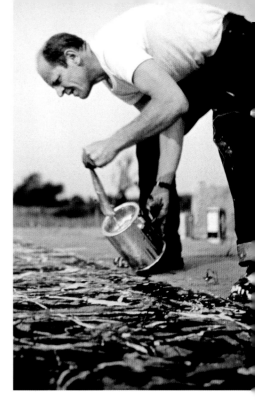

↑ **Bipolar disorder is often associated with creativity, as in the artist Jackson Pollock, who is thought to have suffered from the condition.**

Treatment of depression

Treatment of depression depends on the type and severity of the mood disorder. For milder depression, lifestyle change, exercise, stress reduction, and social support are of benefit. Various forms of psychological therapy (cognitive behavior therapy and interpersonal therapy) are also of help. Psychiatric medication may use a range of drugs including selective serotonin reuptake inhibitors (SSRI) that make more serotonin available at synapses in the cortex. For more severe depression with strong suicidal thoughts, electro-convulsive therapy may be necessary. Bipolar disorder requires treatment with mood-stabilizer drugs such as Lithium salts to control the mania.

↓ **One type of antidepressant (SSRIs, or selective serotonin reuptake inhibitors) works by blocking the removal of serotonin from cortical synapses, thereby making more serotonin available for longer.**

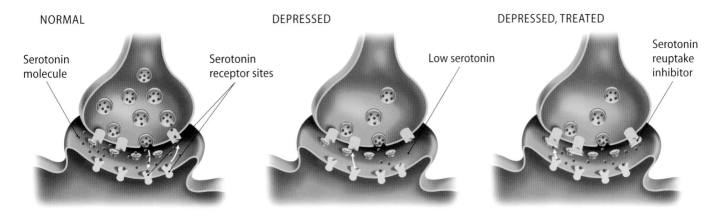

NORMAL

Serotonin molecule

Serotonin receptor sites

DEPRESSED

Low serotonin

DEPRESSED, TREATED

Serotonin reuptake inhibitor

Schizophrenia

Schizophrenia is a complex brain disorder characterized by a breakdown of thinking and emotions, and a loss of contact with reality. Its symptoms may affect every attribute of character and personality.

Occurring in about 1 percent of the population, schizophrenia usually makes itself known in a person's late teens and early 20s, equally affecting all races, cultures, classes, and sexes. Between 20 and 30 percent of people with schizophrenia experience only a few brief episodes, but for others it may become a chronic condition, and about 10 percent of people with schizophrenia commit suicide. Neuroscientists still do not know what causes this illness, although there is undoubtedly a genetic component.

Symptoms of schizophrenia

One of the principal symptoms of schizophrenia is experiencing hallucinations—mainly hearing, but also seeing, feeling, smelling, or even tasting something that is not actually there. A person with schizophrenia often hears disembodied voices that may be derogatory or accusatory, telling the individual that they are bad or worthless. Very commonly, schizophrenic people experience delusions of self-reference—a false belief that something in the news or on a billboard is "about"

→ **In this early 1800s engraving, various demonic creatures torment a mentally ill woman. Most hallucinations experienced by schizophrenic patients are auditory.**

them—and often experience confused thinking so that everyday thoughts become disjointed. A person with schizophrenia will also have social problems, including social withdrawal, a lack of motivation, blunting of emotions, inappropriate responses in social settings, and a lack of insight into the consequences of their actions. Not all people affected by schizophrenia have all these symptoms, and some symptoms appear only for short periods or episodes.

What causes schizophrenia?

The causes of schizophrenia are not fully understood but are likely to be a combination of hereditary and other factors. It seems that some people are born with a tendency to develop this illness. Certain things, like stress or the use of drugs such as marijuana or LSD, can

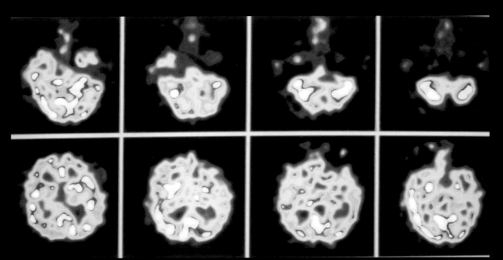

← **A series of PET scans records the brain activity patterns of a schizophrenic patient experiencing a hallucination. Intense activity is shown as yellow in the sensory areas at the back of the brain.**

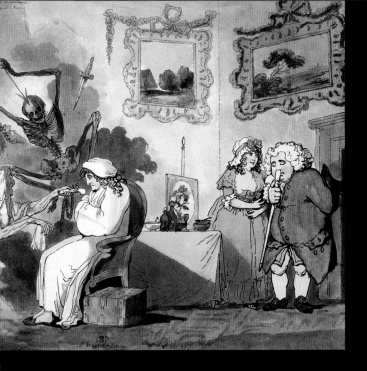

trigger the first episode in susceptible people. Brain abnormalities are thought to play a role; these may include neurotransmitter, structural, behavioral, neurophysiological, and cognitive abnormalities.

Among the theories that try to explain schizophrenia is the neurodevelopmental model, which suggests that disordered developmental processes underlie the disease. This is based on observations of abnormal layering of nerve cells in the hippocampus, suggesting that disordered migration of nerve cells is a cause. Other evidence suggests that organization of synaptic circuits, particularly in the prefrontal cortex, is responsible. The circuits of the frontal cortex are known to undergo extensive remodeling during adolescence, due in part to a mechanism involving a type of glutamate receptor that is deficient in the brains of schizophrenic patients. Researchers believe that there is an excessive amount of synaptic pruning in the dorsolateral prefrontal cortex of some young people during adolescence. This abnormal pruning process, which involves the elimination of many synapses, may trigger the disease, or predispose affected individuals to it.

The dopamine hypothesis

Drugs that alleviate symptoms of schizophrenia belong to two classes, the phenothiazines and the butyrophenones. Both block receptors of the neurotransmitter

Brain changes in schizophrenia

Schizophrenic patients have enlarged ventricles, the fluid-filled spaces inside the brain. Imaging studies have shown that structures in the temporal lobe (the amygdala, hippocampus, and entorhinal cortex) are reduced in size. Analysis of nerve cell populations has found fewer nerve cells in many of the structures of the limbic system and abnormal arrangements of nerve cells in the cingulate gyrus and entorhinal cortex. These regions are involved in circuits linking the association areas of the cerebral cortex with the septum and hypothalamus, which control the expression of emotions.

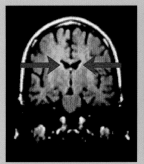 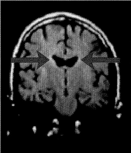

Unaffected   Affected

↑ **MRI scans of identical twins show enlarged lateral ventricles in the twin affected by the disease, compared to his unaffected brother.**

shown to have more dopamine receptors than normal individuals, but it is difficult to determine whether this is a primary cause or due to long-standing medication with phenothiazines or butyrophenones.

It may be that the underlying abnormality in schizophrenia is not an excess of dopamine, but a reduction in the availability or activity of another neurotransmitter, glutamate, in the brain. Dopamine synapses are known to inhibit glutamate release in the limbic parts of the brain, so antipsychotic drugs may

Other behavioral disorders

Reactive depression, bipolar disorder, and schizophrenia account for much of the serious mental illness in our society, but there are a host of other mental, behavioral, and personality disorders that cause problems both for the individual and those around them.

Among the most widely experienced behavioral disorders are obsessive–compulsive disorder, Tourette's syndrome, autism, and psychopathy.

Obsessive–compulsive disorder

Characterized by recurrent intrusive thoughts (obsessions) and ritualistic behaviors (compulsions) that take up much of the individual's time, obsessive–compulsive disorder (OCD) is usually classified as an anxiety disorder because of the distress produced by the obsessions and compulsions. The age of onset of OCD is usually late childhood to early adulthood.

Common obsessions include thoughts of being contaminated with germs, being affected by illness, or harming oneself or others. Compulsions often occur in response to the obsessive thoughts (e.g., hand-washing in response to thoughts of germs), or may be repetitive rituals performed according to some arbitrary internal rule (e.g., counting your footsteps to avoid ending on an odd number).

Functional brain imaging studies have provided evidence that OCD is due to abnormal function in the pathways involving the prefrontal cortex and the striatum, part of the basal ganglia. In patients with OCD there is increased blood flow in the orbitofrontal cortex (the underside of the frontal lobe) and the caudate nucleus of the striatum, particularly when the patient is engaged in an obsessive thought or compulsive action.

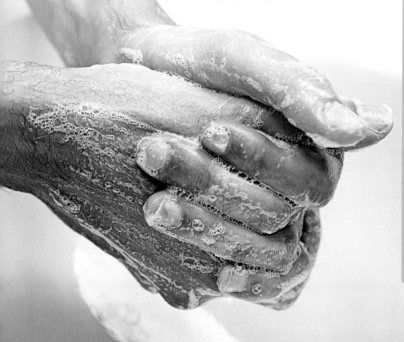

↓ **A common symptom of obsessive–compulsive disorder is the compulsion to repeatedly wash one's hands, sometimes until the skin is raw.**

Treating OCD

OCD may be treated with drugs that reduce reuptake of the neurotransmitter serotonin. These medications cut down the time that the person engages in obsessions and compulsions. Behavioral therapy that exposes patients to "dirty" objects while preventing them from engaging in the usually ensuing compulsion (e.g., hand-washing), may help to extinguish the anxiety that drives their compulsive behavior. Functional imaging studies of patients who have undergone such behavioral therapy show levels of metabolic activity in the orbitofrontal cortex and caudate returning to normal levels.

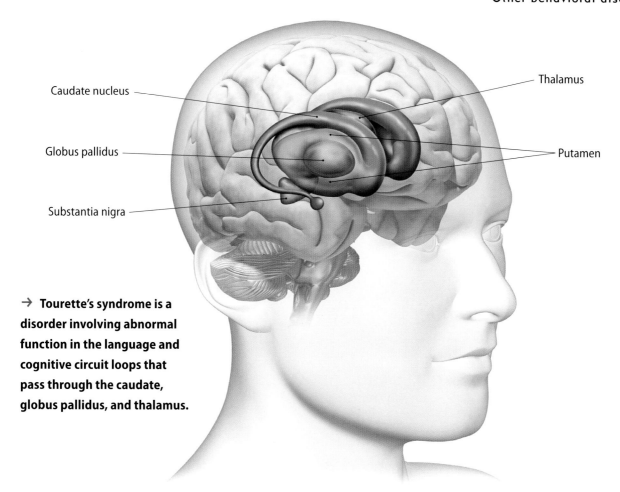

Caudate nucleus

Globus pallidus

Substantia nigra

Thalamus

Putamen

→ **Tourette's syndrome is a disorder involving abnormal function in the language and cognitive circuit loops that pass through the caudate, globus pallidus, and thalamus.**

Tourette's syndrome

Tourette's syndrome (TS) affects 0.1 to 1 percent of the population, with about three and a half times as many males being affected as females. People with TS show persistent tics, which are sudden, rapid, stereotyped behaviors. Tics may be a movement (motor tic), or a sound (phonic tic). The movements are purposeless and generally recur many times in a day. Phonic tics may consist of inappropriate or offensive words. About 40 percent of patients with TS have OCD and a similar number also have symptoms of attention deficit hyperactivity disorder (ADHD). The condition usually begins during childhood and often improves early in the third decade of life, although some patients continue to have symptoms and signs.

Sensory or mental states are also associated with the tics. Patients may experience a sensory tic, which is a recurrent sensation on, or near, the skin. They may also experience a premonitory urge, a feeling of sensory or mental discomfort that may be relieved by a physical tic. In fact, there appears to be a sequence of events in the brain that make up the tic cycle: A) a premonitory urge; B) a state of inner conflict over whether to give in to the urge; C) the production of the motor or phonic tic; and D) a temporary feeling of relief.

There is a strong genetic component to TS. The chance of the identical twin of someone with TS also developing TS is 80 to 90 percent and the first-degree relatives (i.e., brother, sister, child) of patients with TS have 20 to 150 times the risk of developing the condition as the general population.

Studies have suggested that the underlying abnormality in TS is dysfunction in the loop pathway that connects the cerebral cortex, striatum, pallidum, and thalamus. Other imaging studies have reported an enlarged corpus callosum, the pathway that connects the two cerebral hemispheres, and a reduction in the volume of the caudate part of the striatum.

Treatment for TS is based on education of the patient and their family members, treatment of any associated OCD or ADHD, and suppression of the tics by drugs that block receptors of the neurotransmitter dopamine.

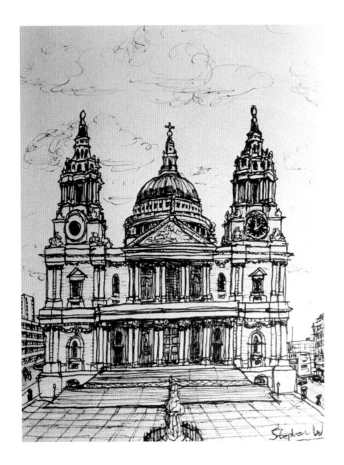

← **Autistic savant artist Stephen Wiltshire, at age 17, did this pen-and-ink drawing of St. Paul's Cathedral by memory even though he has a mental age of ten.**

syndrome (high-level functioning autism) is used for those autistic patients with normal intelligence. Some autistic people develop extraordinary skills in musical, linguistic, and artistic areas, and are sometimes known as autistic savants.

No one knows for sure what causes autism. Autistic patients are said to lack a "theory of mind." In other words, they do not seem to realize that other people have ideas and beliefs different from their own. Children normally develop a theory of mind at about the age of four, and some neuroscientists have argued that of all the primates, it is only fully developed in humans. Other scientists have proposed that many of the signs of autism (lack of empathy, language deficits, and poor imitation skills) may be the consequence of a deficiency or abnormal function of the mirror neurons, special nerve cells in the cortex that allow us to empathize and model the feelings of other people. On the other hand, autistic features such as repetitive movements, hyper-sensitivity, aversion to certain sounds, and avoidance of eye contact are less readily explained by the mirror neuron hypothesis. These features might be explained by abnormal function in the amygdala, the prefrontal cortex, or links between the visual cortex and amygdala.

There is no cure for autism, and no medications have been found to make a difference. Treatment includes speech, language, and behavioral therapy.

Autism

Three main symptom categories define autism:

- A profound impairment of social relationships, including lack of eye contact and poor facial recognition.
- A profound impairment in communication skills, such as limited use of speech.
- Restricted, repetitive, and stereotyped patterns of behavior, with an inability to cope with change and a fixation on detail.

Autism affects four or five in every 10,000 children and seems to have a genetic component—identical twins of an affected child have a 70 to 90 percent chance of also developing the condition. About 75 percent of children with autism are also intellectually disabled. The term Asperger's

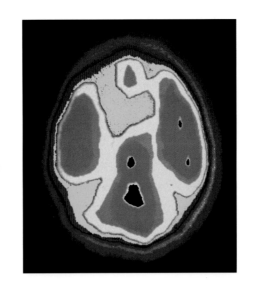

← **In this PET scan of the brain of a child with autism there is low activity in the frontal cortex (top of the scan), involved with language and conscious thought, and the visual processing cortex at the rear of the brain (bottom).**

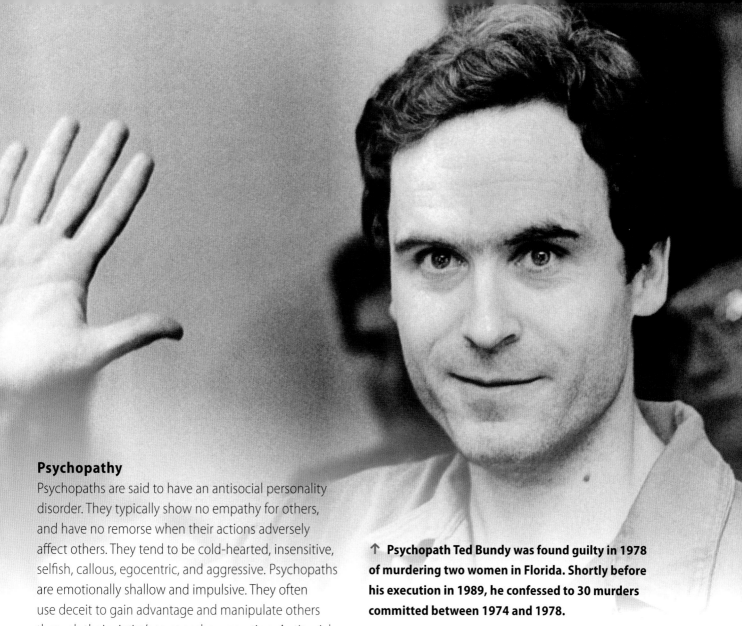

Psychopathy

Psychopaths are said to have an antisocial personality disorder. They typically show no empathy for others, and have no remorse when their actions adversely affect others. They tend to be cold-hearted, insensitive, selfish, callous, egocentric, and aggressive. Psychopaths are emotionally shallow and impulsive. They often use deceit to gain advantage and manipulate others through their victim's trust and cooperation. Antisocial personality disorder is more common in males (about 3 percent) than in females (1 percent). Psychopathy naturally predisposes to crime, particularly those crimes involving trust, such as fraud and bigamy, and it is estimated that psychopaths make up about 20 percent of prison inmates.

Psychopathy is traditionally regarded as a behavioral impairment. In this point of view, psychopathy is seen as a disorder of the prefrontal cortex caused by genetic or early life environmental factors. Certainly there is a strong genetic basis for psychopathy, and criminality and psychopathy share common heredity. On the other hand, psychologists have shown that, as babies, psychopaths have fewer birth complications than the rest of the population, so it seems that adverse events during prenatal life are not responsible for psychopathy.

↑ **Psychopath Ted Bundy was found guilty in 1978 of murdering two women in Florida. Shortly before his execution in 1989, he confessed to 30 murders committed between 1974 and 1978.**

Psychopathy as an evolutionary strategy

Evolutionary psychologists see psychopathy not as an impairment, but as a genetically based adaptation, albeit one that causes problems for society. If psychopaths make up only a small percentage of the population, they may enjoy benefits by exploiting those around them, because detecting their deception may be costly and time-consuming for the bulk of the cooperative population. Of course, if psychopaths made up more than a few percent of the population, then a cooperative society would be impossible.

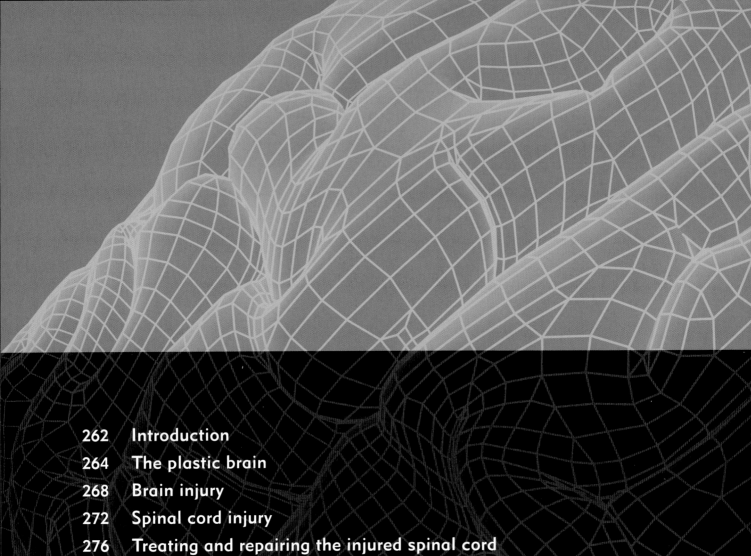

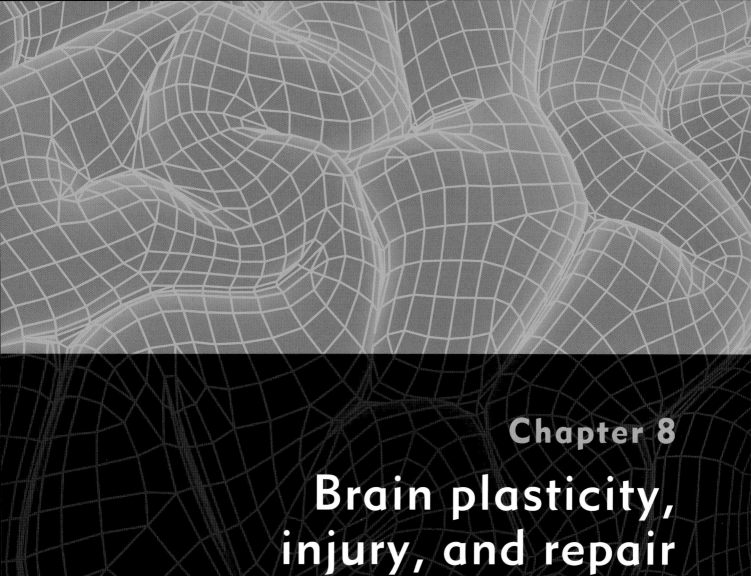

Chapter 8

Brain plasticity,
injury, and repair

Introduction

Plasticity is the ability of the nervous system to change its structure in response to experience. It is best seen during early development, but persists into adult life. Plasticity enables a degree of recovery from brain injury and offers hope for effective treatment for spinal injuries in the future.

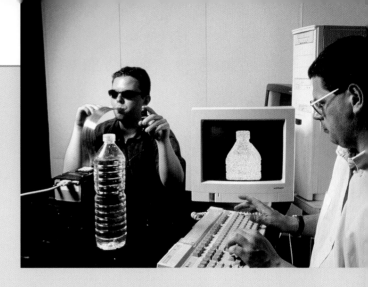

↑ **The blind can learn to use other senses to experience a sort of vision. Here, input from a video camera (held in the left hand) is converted into output to an electro-tactile tongue pad. The patterns felt on the tongue allow the blind person to "see" by "touch at a distance."**

It would be impossible for the human genome to contain the code for the detailed structure of all nerve cells in the body. The genetic code sets in place a series of rules about how the broad structure of the nervous system should be built, but its final form depends on a combination of interactions: those between nerve cell populations in the brain; those between nerve cells and the rest of the body (e.g., in motor systems); and the effects of sensory stimuli from the external environment on nerve cells (e.g., in sensory systems).

Plasticity is central to the process of brain development. It means the developing brain can be molded and stimulated by rich sensory experiences, as when a young child is inspired and stimulated by social and learning interactions with parents, grandparents, and siblings. On the other hand, the plastic nature of the developing brain means that adverse events in the environment, whether chemical, physical, or social, can impair brain development.

Plasticity underlies learning and memory

One particular type of plasticity that extends into maturity is the ability to adjust synaptic connections in response to experience. This may involve either very short-term adjustments of only a few seconds to minutes in duration, or alterations that last for years and underlie long-term memory. Memory systems in the mature brain are critically dependent on this ability to strengthen some synapses, while others become less effective. At a larger scale, sensory experience or practice of motor tasks adjusts the maps of sensory information or motor programs on the cerebral cortex, suggesting that axonal connections are being changed.

← **The pattern of nerve impulses (red arrows) arising from experience leads to the rearrangement of neural connections by removing those that are underutilized (blue arrow, far left) while increasing the number of contacts elsewhere (purple arrow, left).**

Plasticity declines with age

The ability of nerve cells to adjust their shape in response to their environment declines significantly with maturity. This means that the mature nervous system is relatively stable and allows us to rely on tried and tested strategies for handling life's problems. However, reduced plasticity greatly limits the ability of the nervous system to repair itself after injury or disease and restricts our ability to learn new skills in old age.

Could the nose fix the spine?

Nerve cells in the central nervous system do not regrow their axons after damage, with the result that brain and spinal cord injury has catastrophic effects on daily function. One part of the nervous system may provide the key to discovering how to regrow central axons. That is the nose, where olfactory receptor nerve cells are continuously replaced throughout life and new receptor cells grow axons into the brain every day of our lives (see p. 279). This amazing feat may be due to the environment provided by the olfactory ensheathing cells that help new axons grow into the brain from the olfactory area.

Brain and spinal cord injury

The densely packed nerve networks of the central nervous system are vulnerable to tearing or crushing by sudden acceleration or compression forces. Often the eventual area of nerve cell death far exceeds the initial volume of damage, because damage to nerve cells and blood vessels in one site leads to a cascade of damaging effects in the surrounding brain tissue. Some of these effects are due to the release of chemicals that excite surrounding cells, others are due to damage to the rich vascular networks in the brain, or the damaging activities of invading inflammatory cells and their chemicals.

Plasticity repairs

Nerve cells in the developing brain and spinal cord have an extraordinary ability to grow axons to the correct target and to adjust their shape in response to the environment. If we could return the nerve cells of the mature brain or spinal cord to this developmental state and coax them to reacquire the ability to grow new connections, we could repair damage from trauma and reverse the effects of degenerative brain disease.

↓ **Childhood is a time of intense experiences as the young brain is molded by its exposure to the sensory world. Rich sensory experiences and good nutrition are key to healthy brain growth.**

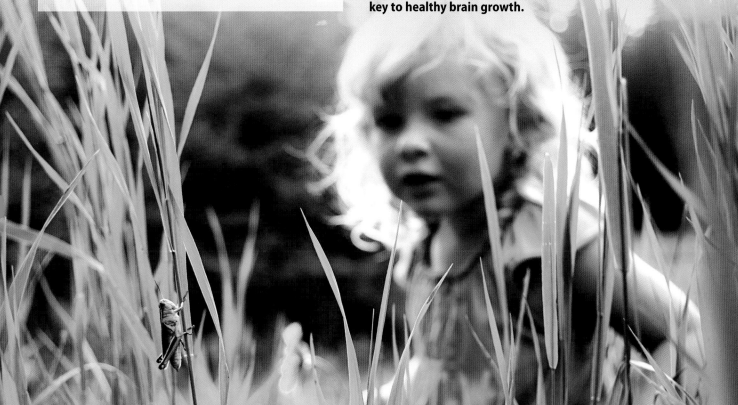

The plastic brain

The brain's ability to remake itself in the light of experience is an amazing process that underlies the changing nature of our lives from babyhood to old age. The two most important processes behind that plasticity are the ability of nerve cells to grow new axon branches and competition between nerve fibers.

There are two developmental processes that underlie plasticity in the young nervous system. For nerve connections at the rim of the nervous system—where sensory pathways start from the eye or body surface, or where motor pathways contact muscles—the overproduction of nerve cells during development is the mechanism that matches nerve cells to their role. For example, many more motor nerve cells are produced than normally survive to adulthood, but some of the motor nerve cells that would usually die can be rescued if additional muscle is made available for them to contact. Developing nerve cells that are subject to this sort of developmental death must compete for special chemicals (neurotrophic factors) that the skin or muscles produce.

Deeper inside the nervous system, it is the overproduction of nerve connections that helps shape the nervous system. Developing nerve cells in the cerebral cortex produce axons to many different parts of the brain that they would not normally contact in adult life. The connections that are reinforced by effective function are retained and strengthened, whereas those that are less effective are withdrawn.

Critical periods

The opportunity to adjust connections in the brain during development is greatest at a span of time called the critical period. This is usually shortly after the sense or motor function begins to be used, typically during early postnatal life. Once the critical period has passed, the wiring of the sensory or motor pathway is relatively fixed, but the critical period is different for various senses or skills.

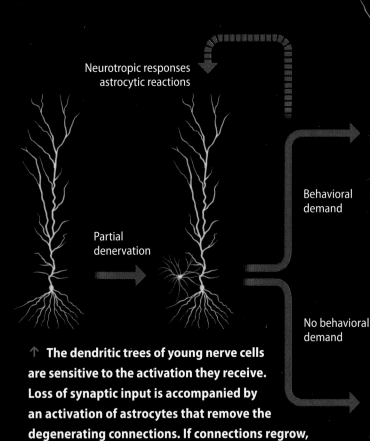

Neurotropic responses
astrocytic reactions

Partial denervation

Behavioral demand

No behavioral demand

↑ **The dendritic trees of young nerve cells are sensitive to the activation they receive. Loss of synaptic input is accompanied by an activation of astrocytes that remove the degenerating connections. If connections regrow, then the greater the behavioral demand, the more complex the dendritic tree becomes.**

→ **People born disabled or injured during early life can train parts of their brain to take on unusual roles. Chinese artist Huang Guofu draws with paintbrushes held by mouth and foot.**

The adaptable cortex

People who have lost a limb often achieve extraordinary feats with their remaining limbs. Upper limb amputees often develop the ability to perform fine motor tasks with their feet to a level of skill usually associated with the hand. Functional MRI scanning of the motor cortex of these people while they perform fine motor tasks with their toes shows activation of not only the cortical region that controls the lower limb, but also of the cortical region that usually controls the hand. The extent to which cortical maps can be adjusted is critically dependent on the age of injury. If amputation occurs early in life, before plasticity has declined to adult levels, the changes will be much more extensive than if amputation occurs during adulthood.

Critical periods have been studied best in the visual pathways, by experiments that alter the visual input from one or both eyes. In mammals with binocular vision (meaning they view most of the visual field with both eyes, e.g., in humans, monkeys, cats) visual input from both eyes is processed in the primary visual cortex of each hemisphere, with the two eyes stimulating nerve cells in distinct areas called ocular dominance columns. Covering one eye of a kitten for the first few months of life deprives the visual cortex of input from that eye. In the primary visual cortex of these animals, the ocular dominance column of the uncovered eye expands into the region of the covered eye. Even after the cover is removed from the eye, the kitten will continue to behave as if it were blind in that eye. Covering the eye of a cat older than four months has no effect on the ocular dominance columns in the cortex. Experiments like this show that many of the sensory connections of the brain are established by competition between sensory inputs: when one input is placed at a disadvantage, the other inputs will dominate.

Critical periods are also found for the senses of touch and hearing. They also apply for motor tasks, so if splinting prevents the use of a limb in early life, the subject may never attain proper control of the limb. Even higher forms of cortical function are subject to critical periods: learning a language is much easier during childhood than in young adulthood. As a general rule, critical periods for primary senses like vision are earlier than those for sensory interpretation tasks that involve input from many senses such as language. This reflects the longer period of time that the brain needs to complete the wiring of higher brain centers.

Stimulating plasticity?

Our lives would be much richer if we could retain the ability to learn new skills into old age, and many of the adverse effects of brain disease and injury might be overcome or at least minimized if we could reactivate plasticity. So, learning how to stimulate plasticity in old brains is a worthy goal, but the task is not easy. In the natural course of ageing there is a steady decline in brain weight from age 25, probably due to the pruning of infrequently used connections, because the number of nerve cells stays fairly stable for much of maturity. This suggests that the natural course of ageing is to reduce nerve connections, a normal process that consolidates experience and reduces impetuous actions, but also limits behavioral flexibility.

The task of stimulating plasticity requires not only that we understand the chemical (neurotrophic) factors that promote the outgrowth of axons, but also that we determine how that outgrowth can be directed to produce functionally beneficial new connections. A variety of neurotrophic factors that act during development have already been identified (nerve growth factor—NGF; brain-derived neurotrophic factor—BDNF; neurotrophic factors 3 and 4/5—NT-3 and NT-4/5), but the task of delivering these or other trophic compounds into the ageing brain in a way that is both effective and does not cause damage is an ongoing challenge.

Increasing plasticity in older brains may have undesirable side effects. The impulsivity and poor judgment of adolescents may be due to plasticity in their prefrontal cortex. It is no accident that every society has developed conventions and institutions that protect adolescents from the consequences of their actions while they learn. Enhancing plasticity in older people would have to be focused on particular skills rather than a global effect that might create a population of rash and impetuous elderly.

→ **Children learn foreign languages with relative ease. The ability to acquire a language other than your native tongue declines during adolescence and becomes very difficult during adult life.**

Learning language

Everyone recognizes the difficulty of learning a new language when we are older, whereas young children acquire language apparently by osmosis. Linguist Noam Chomsky recognized that children aged between six months and four years rapidly acquire the language they hear spoken around them without any instruction in grammar and minimal correction of pronunciation. This ability is universal for all human populations and so similar in nature across the world that it appears to be programmed into our genes. The ability to acquire language declines markedly after the age of eight and is particularly difficult after 16 years. Familiarity is critically important to the retention of skills in a particular language. Exposing children from an English-speaking background to Chinese sounds during babyhood (up to about nine months of age) greatly improves their ability to understand Chinese and retain Chinese language skills into older life.

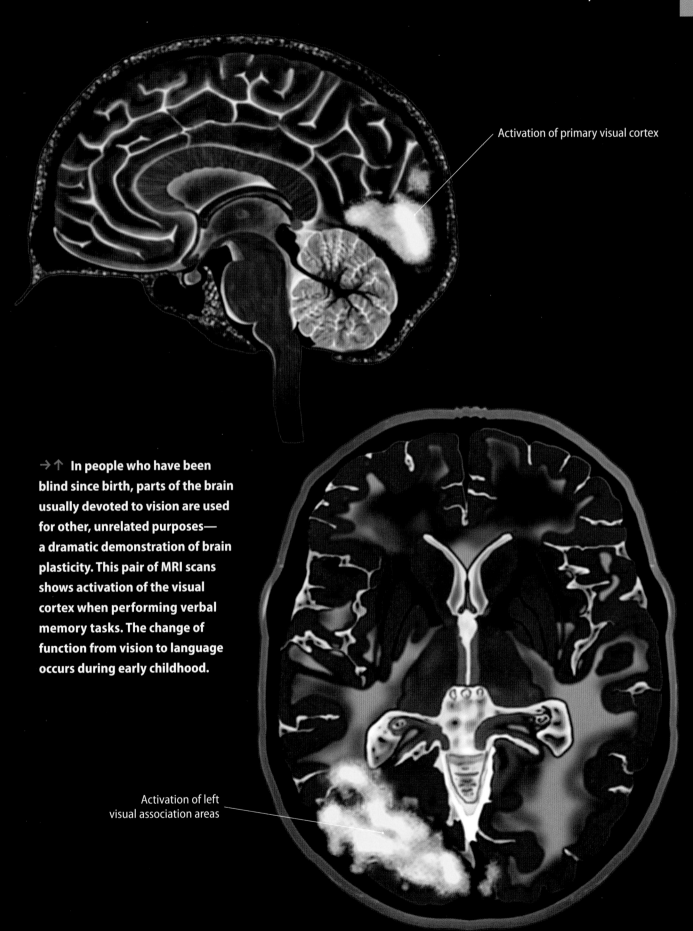

Activation of primary visual cortex

→ ↑ **In people who have been blind since birth, parts of the brain usually devoted to vision are used for other, unrelated purposes— a dramatic demonstration of brain plasticity. This pair of MRI scans shows activation of the visual cortex when performing verbal memory tasks. The change of function from vision to language occurs during early childhood.**

Activation of left visual association areas

Brain injury

The brain is extremely vulnerable to both external acceleration or compressive forces, and internal disruption by blood or foreign material forcing its way through the delicate tissue.

The brain has very little structural strength. Freshly removed from the skull it has the consistency of jelly and will sag and deform if removed from its protective bath of cerebrospinal fluid. Furthermore, the nerve cells of the central nervous system are densely packed, with little intervening space, meaning the brain can be easily damaged by a rise in pressure inside the skull.

Acceleration damage

A sudden change in the velocity of the body, such as when a fast-moving motor vehicle is suddenly decelerated by striking a tree, throws the brain forward against the inside of the frontal bone. The brain then rebounds from the initial blow to strike the interior of the back of the skull (a *contre coup* injury), producing paired bruising of the frontal and occipital poles of the brain. Rotational movements, twisting the brain on the midbrain, may also occur. In addition, the sharp border between the front and middle cavities of the skull base can bruise and tear the tissue at the front of the temporal lobe.

While these forces are damaging the brain surface, flexing and deformation of the brain interior tears the axons that connect brain regions. Compressive forces where the brain surface contacts the skull also squeeze delicate axons, disrupting the neurotubules that transport essential chemicals between the cell body and axon terminal and stopping nerve impulse conduction.

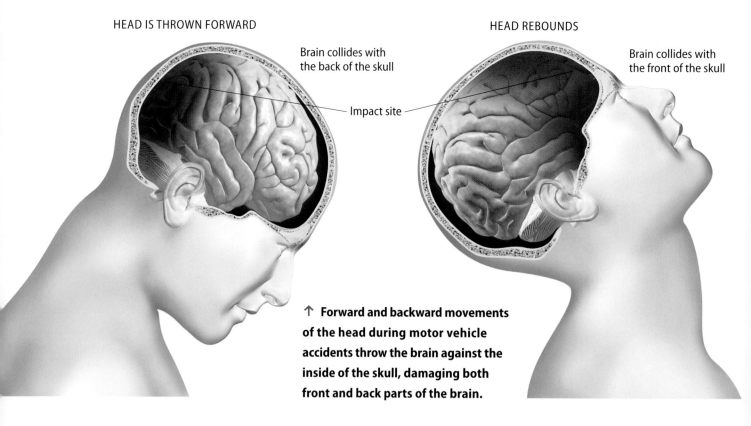

HEAD IS THROWN FORWARD

Brain collides with the back of the skull

Impact site

HEAD REBOUNDS

Brain collides with the front of the skull

↑ **Forward and backward movements of the head during motor vehicle accidents throw the brain against the inside of the skull, damaging both front and back parts of the brain.**

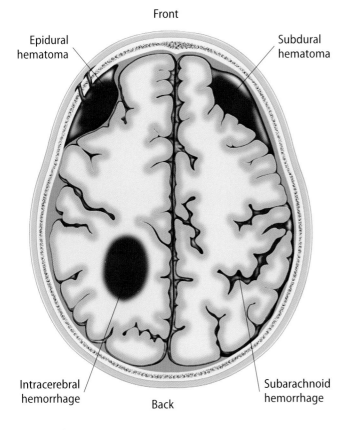

Front

Epidural
hematoma

Subdural
hematoma

Intracerebral
hemorrhage

Back

Subarachnoid
hemorrhage

↑ **Bleeding can occur into the space outside the dura (epidural hematoma), between the dura and arachnoid (subdural hematoma), in the subarachnoid space, or within the brain tissue itself (intracerebral hemorrhage).**

Apart from the direct damage to nerve cells, physical forces can damage the rich network of blood vessels that keep the brain supplied with oxygen and glucose. Fine blood vessels often tear where the brain is thrown against the skull and leak red blood cells. These blood cells split the fine axons and dendrites of the brain tissue and the damage to the vessel network deprives the surviving cells of essential oxygen and nutrients.

Blood on the brain

The skulls of adults and older children are enclosed spaces. Any blood that escapes from either arteries or veins into the spaces around the brain compresses the brain and raises intracranial pressure.

A blow to the side of the head can fracture the thin skull of the temple and tear the arteries supplying the dura mater of the meninges, the three membranes that

What is concussion?

Concussion, or mild traumatic brain injury, is a temporary state of disordered brain function following injury. A period of unconsciousness often follows a blow to the head or acceleration forces. This may be followed by confusion and disorientation in space and time and a post-traumatic amnesia. Other symptoms include difficulty balancing, problems with coordination, dizziness, vomiting, nausea, double vision, blurred vision, sensitivity to light, and ringing in the ears. Longer-term effects may include sleep disorders, problems with reasoning and concentration, and emotional disturbances.

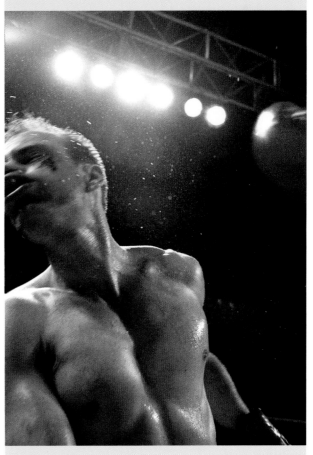

↑ **People who have experienced repeated concussions (such as boxers) may be at risk of related neurodegenerative disease later in life.**

enclose the skull. Arterial blood is under high pressure so these tears produce a rapidly expanding collection of blood (epidural hematoma) that forces brain tissue across the midline and down toward the skull base. The shifting of the brain squeezes the delicate tissues against the skull interior and dural membranes, crushing and tearing the nerve cells and their axons.

Rapid acceleration or deceleration of the head can also tear the delicate veins that enter the dural venous sinuses. Veins are low-pressure vessels, so the rate of bleeding may be slow or fast depending on the size of the tear. Shifting of the brain by the expanding mass of blood may squeeze brain tissue against hard parts of the skull interior.

Brainstem compression

The most life-threatening consequence of brain injury is often the downward shifting of the brainstem against the skull base. The medulla is the most vulnerable part because it is the closest to the skull base and contains the nerve cell groups that control the rate and rhythm of breathing. Other nerve cell groups in this region control blood pressure and heart rate. Compression of the medulla against the skull base can completely destroy these circulatory and respiratory centers, causing breathing and blood pressure control to stop.

Can axons regrow?

Axons in the central and peripheral nervous systems have very different abilities to regrow when cut. When a peripheral nerve is cut, the axon degenerates over a week or two. Provided the two ends of the nerve are kept in contact, the axon can regrow at the rate of about 0.04 inches (1 mm) per day. This is possible because Schwann cells that make the myelin coat of peripheral nerves are able to signal the nerve cell to activate growth-related genes to rebuild the axon end.

Cut or compressed axons in the central nervous system do not have the ability to regrow, because the cell types there are very different from Schwann cells. Central glial cells do not make the trophic factors that stimulate axon regrowth. Axon injury may even cause the cell body to die and give rise to effects in other nerve cells that connect with the damaged nerve cell. Nevertheless, central nerve cells do have the ability to grow new axons if they are transplanted to an environment similar to the peripheral nervous system (see pp. 277–9).

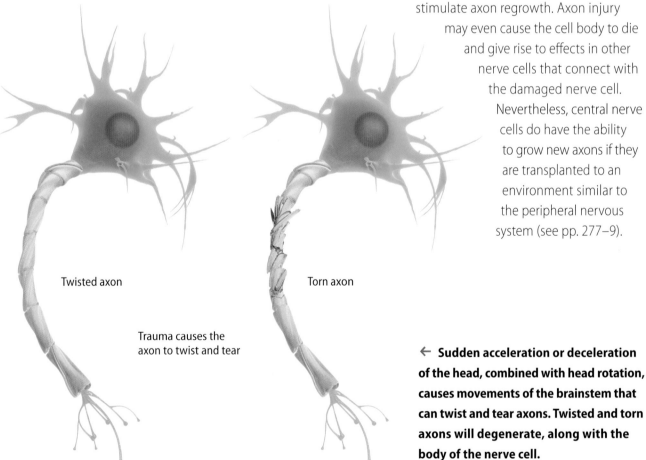

Twisted axon

Torn axon

Trauma causes the axon to twist and tear

← Sudden acceleration or deceleration of the head, combined with head rotation, causes movements of the brainstem that can twist and tear axons. Twisted and torn axons will degenerate, along with the body of the nerve cell.

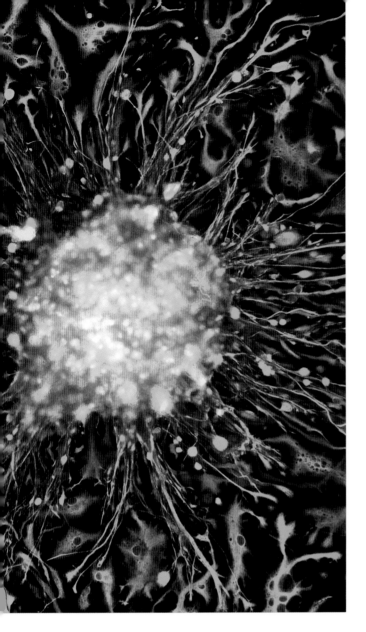

← **In this fluorescent light microscope image of a group of neural stem cells in culture, the stem cells are differentiating into nerve cells (red) and glia (green), which can be seen migrating out of the central clump.**

Stem cells

Most nerve cells are made during embryonic and fetal life, but the sites around the brain ventricles where nerve cells are produced retain a limited ability to make new nerve cells into adult life. These proliferative sites contain undifferentiated, self-renewing neural stem cells that might be coaxed into the production of new nerve cells with the appropriate stimulus, with the potential to replenish nerve cells lost to injury or disease.

There are two sites in the brain where stem cells naturally give rise to new nerve cells during life. One of these is the subgranular zone of the dentate gyrus of the hippocampus. The other site is in the subventricular zone of the front end of the lateral ventricle that gives rise to the sensory cells in the olfactory bulb. The continuous production of nerve cells in these two sites provides a limited but steady stream of new nerve cells, perhaps to facilitate learning. A lot of research effort is being directed at understanding how these regions retain the ability to make new nerve cells and to develop new technologies to stimulate the process.

Roadblocks to repair

When central nervous tissue is damaged, astrocytes and oligodendrocytes (see pp. 78–9) do not produce trophic factors to stimulate axon growth. Instead, astrocytes form a scar to wall off the injured site, a response that contains the injury, but also prevents the regrowth of axons. Astrocytes also produce molecules (chondroitin sulfate proteogly-cans) in the space between cells, which inhibit the growth of nerve cell processes. Oligodendrocytes also produce growth-inhibiting molecules and do not clear myelin debris as effectively as Schwann cells do in the peripheral nervous system.

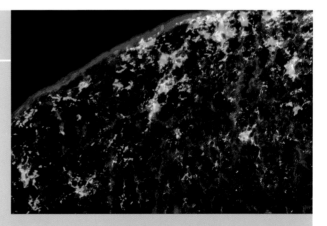

↑ **Reactive astrocytes act to protect other nerve cells, but they can also form destructive scar tissue. In this fluorescent light microscope image through an injured brain, the astrocytes are visible in red.**

Spinal cord injury

Damage to the spinal cord is one of the worst types of traumatic injury. It disproportionately affects young people, especially otherwise healthy males in their teens or twenties, and can lead to a life sentence of paralysis in a wheelchair.

Approximately 10,000 people sustain a spinal cord injury in the United States each year. With modern medical intervention, those affected can live for many years after injury, so there are more than 230,000 people in the United States living with the consequences of spinal cord injury. The main causes of spinal cord injury (based on US statistics) are motor vehicle accidents (about 41 percent of all cases), violence (22 percent, mainly gunshot wounds), falls (21 percent), and sports injuries (8 percent). Rarer, nontraumatic causes are tumors, infections, damage to the blood supply to the cord, and the demyelinating disease known as multiple sclerosis. People with spinal cord injury must cope not just with an inability to walk or use their upper limbs, but also with loss of control of the bowel, urinary bladder, and sexual organs.

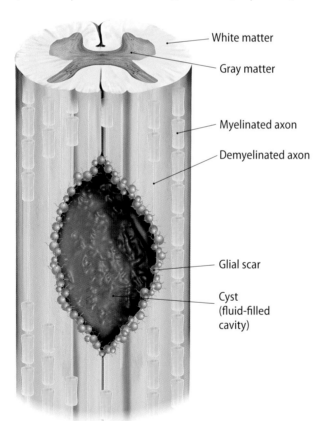

White matter

Gray matter

Myelinated axon

Demyelinated axon

Glial scar

Cyst (fluid-filled cavity)

↑ **When a spinal cord is injured, there is a central zone where axons and nerve cell bodies are destroyed by hemorrhage and loss of oxygen. This eventually turns into a fluid-filled cyst surrounded by a glial scar.**

The cellular effects of spinal cord injury

When a fall or some other force fractures or dislocates the bones of the vertebral column, the bones—which normally enclose and protect the spinal cord—may crush its soft tissue, damaging the nerve cell bodies and their axons. Occasionally, only the gray matter in the center of the cord is significantly damaged, but often the white matter is also affected. The crushing usually tears blood vessels, releasing blood into the tissue spaces and causing more damage as the blood cells force their way through the delicate processes of the spinal cord's nerve cells.

Mechanical damage to blood vessels usually triggers a second wave of damage due to disrupted oxygen delivery to tissue. This in turn causes injured spinal axons, nerve cell bodies, and astrocytes (a type of support cell for nerve cells) to release chemicals like glutamate. Glutamate is an excitatory neurotransmitter in normal central nervous system tissue, but its release in high levels overexcites nerve cells, inducing them to admit ions that in turn trigger the production of damaging molecules within the nerve cells called free radicals. This process is known as excitotoxicity.

This cascade of excitotoxic damage and free radical production enlarges the area of damage over a period

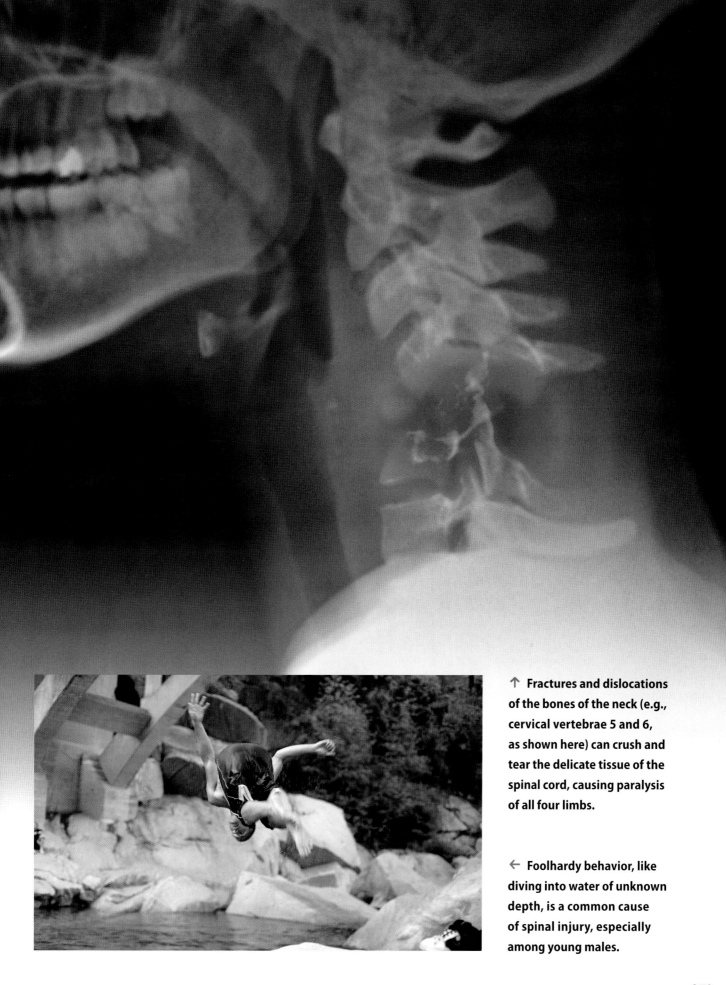

↑ **Fractures and dislocations of the bones of the neck (e.g., cervical vertebrae 5 and 6, as shown here) can crush and tear the delicate tissue of the spinal cord, causing paralysis of all four limbs.**

← **Foolhardy behavior, like diving into water of unknown depth, is a common cause of spinal injury, especially among young males.**

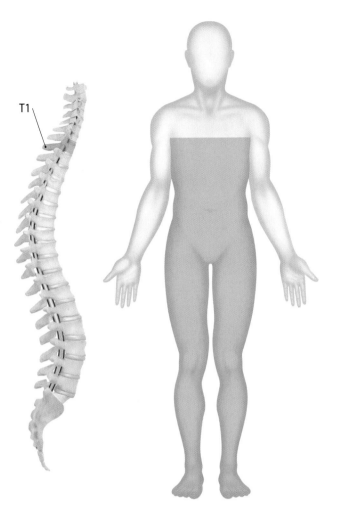

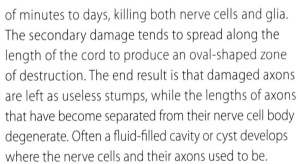

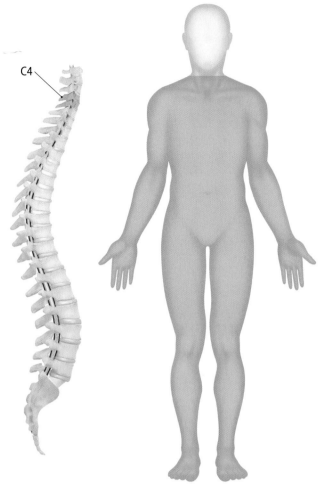

↑ **Injury to the spinal cord at upper thoracic levels (left) causes paralysis of the trunk and lower limbs (including urinary bladder and lower bowel). Injury in the middle neck (above) can cause paralysis of all four limbs, trunk, urinary bladder and lower bowel.**

of minutes to days, killing both nerve cells and glia. The secondary damage tends to spread along the length of the cord to produce an oval-shaped zone of destruction. The end result is that damaged axons are left as useless stumps, while the lengths of axons that have become separated from their nerve cell body degenerate. Often a fluid-filled cavity or cyst develops where the nerve cells and their axons used to be.

The functional effects of spinal cord injury

The effects of spinal cord injury consist of not only damage to nerve cells at the level of injury, but also interruption of the nerve pathways that must pass through the level of injury and connect the brain and lower levels of the spinal cord. If the disruption is complete, then voluntary movements are lost below the level of the injury. Damage to ascending sensory pathways can cause complete or partial loss of sensation below the level of injury. Damage to the

pathways in the white matter has far greater impact than damage to nerve cells at the level of injury.

The extent of functional loss depends on the site of injury. Lower level injury (e.g., below the first chest segment of the spinal cord) leads to paraplegia, a paralysis affecting only the legs, and loss of control of the pelvic organs (including the urinary bladder and anal sphincter). Interruption of the pathways to the urinary bladder can cause problems with control of urination. Bacteria can multiply in pooled urine within the bladder leading to urinary tract infections that may ascend to the kidney, resulting in kidney failure and possibly death.

Damage higher up the spinal cord (e.g., the middle levels of the neck) can cause loss of control of the arms and chest, as well as the lower limbs (quadriplegia, or paralysis of four limbs). Quadriplegic patients also experience the problems with bladder and bowel control that are found in paraplegics.

Spinal cord damage at very high levels (e.g., the highest level of the neck) has the most profound effects, because this can interrupt the descending pathways to the motor nerve cells in the spinal cord that control movements of the muscular diaphragm between the chest and abdominal cavities. Paralysis of the diaphragm is life-threatening: death will rapidly follow unless the patient receives artificial ventilation of the lungs.

Spinal shock

Injury of descending motor pathways in the spinal cord eventually leads to increased tone or tightness of muscles and more powerful deep tendon reflex responses below the level of damage, but the initial effect of spinal cord injury is a stage known as spinal shock.

Spinal shock may last for weeks and is a period when the muscles of the body below the level of injury are

Spinal cord injury and the autonomic nervous system

Loss of voluntary muscle control is not the only problem of spinal cord injury. Important pathways from the brainstem to the spinal cord control the functions of the autonomic nervous system. Although some parts of the autonomic nervous system (like the enteric nervous system of the gut, or the cardiac muscle) can continue to function without commands passing through the spinal cord, some internal organs are dependent on the brainstem and its pathways through the spinal cord for their coordinated function. This can cause a problem with control of the blood pressure when the brainstem cardiovascular centers are separated from sympathetic nerve cells in the spinal cord.

limp and flaccid and show no reflex responses. The reason for this shock is poorly understood, but it may be due to changes in the sensitivity of motor nerve cells below the injury to the remaining sources of sensory input. With the loss of descending control from the brainstem, motor nerve cells of the lower spinal cord become much more sensitive to the sensory information arriving from muscle spindles. This increased activity in the stretch reflex circuit makes muscles more rigid (increased tone) and may impair the patient's recovery of movement.

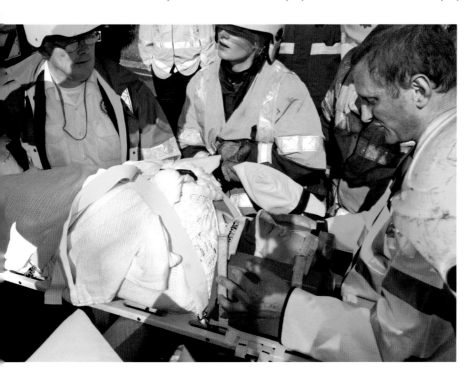

← **When the vertebral column is fractured, even slight movements may crush the spinal cord. Paramedics know to keep the necks of patients immobilized with a spinal board and neck brace.**

Treating and repairing the injured spinal cord

There are two broad approaches to the challenge of giving people with spinal cord injuries the best possible quality of life. The first is to minimize the spread of the devastating cascade of events that results from the initial injury. The second is to repair injured nerve pathways after the damage is done—a still-distant prospect that is the subject of promising research.

If movement or sensation returns within a week after a spinal cord injury, then most function will eventually be recovered. Losses remaining after six months are likely to be permanent.

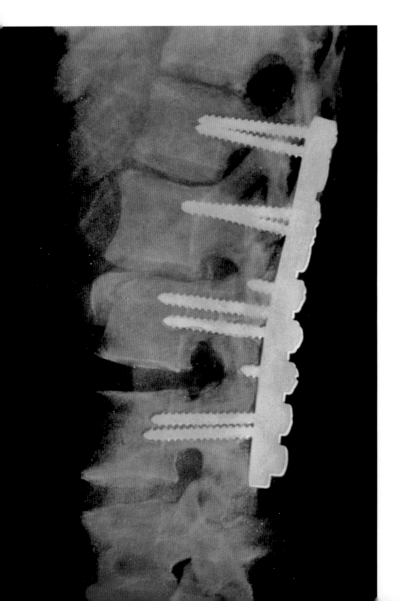

Containing the damage

The healthy spinal cord has millions of axons in the sensory and motor pathways that run through its white matter, but there is some redundancy built into those pathways. This means that limiting the amount of damage from a spinal cord injury can have profound effects on the ability of the patient to lead a normal life. For example, saving just 10 percent of the normal complement of axons that run from the brainstem to the spinal cord can mean the difference between a patient being mobile or wheelchair bound, or being able to pass urine normally rather than with a catheter.

Even lowering the segment of spinal cord affected by an injury by just one level can make a huge difference to the patient's quality of life. A patient whose spinal cord injury is kept below the level of the seventh neck segment will retain some ability to grasp objects, but if the damaged area is allowed to extend to the sixth or fifth neck segment, this function may be lost. So the primary goal for the clinical management of spinal cord injury is to minimize the spread of damage and preserve as much function as possible.

← **Spinal cord injury usually involves some fracture or dislocation of the protective bony vertebral column that surrounds it. The first rule of treatment is to stabilize the fracture site to protect the spinal cord. This X-ray shows four vertebrae fixed with metal screws and plates to promote healing.**

1. FLUID PHASE

Accumulation of neurotrophic factors and extracellular matrix molecules

2. CELLULAR PHASE

Cell migration, proliferation and alignment, and axon formation

3. AXONAL PHASE

Growth of axons

4. MYELINATION PHASE

Myelination of regenerated immature axons forming mature axonal fibers

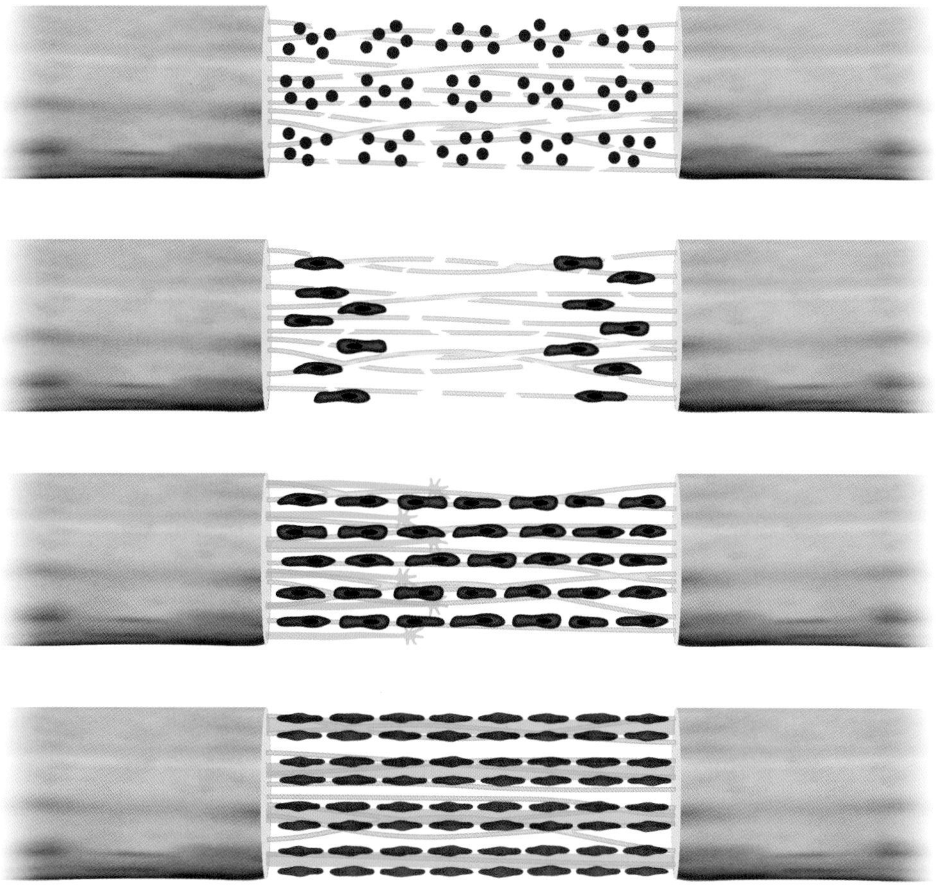

↑ **A future goal of spinal cord repair is to induce nerve cells to regrow axons through injury sites or artificial conduits. This illustration shows the four stages by which an artificial conduit bridging the gap between two ends of a severed nerve could encourage axon regrowth and restore motor function. Red spheres at Stage 1 represent introduced support cells, which migrate to line up along the degenerated axons (beige) and encourage new axon growth (green).**

Some of the damage that spinal cord injury produces is due to an excessive response by immune system cells and molecules. Drugs like methylprednisolone help reduce the swelling and inflammation that follow injury. Anti-inflammatory drugs may also reduce the release of excitotoxic glutamate and the accumulation of damaging free radical molecules in the tissue. Drugs that block the receptors for glutamate on nerve cell membranes (AMPA receptor antagonists) may reduce the excitotoxic injury.

Regenerating damaged nerve pathways

Research over the last 30 years has started to raise hopes for central nervous tissue repair. While this is still a long way from being an effective treatment in the clinical setting, encouraging studies in animals show that axons from the brain can regrow if given the right environment.

Peripheral nerves have the ability to regrow, but central nerves do not. This is because the two parts of the nervous system have different types of supporting cells. Studies in animals have demonstrated central axon regrowth along a graft of peripheral nerves transplanted to a site of central nervous system damage. Grafting peripheral nerves is a cumbersome way to repair central connections, but these experiments naturally raise the question of what it is about the central environment that prevents axon regrowth. The four key problems are: glial scarring, the presence of inhibitory chemicals, the lack of trophic support chemicals, and the lack of guidance for regenerating axons.

Controlling glial scarring

In the central nervous system, support cells (astrocytes and microglia) and blood vessel cells contribute to scar tissue that walls off sites of damage, but also produces a mechanical and chemical barrier that impedes regrowth of axons. One strategy to reduce scarring and improve axon regrowth is to use enzymes like chondroitinase ABC that break down these components of scar tissue.

Bad molecules and good chemistry

The myelin debris produced by central nervous tissue damage and the natural products of oligodendrocytes (myelin-producing cells) can inhibit the regrowth of axons. Some of these molecules (e.g., Nogo) are anchored to the cell membranes of oligodendrocytes and inhibit the growth of new axons through the spaces between these cells. Strategies for overcoming this problem involve using antibodies to attach to and block the effects of Nogo and the use of special molecules like CREB (cyclic AMP response element binding protein) to overcome the inhibitory effects of myelin on axonal growth.

Neurotrophic chemicals are present during nervous system development to promote natural axon growth and to maintain nerve cell populations. Their absence from, or low concentration in, the mature spinal cord is a major impediment to regrowth of axons. Methods to address this deficiency include the introduction of neurotrophic factors to the damaged tissue using minipumps or cells genetically modified to express the factor. Transfer of genes for making brain-derived neurotrophic factor (BDNF) into spinal cord cells has been shown in animals to promote the regrowth of the pathway from the red nucleus of the midbrain to the spinal cord. Most importantly, these treatments have been shown to result in functional improvements in hind limb movement and locomotion.

Supporting and guiding regenerating axons

Stimulating the regrowth of axons is of little benefit unless that new growth produces effective functional connections, and a major part of that problem is ensuring that regrowing axons reach the correct target. Approaches to support and guide regenerating axons

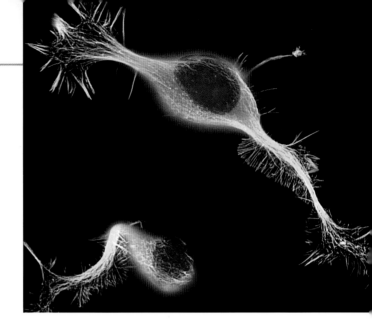

↑ **This fluorescent micrograph of nerve cells growing in tissue culture shows them forming the axons and dendrites that connect with other nerve cells. In the future, clinicians may be able to use cultured nerve cells to help heal spinal cord damage.**

include the use of peripheral nerve grafts, insertion of artificial scaffolds for axon growth, and transplantation of fetal stem, Schwann, or olfactory ensheathing cells (OECs). The goal of many of these approaches is to provide an environment that is known to support axon regrowth in another part of the body (e.g., peripheral nerves, Schwann, or OECs), or replenish nerve cells that can fulfill the role of lost cells.

What way forward?

The challenge for spinal cord repair is that many factors act together against axon regrowth. It is therefore highly likely that any successful intervention for human spinal cord repair will consist of several therapies in a simultaneous or sequential combination. At present, clinicians are reluctant to permit the testing of novel therapies in patients with recent spinal cord injury, when the primary goal is to limit the spread of damage. Rigorous testing of single and combination therapies in animal models is essential before application to acutely injured patients can be permitted. Until the clear benefits of novel therapies have been demonstrated, human trials of new treatments will be confined to patients who have been injured months to years ago.

An olfactory cell solution?

Olfactory nerve cells at the top of the nasal cavity are continuously exposed to the damaging effects of dry air and bacteria. These central nervous system cells have a limited lifespan and both the cell body itself and its axon into the brain must be regularly replaced. The olfactory ensheathing cell is a special type of support cell in the olfactory pathway that makes this regrowth possible. Many researchers believe that OECs could be a key to regrowing spinal cord axons.

The particular beauty of using OECs is that the patient's own nose can provide the cells, thereby avoiding tissue rejection. The challenge is to get OECs from the nose to survive and flourish in the foreign environment of the injured spinal cord, where blood supply may be poor and scar tissue common.

→ **One promising strategy for spinal cord repair is to use cultured olfactory ensheathing cells taken from the nose.**

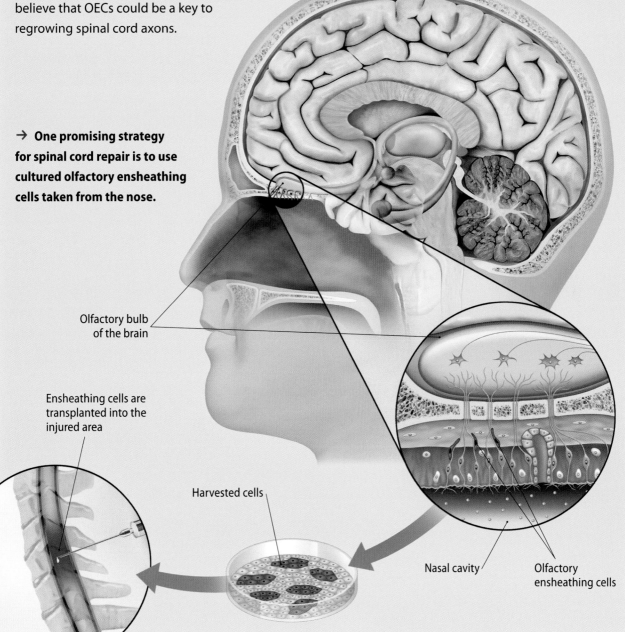

Olfactory bulb of the brain

Ensheathing cells are transplanted into the injured area

Harvested cells

Nasal cavity

Olfactory ensheathing cells

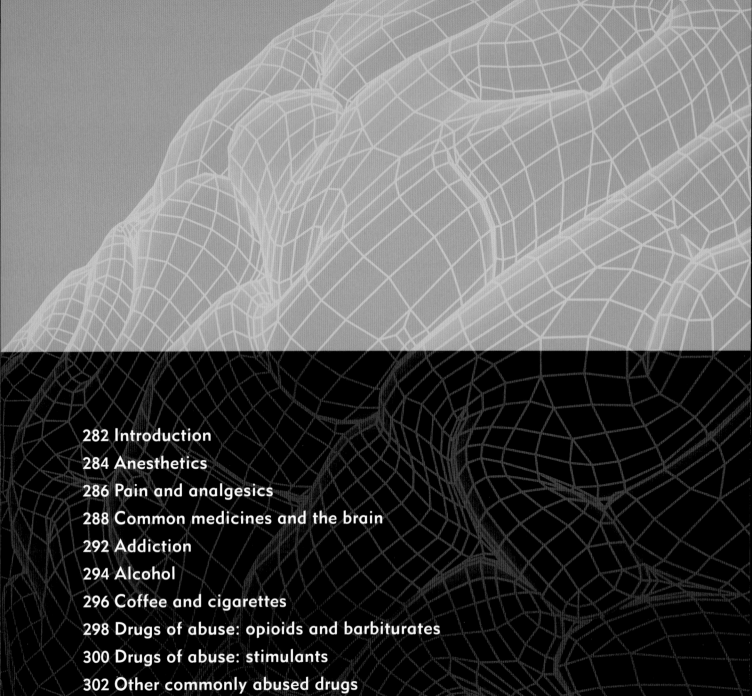

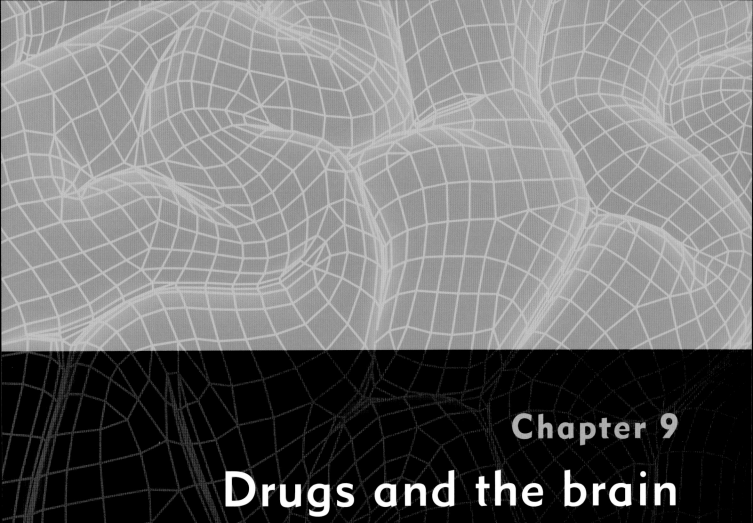

Chapter 9

Drugs and the brain

Introduction

From aspirin and alcohol to cannabis and caffeine, drugs are a part of everyday life. Some are used for medical purposes, others for pleasure or to relieve a craving. This chapter focuses on drugs that affect the brain's communications system, and thus alter its function.

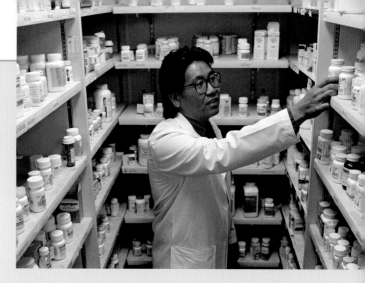

↑ **Pharmaceutical research has provided a wide array of drugs for the nervous system, with a multitude of effects, from subtle to substantial.**

Medicinal drugs are chemicals designed to alter the processes of the body in order to prevent, treat, or manage disorders and to relieve symptoms or pain. Other drugs, some of them classified as illegal because of their perceived ill effects on health and society, are used for their mood- or mind-altering properties.

The brain is the target

Nerve cells communicate by the release and detection of chemical substances, most of which are neurotransmitters. Connections between nerve cells, called synapses, are tiny spaces into which the cell on one side of the synapse releases neurotransmitters, and within which the cell on the other side detects those substances by means of protein molecules called receptors.

This chemical interaction provides an opportunity for doctors to modify the behavior and responses of the nervous system, by administering drugs which interact with neurotransmitters, receptors, or other aspects of synaptic communication. This chapter discusses a range of these drugs, which may be prescribed by medical professionals to treat disorders or illnesses, or self-administered for pleasurable effects or to ease the cravings of addiction. The latter category includes illegal drugs; common socially accepted drugs such as alcohol, caffeine, and nicotine; and drugs which may be legally prescribed but which are illegally abused. All of these substances affect the functioning of the nervous system

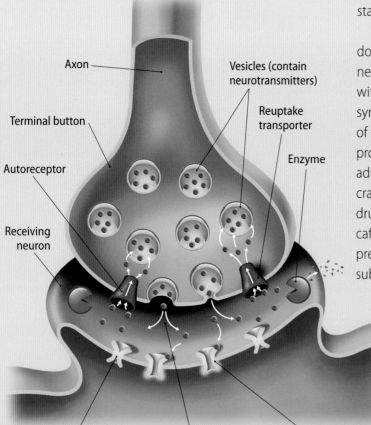

Axon

Vesicles (contain neurotransmitters)

Reuptake transporter

Terminal button

Enzyme

Autoreceptor

Receiving neuron

Closed receptor   Synaptic cleft   Open receptor

← **Neurotransmission from one nerve cell to another may involve release, recycling, and breakdown of neurotransmitter chemicals. Drugs that affect the brain may do so by intervening at any point in this process.**

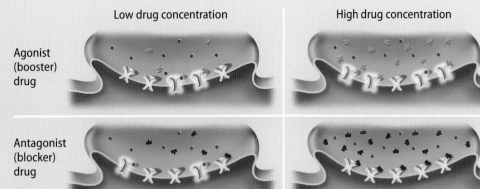

→ **Drugs may boost or block neurotransmitter receptors. Top: increasing levels of an agonist drug activates more receptors. Bottom: adding an antagonist drug blocks receptors, stopping the activation of the synapse.**

Low drug concentration

High drug concentration

Agonist (booster) drug

Antagonist (blocker) drug

by interacting with synaptic communication or cellular functions. Many other drugs, not covered by this chapter, are used to treat diseases such as cancer or infections in the nervous system. These drugs do not usually affect behavior or mental state, since they do not interact with cellular communication.

Drugs by accident

Most drugs that affect the brain have been discovered by accident or are derived from cultural practices. For example, chlorpromazine, an antipsychotic, was originally used as a decongestant during recovery from anesthesia before its calming properties were noticed, and acetaminophen (paracetamol) was ordered by mistake for use in an experiment, in which it turned out to be much better at reducing fever than the drug originally under test. Willow bark and coca leaf were chewed for centuries before their active compounds (aspirin and cocaine) were isolated for use in Western medicine.

↓ **Villagers in Peru chew leaves of the coca plant —from which cocaine is derived—as a stimulant.**

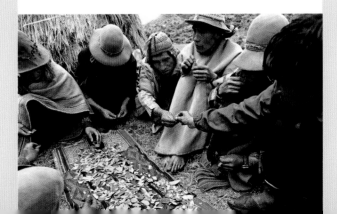

Neurotransmitters and drugs

Neurotransmitters can be divided by general function: excitatory (e.g., glutamate, acetylcholine), inhibitory (e.g., GABA), and modulatory. Excitatory and inhibitory transmission deals with things we might consider "factual" information in the nervous system: the position of limbs, how far to move a muscle, or where a sound is coming from. Modulatory neurotransmitters alter the quality of neural activity—e.g., adrenaline (epinephrine) changes the style of our thinking, and dopamine can add a gloss of pleasure to an otherwise ordinary sensory experience. Neurotransmitters (including serotonin, dopamine, and adrenaline) are closely associated with emotional states and the desires and rewards that cause us to seek the things we need, such as food and shelter, as well as more abstract pleasures such as maintaining friendships and planning for the future.

Neurotransmitters are potent messengers in the nervous system, and their manufacture, distribution, and processing are very carefully regulated by nerve cells and their support cells, glia. Rather than directly activate or block the receptors for a particular neurotransmitter, sophisticated techniques of drug discovery and design allow for much more subtle effects. A single type or subtype of receptor may be targeted, confining the drug's action to a specific part of the nervous system, or a particular aspect of function, while leaving others unaffected.

Other ways of achieving subtle effects include changing the processing of neurotransmitters, such as the way they are handled at the synapse. Nerve cells retain control of when the neurotransmitter is released, but it has a slightly stronger or weaker effect.

283

Anesthetics

We take for granted that surgical procedures, both large and small, can be performed without pain or distress—thanks to anesthetics. But how does this medical miracle happen?

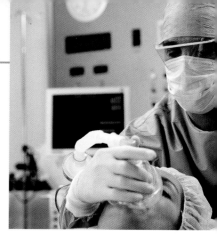

The word "anesthesia" comes from the Greek for "without feeling." The two categories of anesthetics—local and general—achieve this in completely different ways. Another class of drugs, analgesics, reduces the perception of pain without causing anesthesia (see pp. 286–7).

Blocking damage signals: local anesthetics

Local anesthetics act to block nerves from firing, including nociceptors—specialized nerve cells which signal tissue damage—so the brain has no "damage reports" to interpret as pain. They do this by preventing nerve impulses (action potentials), usually by disabling sodium channels. Novocaine, lignocaine, and even cocaine act in this way, although other methods such as ice and clove oil can prevent or reduce the frequency of action potentials as well.

↗ **Unlike sleep, general anesthesia shuts down large parts of the nervous system, requiring very careful monitoring to ensure patient safety.**

Blocking consciousness: general anesthetics

General anesthetics are consciousness blockers. Under a general anesthetic, most nerve cells function quite normally, reporting damage and other sensory events, but the person is unconscious and thus unable to interpret these reports, or feel anything. Doctors commonly use local anesthesia in combination with general anesthesia, to prevent reflexes triggered by surgical cuts, even though the unconscious patient would not object. Conversely, it is possible to perform brain surgery with just local anesthesia of the scalp, bone, and vessels, since the brain has no nociceptors. This is essential in testing functions during surgery, to make sure they are not damaged by the operation.

The range of chemical substances that act as general anesthetics is very broad, and includes solvents such as chloroform and ether, the inert gas xenon, and drugs thought to interact with neurotransmitter systems, such as barbiturates, ketamine, or propofol.

↓ **Pain depends on signals coming from nociceptors. Local anesthetics jam the mechanism that allows signals to travel along nerve fibers, stopping messages getting through. The anesthetic must be injected near the nerve fibers to successfully block them, although some ointments can deactivate surface receptors.**

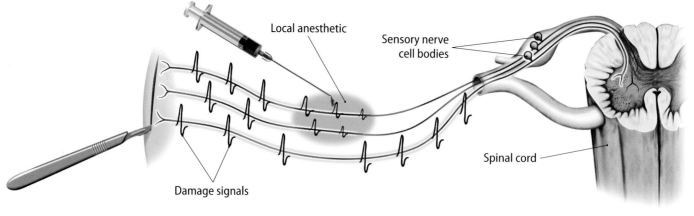

Local anesthetic

Sensory nerve cell bodies

Damage signals

Spinal cord

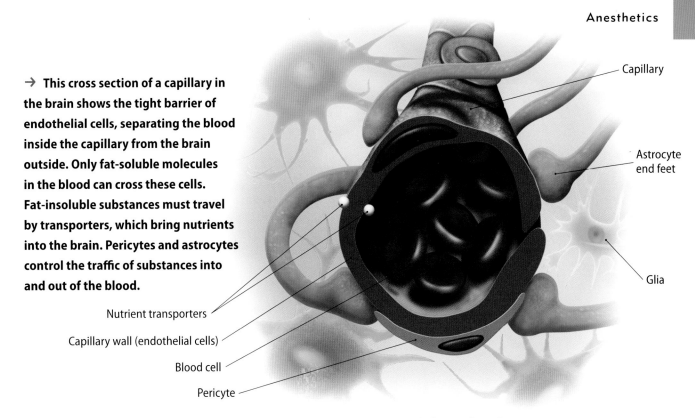

→ **This cross section of a capillary in the brain shows the tight barrier of endothelial cells, separating the blood inside the capillary from the brain outside. Only fat-soluble molecules in the blood can cross these cells. Fat-insoluble substances must travel by transporters, which bring nutrients into the brain. Pericytes and astrocytes control the traffic of substances into and out of the blood.**

Capillary

Astrocyte end feet

Glia

Nutrient transporters

Capillary wall (endothelial cells)

Blood cell

Pericyte

The only common factor is that they must be at least partly soluble in fat.

How general anesthesia works is still not fully understood. It may be that the same effect is achieved by different drugs in different ways, since there is no one explanation that accounts for the full range of substances which can produce general anesthesia. Despite these gaps in our knowledge, careful testing and widespread usage ensure the safety of anesthetics administered by specialist doctors.

Breaching the barrier

If a drug is fat soluble, it can dissolve through membranes and bypass the blood–brain barrier. Many psychoactive compounds (those that affect brain states) are fat-soluble molecules such as alcohol and delta-9-tetrahydrocannabinol (THC, an active component of cannabis). Heroin is a more fat-soluble form of morphine, so that when it is injected it readily crosses the blood–brain barrier to deliver a stronger dose more quickly. Other methods are under study to allow drugs to cross the barrier more easily.

The blood–brain barrier

Unless injected directly into the brain—which is sometimes done for specific, often life-saving reasons—drugs reach the nervous system via the bloodstream regardless of whether they are injected, inhaled, swallowed, or delivered by skin patches. Swallowed drugs are processed first by the liver, which is not the case for the other routes.

Every drug that affects the central nervous system (CNS), therefore, has to cross from the circulation to the CNS through the blood–brain barrier, a system of protective walls and cellular defenses surrounding every capillary in the brain. The CNS environment is a protected and insulated place, carefully maintained for the health of nerve cells and glia; substances passing in and out are subject to tight controls. Introduced substances have difficulty gaining access, and this is a major factor in designing drugs intended to act in the brain and spinal cord. Substances that affect nerve cells, but which cannot cross the blood–brain barrier, can affect peripheral nerves without affecting the brain. For example, beta-blockers, which mask many of adrenaline's effects during episodes of anxiety, can make people very drowsy (among other side effects) if they enter the brain in significant amounts. For this reason, most beta-blockers in use are relatively insoluble in fat.

Pain and analgesics

Pain is one of the most important, and difficult to treat, problems in medicine. Among current approaches to pain management, drugs are by far the most commonly used, and are often the most effective treatment.

The sensory nerve cells that mediate pain sensation are known as nociceptors. Nociception is the detection of tissue damage. Pain is the mental and emotional state that usually follows nociception, and may be acute (lasting no longer than its cause) or chronic (outlasting the initial injury and healing process). Analgesics are drugs that relieve pain. See pp. 152–5 for more information about pain and nociception.

The experience of pain
The experience of pain usually arises from nociception, which often results from tissue damage. Chronic pain states can sometimes alter the handling of sensory information in the spinal cord and the brain, so that the sensation of pain persists when the original nociceptive input is no longer active. Ordinary touch or pressure

may be interpreted as pain, or in the most severe cases, the central nervous system can generate the sensation of pain without requiring any input at all.

Drugs can interact with pain systems in many ways. Local anesthetics (see p. 284) can prevent nerve signaling by blocking nerve impulses (action potentials). Analgesics, discussed here, can act to block the chemical distress signals given off by damaged tissue, or they can impair the transmission of this information at synapses inside the nervous system.

Acetaminophen
Also known as paracetamol, acetaminophen (e.g., Tylenol, Panadol) is an antipyretic (fever reducer) and an analgesic, but even after 60 years of use, relatively little is known about how it works. There is evidence that it alters fever- and pain-related signaling in the hypothalamus, and its pain-relieving effects may be related to cannabinoid receptors (which also respond to the active compounds in cannabis). Although safe in recommended doses, acetaminophen in high doses generates a toxic byproduct which irreparably damages the liver.

Anti-inflammatories
Ibuprofen and aspirin are examples of anti-inflammatory drugs, which reduce inflammatory signaling by damaged cells. Ibuprofen (e.g., Advil, Nurofen) has its analgesic effect by interfering with pain-related signaling. Damaged and inflamed tissues produce chemical distress signals, which are detected by

← **Pain is an important signal of damage, and its cause should always be located and treated.**

Pain relief without drugs

Aside from liniments and massage, which clear chemical distress signals by increasing blood flow to injured tissues, there are other treatments for pain which do not use drugs. Transcutaneous electrical nerve stimulation (TENS) uses electric currents passing through the skin near the spinal cord in order to stimulate non-nociceptor nerve fibers, adding large quantities of sensory information in an attempt to mask nociceptor activity by flooding the spinal cord with stimuli. At the other extreme, hypnosis can detach a patient's mental state from the experience of pain, enabling surgery for people who are allergic to anesthetics.

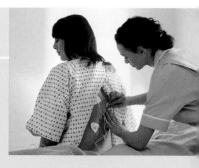

↑ **A TENS machine can help reduce the pain of childbirth.**

nociceptors and interpreted as pain by the brain. Analgesics impair the production of distress signals, which reduces the painful feeling and also reduces swelling, which can help injuries heal more quickly.

Like ibuprofen, aspirin impairs the production of chemical distress agents, reducing nociception and swelling. Aspirin's analgesic properties are particularly effective in some cases of migraine. This drug is increasingly used for its blood-thinning properties as a cardiovascular medication.

Other anti-inflammatory analgesic drugs have come into wider use, including indomethacin (e.g., Indocin), celecoxib (e.g., Celebrex), and diclofenac. Some are swallowed as tablets, but some can be applied as ointments that diffuse through the skin and concentrate the dose in the injured area. These anti-inflammatories aim to reduce the activation of nociceptors.

Codeine and other opiates

Opiates are drugs derived from the opium poppy. They interact with the receptor systems that regulate pain transmission and perception, as has been known for centuries—opium tinctures, and later codeine and morphine extracted from opium, were the first widely used potent analgesics. Opioids (synthetic opiates) vary in strength and addictive potential, but codeine is sufficiently mild that in some countries it is available without prescription in the "forte" or "extra strength" versions of common analgesics. Opioids are discussed further on pp. 298–9.

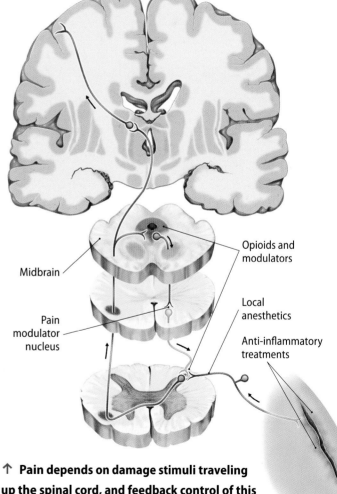

Midbrain

Pain modulator nucleus

Opioids and modulators

Local anesthetics

Anti-inflammatory treatments

↑ **Pain depends on damage stimuli traveling up the spinal cord, and feedback control of this signaling. Incoming stimuli trigger descending feedback to regulate how much signaling gets through (blue line), which opioids and other modulators can alter. Anesthetics and anti-inflammatories reduce the damage signaling coming in.**

Common medicines and the brain

Medical practitioners and the general public alike are able to draw on an impressive armory of medicines to treat both serious disease and everyday ailments. Some of these medicines affect the brain's functions, and a number of the most commonly used ones are described here.

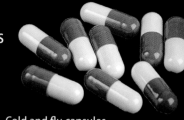

Cold and flu capsules

Drugs that restore or adjust the balance of chemicals and electrical impulses in the brain can be used to modify or control brain activity and to treat disorders of the central nervous system.

Benzodiazepines

Benzodiazepines (e.g., Valium and Midazolam) enhance the natural inhibition provided by the neurotransmitter GABA. They do this by boosting GABA receptors to provide a stronger effect. Different benzodiazepines affect different parts of the brain, so their effects may be sedative, anticonvulsant, calming, or dissociative (producing a sense of detachment from the real world), depending on the particular drug.

Because benzodiazepines share many of their effects with alcohol, they are often used to reduce the unpleasant effects of withdrawal in alcoholics. Their shared effects also mean that combining alcohol and benzodiazepines, or other sedatives, can have unpredictable, potent, and dangerous effects.

Hypnotics

Hypnotics are sedative drugs often used to treat insomnia. Although "hypnotic" means "causing sleep," they induce unconsciousness rather than sleep—meaning that they slow the person down enough for natural sleep cycles to begin.

Sedative-type benzodiazepines (e.g. Temazepam) are often used as hypnotics. Another common hypnotic is flunitrazepam (Rohypnol), which also boosts GABA action but by a different method. Rohypnol and similar drugs have been used illegally as so-called "date rape"

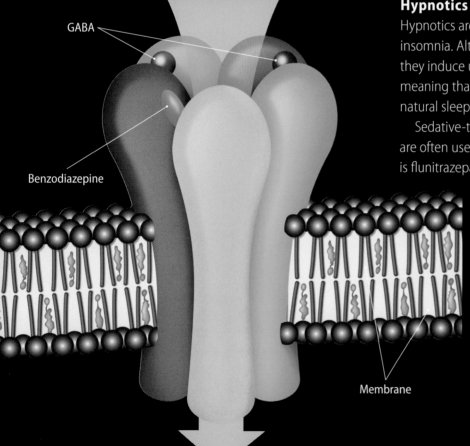

GABA

Benzodiazepine

Membrane

← **Molecules of the neurotransmitter GABA slot into sites on each GABA receptor in the synapse, thereby opening a channel in the membrane. Benzodiazepines, whose molecules have their own sites on GABA receptors, boost the calming effect of GABA.**

drugs when they are surreptitiously added to alcoholic drinks. The effects of the hypnotic feel like alcohol at first, but go on to cause loss of consciousness and memory. Because of this abuse, most hypnotics are now supplied in tablets that are hard to dissolve, and contain dyes that strongly color any drink to which they are added.

Anxiolytics

Anxiolytics are drugs that reduce anxiety. They include benzodiazepines (e.g., Xanax, Valium, Klonopin, Librium, and Ativan), and drugs with similar effects, such as zolpidem (Stilnox and Ambien). Anxiolytics particularly affect the cerebral cortex and the amygdala, a stress-related structure in the brain. Midazolam, a dissociative

benzodiazepine, is often used for unpleasant but harmless medical procedures, and suspends the formation of new memories so that a patient can comply with a colonoscopy, for example, but have no recollection of it afterward.

Antihistamines

Antihistamines (e.g., Benadryl in the USA) are intended to damp down allergic flare-ups caused by histamine release in the immune system throughout the body. However, histamine is also used as a neurotransmitter in the brain, where it helps to keep the cortex awake. Some antihistamines leak in through the hypothalamus, where the blood–brain barrier is slightly open, and can affect this system, causing drowsiness. Most current antihistamine drugs were chosen for marketing because they lack this effect, but individual responses are quite variable, and it is always a good idea to check the effects of an unfamiliar antihistamine before doing anything potentially hazardous like driving.

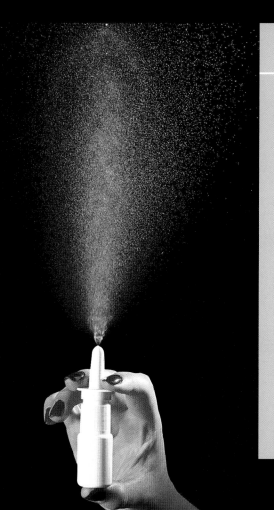

↓ **Antihistamines may alter alertness if they reach the brain. Spraying them directly into the nose can limit unwanted side effects.**

The placebo effect

Among all the challenges of understanding a drug's effect, one of the most important is the complex interaction between the nervous system and every other system of the body. If a drug is *perceived* as being effective, this is often a significant factor in the benefits it provides. This ability to treat by persuasion is called the placebo effect and forms a component of any treatment— and is sometimes deliberately engaged by prescribing harmless medications, which are also called placebos. Often, to scientifically demonstrate that a medication is effective, researchers must show that it has a significantly greater effect than a placebo.

The human nervous system is highly self-regulated and actively resists manipulation of neurotransmission and other functions, so disentangling placebo, drug, and self-regulatory effects is very difficult, and often irrelevant when deciding if a drug is worthwhile. A drug that triggers a helpful placebo response without harmful side effects could be viewed as beneficial, even if it has little pharmacological action.

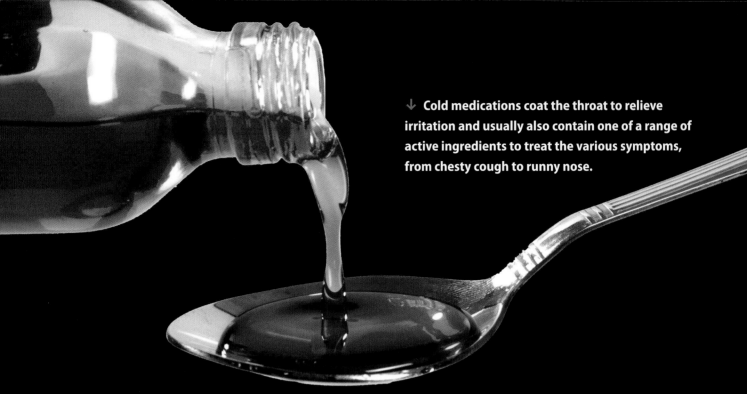

Cold medications coat the throat to relieve irritation and usually also contain one of a range of active ingredients to treat the various symptoms, from chesty cough to runny nose.

Cold and sinus medications

Many medications for colds and flu contain drugs such as pseudoephedrine (Sudafed) and phenylephrine (Sudafed PE), which reduce the secretion of mucus in the nasal cavity by reducing blood supply to the membranes. Although it is more effective as a decongestant, pseudoephedrine can be used to manufacture illegal amphetamines, and lawmakers have therefore made it less widely available. Pseudo-ephedrine itself is a stimulant of the central nervous system, and may disrupt sleep if used later in the day. For this reason antihistamines are often used to alleviate cold symptoms at night.

Antidepressants and antipsychotics

Depression and other mental illnesses are relatively common, and medication is a common treatment approach. Antidepressants are drugs that alleviate depression; antipsychotic drugs reduce many of the symptoms of schizophrenia and bipolar disorder, among other mental illnesses.

The range of antidepressant and antipsychotic medications is very broad, and they operate by very different mechanisms, which are incompletely under-stood. Responses to these medications are highly individual, and a prescription that is safe and effective for one person might be detrimental and dangerous to someone else. A range of side effects can be expected

when trying to adjust the subtleties of cognition and mood, and there is often a long period of frustration on the part of the patient in finding an effective medication with tolerable side effects. Most such medications take several weeks to reach their full effectiveness, due to gradual adjustment processes in the brain.

Drugs for epilepsy and other seizures

Epilepsy, as well as the aftermath of brain surgery, injury, or infections, can make individuals prone to seizures. These may be partial or generalized, affecting part or all of the brain respec-tively. Seizure activity in the brain can be detected by electroencephalography (EEG), and exhibits characteristic patterns for each type of seizure. Generalized seizures may involve convulsions or synchronous movements of the body, whereas absence seizures cause people to abruptly lose awareness of their surroundings, stare for several seconds, then resume normal behavior. Epilepsy is mainly treated by drugs, although in some cases surgery or deep brain stimulation may be effective. In some types of childhood epilepsy, dietary changes may be effective.

The drugs used to control seizures generally work via three mechanisms: enhancement of the inhibitory neurotransmitter GABA; inhibition of sodium channels, which slows the firing of nerve cells; or inhibition of calcium channel function. Some drugs also dampen the actions of the excitatory neurotransmitter glutamate. Many antiseizure drugs have side effects, including drowsiness or lack of mental clarity, and there is a lot of research aimed at developing better drugs. Some antiepileptic drugs are also used for anxiety disorders or bipolar disorder, due to their mood-stabilizing actions.

↓ **This EEG recording shows the major disruption to the brain caused by an epileptic seizure. The delicate balance between excitation and inhibition in the brain is difficult to control with medication.**

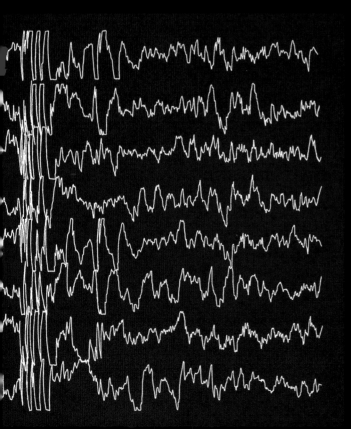

↓ **St. John's wort flowers are made into remedies to alleviate minor depression and anxiety.**

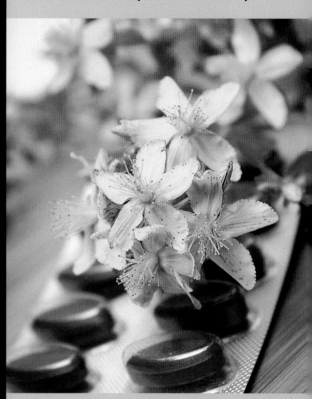

Herbal medicines

Many herbal extracts and preparations are sold by supermarkets and drugstores as alternative treatments for a range of health issues. Some, such as St. John's wort, have shown measurable effects when subjected to scientific trials, while others are essentially foods with no established effect on disease. Many people assume that products derived from natural sources such as plants are beneficial, but many plant-derived compounds are toxic, and evolved to harm animals that might otherwise eat those plants.

It is important to seek good quality advice about herbal medicines before taking them. This includes talking to medical professionals and seeking peer-reviewed evidence rather than relying on the manufacturer's or retailer's claims, or Internet hearsay.

Addiction

Drug addiction is often defined as physical and psychological dependence on a drug. This dependence causes drug-seeking to alter or replace the priorities of normal behavior, so that the addicted person's free will is compromised by meeting an artificial need.

In order to survive, we need motivation to seek out things we need, such as food, shelter, and safety. The motivational system in the nervous system is used to create behaviors that meet our needs. For example, dehydration will cause us to seek drinking water as a matter of urgency.

Drugs that interfere with this motivation system end up altering our behavior patterns, replacing survival behavior with drug-seeking behavior. The latter can be a mild preference or can build up to the point where safety and genuine needs are ignored. This harmful state of drug-seeking is referred to as addiction, but it is difficult to precisely define.

What is addiction?

The concept of addiction is a subjective one. One person's manageable habit, or personal freedom, may seem like chronic drug abuse to another person, and the various psychological and psychiatric professional bodies offer a range of definitions. However, a person may be said to be addicted to a drug if the drug use has a negative impact on their health or social life, and the person is unable to reduce their drug intake despite a desire to do so.

Addiction is usually considered to involve both psychological and physical dependency. Physical dependence arises as the user's body adapts to the

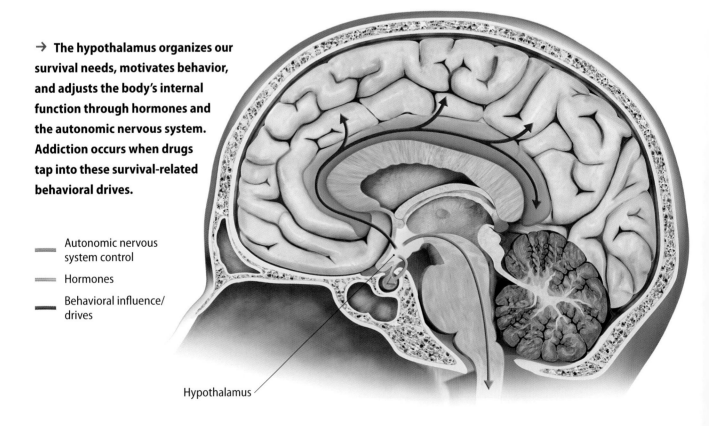

→ **The hypothalamus organizes our survival needs, motivates behavior, and adjusts the body's internal function through hormones and the autonomic nervous system. Addiction occurs when drugs tap into these survival-related behavioral drives.**

—— Autonomic nervous system control

—— Hormones

—— Behavioral influence/ drives

Hypothalamus

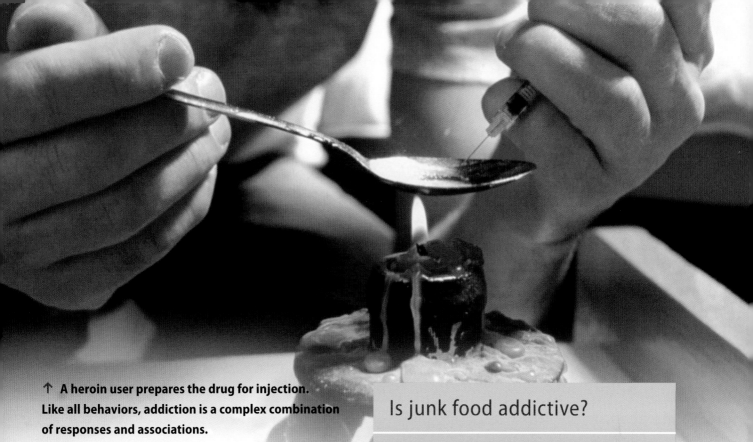

↑ **A heroin user prepares the drug for injection. Like all behaviors, addiction is a complex combination of responses and associations.**

repeated use of the drug, a process called tolerance—a need to continually increase the dose to obtain the original effect. Psychological dependence refers to a user's belief that they cannot cope without the drug, and may occur without physical dependence.

Treatment and causes

Because the nervous system exists to enhance our survival, these reward and motivation pathways are woven deeply into every function: for example, our sensory perception is affected by our current needs, such as noticing water more when we are thirsty. This makes addiction a very difficult problem to treat, and makes it difficult to study as well. In addition, the excess consumption characteristic of drug addiction has a significant effect on the neurotransmitter systems involved, so that treating the addiction may involve restoring receptor systems to normal, as well as changing behavioral motivation.

The factors underpinning drug addiction are complex. Whether a person is vulnerable depends on their genetic makeup, mental health, family support, and environment, as well as the specific qualities of the drug itself.

Is junk food addictive?

The satisfaction of eating when you are hungry is a powerful reward. Some foods are particularly pleasurable (e.g., chocolate, or fatty foods) and we seek them out at times of stress. This can lead to eating habits which closely resemble drug addiction, and share the same biological circuitry. Dopamine, one of the strongest signals of pleasure involved in these behaviors, performs a similar role in obesity and drug addiction. Excessive intake of foods high in fats and sugars follows a classic addiction pattern: an inability to reduce consumption despite a strong desire to do so, maintaining the habit despite negative health and social consequences, and an unpleasant withdrawal-type feeling when unable to consume. Although this view is controversial, the difficulties and cravings of overweight people trying to lose weight resemble those of drug users attempting to control their habit. Dietary patterns established during times of stress become increasingly difficult to shake, and temporary relief often requires increasing levels of intake.

293

Alcohol

Along with nicotine and caffeine, alcohol is one of the most widely used, socially acceptable drugs. Arguably, of all drugs, it has the highest levels of abuse.

Alcohol has complex effects on the nervous system and other parts of the body, ranging from metabolic to mental. In the central nervous system, most alcohol effects are thought to be due to its influence on inhibition of the neurotransmitter GABA, which affects the brain much more than the spinal cord. Some of the brain's GABA receptors are more alcohol-susceptible than others, and those that are most affected are in the frontal cortex and the cerebellum.

→ **The effects of alcohol change with increasing consumption, from euphoria to depression.**

Effects on the brain

Boosting inhibition in the frontal cortex reduces our ability to plan for, and worry about, the future—which is the reason that people enjoy consuming alcohol and find it relaxing. This impairs judgment and decision making, so that people may behave more freely without considering the consequences.

At higher doses the cerebellum loses its ability to fine-tune our movements, and coordination is affected. The combination of distorted judgment and impaired coordination is particularly serious for driving, which requires both abilities, hence the legal restrictions about alcohol consumption levels for driving.

Alcohol in the bloodstream also diffuses into the fluid canals of the inner ear, altering its density and causing the fluid to circulate, which is interpreted by the vestibular system and brain as an unpleasant spinning sensation, which triggers nausea and a loss of balance. At higher doses, alcohol has a much wider depressant effect on the nervous system, causing unconsciousness and even death at very high blood levels.

Hangovers

Alcohol acts as a diuretic and impairs water absorption in the gut, so the tissues become dehydrated. When the brain becomes dehydrated, it shrinks slightly, which is thought to put tension on the blood vessels crossing

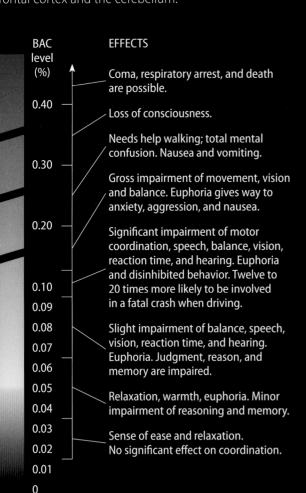

BAC level (%)	EFFECTS
0.40	Coma, respiratory arrest, and death are possible.
	Loss of consciousness.
0.30	Needs help walking; total mental confusion. Nausea and vomiting.
	Gross impairment of movement, vision and balance. Euphoria gives way to anxiety, aggression, and nausea.
0.20	
	Significant impairment of motor coordination, speech, balance, vision, reaction time, and hearing. Euphoria and disinhibited behavior. Twelve to 20 times more likely to be involved in a fatal crash when driving.
0.10	
0.09	
0.08	Slight impairment of balance, speech, vision, reaction time, and hearing. Euphoria. Judgment, reason, and memory are impaired.
0.07	
0.06	
0.05	Relaxation, warmth, euphoria. Minor impairment of reasoning and memory.
0.04	
0.03	Sense of ease and relaxation. No significant effect on coordination.
0.02	
0.01	
0	

← **The amount of alcohol in a person's body is measured by the blood alcohol content (BAC). The table shows the effects of alcohol typically associated with rising levels of BAC.**

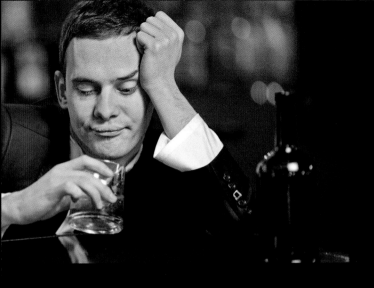

How much can I drink safely?

Medical authorities suggest that consuming no more than two standard drinks on any day reduces the lifetime risk of harm from alcohol-related disease or injury. Drinking large amounts of alcohol in a short space of time can cause greater harm, and it is therefore also recommended to limit intake to four standard drinks on a single occasion.

It is important to realize that safe limits for alcohol intake vary significantly between individuals, and depend strongly on health and other lifestyle and genetic factors. You should consult your doctor for advice that is specific to your own situation.

from the inside of the skull to the brain surface. The brain itself has no nociceptors, but these stretched vessels generate strong sensations of pain and produce the headache effect of an alcohol hangover. In addition, toxic metabolic byproducts of processing a large amount of alcohol, together with other compounds in alcoholic beverages, can linger.

Alcohol dependency

Alcohol dependence is worsened over time by

Coffee and cigarettes

Caffeine (in coffee) and nicotine (in cigarettes) are common "everyday drugs." Although moderate caffeine consumption is safe, smoking cigarettes has a range of potentially deadly consequences.

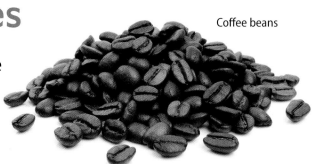

Coffee beans

Breaking the nicotine habit

Nicotine is extremely addictive due to its direct actions on reward systems. Quitting smoking is very difficult, because the behavior is driven by a deeper level of priority setting than rational, logical thought can provide. Although there are a range of therapies which aim to reduce the withdrawal experience by using sustained low doses (nicotine patches) or delivering nicotine via less damaging means (nicotine gum), they can only alleviate the instant discomfort of stopping nicotine intake. The far more complex problem of habit remains: reward systems are used to shape behavior to meet needs, and years of artificially stimulating them with nicotine causes smoking-related behaviors to become deeply ingrained and important to the smoker. The brain is literally wired to seek nicotine, and long after withdrawal effects are eased, it may feel wrong not to smoke, and the desire remains.

Champix, a blocker of nicotinic receptors, has been used to help smokers to quit, although it is associated with a range of side effects related to reducing acetylcholine effects on the brain and the autonomic nervous system.

Caffeine is found in many foods apart from coffee, including tea, soft drinks (especially cola drinks), and chocolate. It has a range of psychoactive and metabolic effects on the body, which are probably due to its blocking of adenosine receptors in the brain. These receptors normally slightly depress brain activity, so blocking them can increase feelings of alertness and clarity of thought. However, excessive caffeine can cause mental confusion and agitation, as well as placing the cardiovascular system under stress.

The effects of caffeine persist for long periods. Caffeine's half-life in the body is five hours or more, meaning that half the dose is still active after that period of time. A coffee consumed in the afternoon can therefore disrupt sleep hours later.

→ **The habit of smoking tobacco, a North American native plant, has spread throughout the world. One in ten adult deaths worldwide is caused by tobacco.**

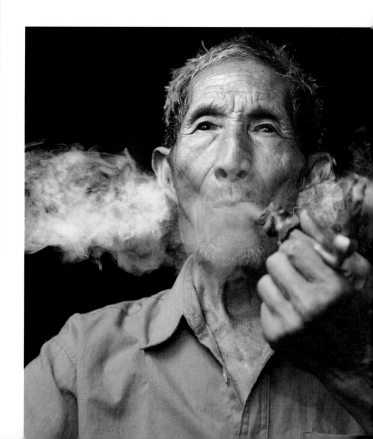

→ **Reward pathways make us feel good when we engage in behaviors that help survival. A pathway from the ventral tegmental area via the nucleus accumbens stirs the cortex to come up with behaviors to meet our needs (purple arrows). When needs are met, the cortex signals back to indicate satiety (lighter arrow). Septal nuclei may also be activated if this is a pleasurable outcome and something we want to do again. Nicotine tampers directly with these pathways, making it strongly addictive.**

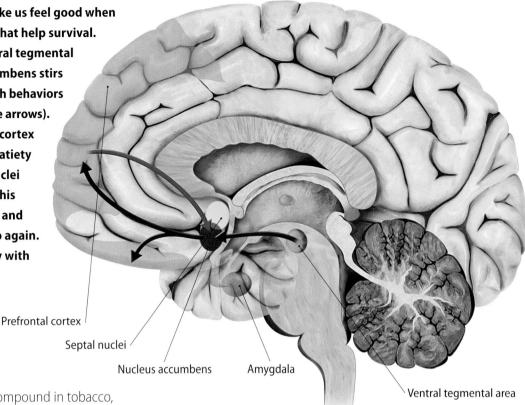

Prefrontal cortex

Septal nuclei

Nucleus accumbens

Amygdala

Ventral tegmental area

Nicotine

The main psychoactive compound in tobacco, nicotine, has been used for centuries. It is a central nervous system stimulant but has a calming effect on chronic users. Nicotine activates an acetylcholine receptor regulating alertness as well as muscular control and regulation of the internal organs, and which directly activates nerve cells in the main reward pathways of the nervous system. Other compounds in tobacco interfere with the breakdown of neurotransmitters such as dopamine and serotonin, producing sensations of pleasure and contributing to its addictive properties.

Chronic, addicted smokers have highly adapted dopamine systems with a particular sensitivity for the effects of nicotine. A dose of nicotine activates the dopamine terminals of the brain, but the receptors involved become desensitized in about the length of time it takes to smoke a cigarette. Once they resensitize, the smoker needs another dose in order to block the unpleasant feelings (withdrawal) that this resensitization produces; this is also pleasurable due to dopamine release, which reinforces the habit. A single dose of nicotine is enough to begin this adaptation process, causing changes in nicotine receptor levels which persist for several weeks.

→ **Nicotine is the cause of tobacco addiction. Other toxic compounds in tobacco cause the cancers and severe lung damage (pictured) that kill smokers.**

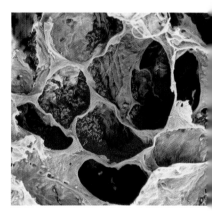

Nicotinic receptors are used by the body's main control systems, including movement and the control of internal organs by the autonomic nervous system. These systems are quite well shielded from ingested nicotine, but the collections of nerve cell bodies (ganglia) of the parasympathetic nervous system can be influenced by smoking. This produces a range of calmative effects on bodily organs.

Smoking is one of the worst things you can do for your health. Among its most common ill effects are cancers of the mouth, throat, and lungs, and severe damage to the cardiovascular system.

Drugs of abuse: opioids and barbiturates

Opiates and related drugs, which affect pain- and pleasure-related systems, are frequently abused for their pleasurable effects. In high doses, opiates suppress the activity of important life-support systems in the brainstem, which can easily be fatal. Barbiturates, another class of depressant, affect inhibitory systems of the brain in a manner somewhat like alcohol.

A range of neurotransmitters such as endorphins, enkephalins, and dynorphins, known collectively as endogenous opioids, are used by the central nervous system to control the perception of damage and pain. Opioids can block the synaptic signaling of nociception and also have a powerful effect on the perception of pain that usually results from nociception. This is useful in normal function, for example to suppress pain during times of stressful demand. Such effects are normally controlled by the nervous system, but they can also be artificially activated by drugs.

Opioids hit the right spot
The best known of these drugs are opiates, which are extracted from the sap of the opium poppy, and opioids, which are chemical modifications of opiates, or may be made entirely artificially, such as methadone, pethidine (Demerol), and fentanyl. The most commonly

↓ **Farmers in Afghanistan harvest opium—the dried sap of the poppy *Papaver somniferum*—which has been used medicinally for thousands of years.**

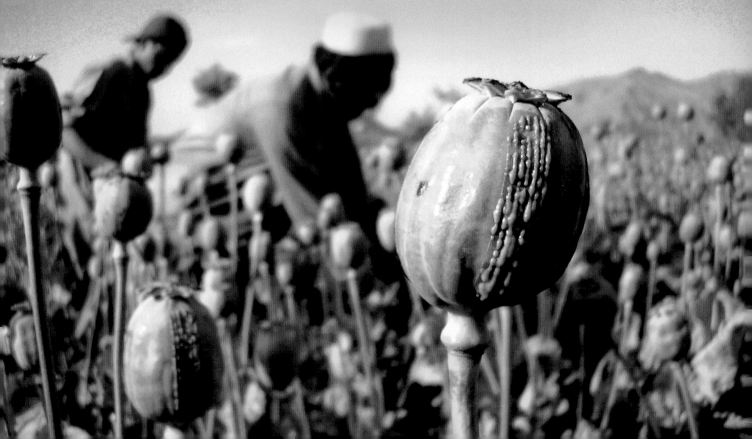

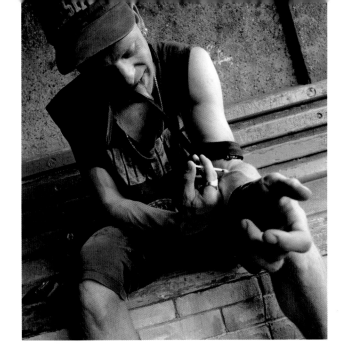

← Many opiates have such powerfully addictive qualities that addicts will tolerate drastic compromises to health, morals, and relationships to continue using.

Like endogenous opioids, opiates have an analgesic (pain-killing) effect by blunting the transmission of damage reports in the nervous system, so that painful sensations become milder or are abolished. Although they are used medically for blocking pain, many opioids also produce feelings of euphoria or well-being, and thus have a strong addictive potential. They also cause changes to the opioid receptor system that produces tolerance, a requirement for higher doses to produce the same effect. This escalating usage makes them dangerous, since overdoses impair breathing.

The search for opioids able to block pain without euphoria, tolerance, or addictive potential is a major goal of the pharmaceutical industry, and finding them would be of great significance in the treatment of pain. As things stand, the prescription and sale of strong opioids is closely monitored.

abused opiate drugs are morphine (MS Contin) and codeine, along with opioid derivatives such as heroin, oxycodone (OxyContin), and hydrocodone. These drugs can be taken orally, which often involves modification by the liver (converting heroin to morphine, for example), or by a range of methods which bypass the liver. Many can be injected, either below the skin or intravenously, and some, such as heroin, can be vaporized for inhalation or snorted for absorption by the linings of the nose.

What are narcotics?

Some people refer to illegal drugs in general as "narcotics," but strictly speaking the term means "causing drowsiness"—so by this definition, opioids and barbiturates are narcotics, and amphetamines (a stimulant) are not. Drug laws have used varying definitions of "narcotic" over the years. For example, cocaine's anesthetic effects were considered to cause numbness, a narcotic effect, when the 1970 US Controlled Substances Act was drafted. However, its main effect is as a stimulant, which is contrary to the previous definition. Such contradictions make "narcotic" an unhelpful term, and it is clearer to refer to drugs by specific type.

Barbiturates

Another frequently used depressant drug class is barbiturates, although these are now much less common than opioid drugs. Drugs such as Nembutal and Seconal, when injected or swallowed in pill form, act at GABA receptors, as does alcohol, and have alcohol-like effects on mood and nervous system function. Since their dosage is often by tablet or injection, the dose is harder to subjectively gauge than is consuming alcohol by drinking. This increases the risk of overdose by suppressing respiration.

→ Barbiturates were once commonly prescribed for insomnia and anxiety, but have fallen from favor because they are habit-forming and, in larger doses, can result in a fatal overdose.

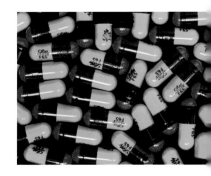

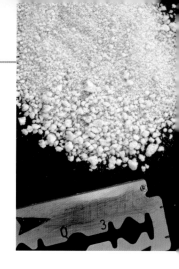

Drugs of abuse: stimulants

Depending on the type and strength of the particular substance, stimulants generally make you more alert and active, help you stay awake, reduce hunger, and elevate mood.

Legal stimulants include caffeine and nicotine, and ephedrine, which is an ingredient in some medicines used for respiratory conditions. Illegal stimulants include cocaine, crack, and amphetamines such as ecstasy, "ice," and methamphetamine.

Cocaine

Cocaine has potent effects on the brain's dopamine, adrenaline, and serotonin systems, which give it a strongly exciting and pleasurable effect, as well as placing considerable stress on the cardiovascular system. Its effects are so powerful that these neurotransmitter systems are forced to readjust to abnormal levels of stimulation, so that chronic intake alters the resting state of the brain and the user may not feel normal without regular use.

↗ **Illegal amphetamines are contaminated with impurities, producing the pink color seen here. Razor blades are used to break the crystals into powder.**

Typically ingested by "snorting" up the nose, cocaine is directly absorbed into the bloodstream by the membranes of the nasal cavity. It can also be injected after dissolving in water, either alone or to alter the effects of another drug in the mixture. When such mixtures allow one drug to mask the effects of another (e.g., cocaine can reduce the drowsiness caused by heroin), the possibility of an overdose is greatly increased.

Crack is a chemical modification of cocaine, which allows it to vaporize for inhalation and rapid absorption in the lungs, producing similar effects to cocaine with a very fast onset. As for heroin, the speed of onset is linked to its highly addictive qualities.

Amphetamines

These drugs and related compounds ("ice," ecstasy, and methamphetamine) have potent effects on many of the modulatory neurotransmitters that affect mood and reward. Their effects on attention, wakefulness, and focus have been used by armed forces and professions such as transport drivers, but their pleasurable effects led to widespread abuse and subsequent prohibition.

Some drugs derived from amphetamines, such as "crystal meth" (also called "ice"), are modified chemically

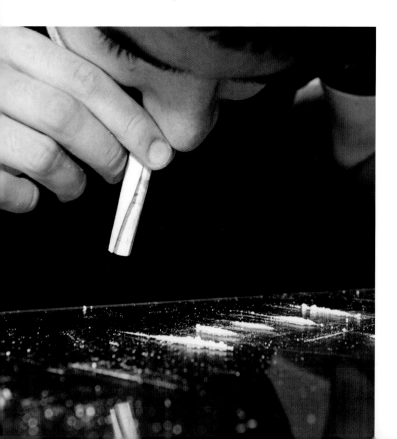

← **Snorting drugs places them in direct contact with the blood-rich membranes inside the nasal cavity, allowing rapid delivery to the brain.**

ADHD medication: prescription use and growing abuse

The widespread diagnosis of attention deficit hyperactivity disorder (ADHD) has led in many cases to the prescription of stimulant drugs such as methylphenidate (Ritalin) and dexedrine/amphetamine mixtures (Adderall) with the aim of improving children's mental focus. The notion of giving stimulants to hyperactive children may seem contradictory, but it is theorized that disruptive behavior results from an inability to concentrate, which is often improved by these stimulant drugs. The nervous system is adjusting and adapting its neurotransmitter systems throughout development, and it is a matter of concern that the regular doses of stimulants will affect this maturation. The adult consequences of this are not well understood.

The widespread availability of these drugs has also led to abuse, most notably by students seeking mental performance enhancement, but also as recreational stimulants. In this context, the negative effects of these drugs become significant, including cardiovascular stress and severe sleep disruption, which may cause delusional thinking.

to allow them to vaporize when heated, allowing absorption by the lungs and rapid delivery of drug effects, which contributes strongly to their addictive potential. These forms are usually inhaled by heating in a glass pipe to vaporize the drug. Other amphetamines can be taken orally as pills, or injected by dissolving in water. Amphetamine-type compounds have strong tolerance effects when abused, and may also produce psychotic states. They also affect thermoregulation, so that ecstasy taken in a hot environment such as a nightclub can lead to dehydration, which can be fatal. Chronic abuse of amphetamine-related drugs can also damage the circulatory system, including the heart, and placental blood vessels during pregnancy.

→ **Dopamine, a powerful signal of significance and excitement in the brain, is sent from one nerve cell to another at synapses. Amphetamines and cocaine alter the amount of dopamine in synapses, either by stimulating release (amphetamines) or preventing reuptake deactivation (cocaine), producing powerful effects on users' mental and emotional states.**

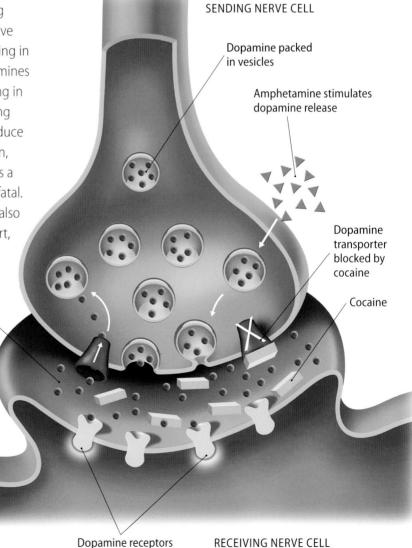

SENDING NERVE CELL

Dopamine packed in vesicles

Amphetamine stimulates dopamine release

Dopamine transporter blocked by cocaine

Cocaine

Dopamine transporter functioning normally

Dopamine receptors

RECEIVING NERVE CELL

Other commonly abused drugs

Cannabis and LSD are among the chemical substances abused for the variety of pleasurable effects they produce. Some medical drugs, such as anesthetics and cough medicines, also have properties that make them attractive for non-medical use.

Dozens of chemical substances—some of them legal and widely available—are used recreationally. Many have serious effects on the mind and body, especially if used heavily over a long period.

Cannabis

The term "cannabis" refers to leaves or other extracts of the hemp plant, *Cannabis sativa*; the active constituents are delta-9-tetrahydrocannabinol (THC) and cannabidiol. The dried leaves and flower buds (marijuana) can be smoked or eaten, while hashish, the extracted resin, can be inhaled by vaporization, added to tobacco cigarettes, or incorporated into food and eaten. Preparations of cannabis contain a range of related cannabinoid chemicals.

The main effects of cannabinoids are euphoria, relaxation, and pain relief, but they also significantly impair memory and motor coordination. Smoking cannabis also poses serious health risks similar to tobacco smoking.

Hallucinogens

Lysergic acid diethylamide (LSD) has strong effects on serotonin neurotransmission in the cortex, producing vivid hallucinations and emotional responses. Effective doses of LSD are extremely small (users only need a few

micrograms) and it is usually taken by direct absorption in the mouth or the eye as drops of LSD solution, or on pieces of paper which have absorbed such a solution and dried out. The effects of the drug are strongly subjective, and some LSD users have "bad trips"—acute panic or paranoid reactions. On the other hand, LSD is so potent that the potential for contamination with other substances (a common risk for other illegal drugs) is very low.

Psilocybin, mescaline, and dimethyltryptamine (DMT) are hallucinogens found in high concentrations in mushrooms, cacti, and leafy plants respectively. Each compound affects many neurotransmitter systems, but all involve some interaction with serotonin systems.

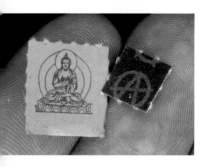

← **Effective doses of LSD are only a few micrograms, and can be absorbed in sheets of paper like these.**

Cannabis in the medicine cabinet

Of the two active constituents of cannabis, the majority of the psychotropic (mind-altering) and painkilling effects of the drug are due to delta-9-tetrahydrocannabinol (THC), whereas cannabidiol is potently effective against nausea, insomnia, anxiety, and inflammation, and can be used clinically in treating these ailments. For this reason, therapeutic cannabis (also called medical marijuana) has been decriminalized in some countries and US states. Synthetic cannabinoid drugs are also under development and evaluation in the hope of separating therapeutic from psychotropic effects more cleanly.

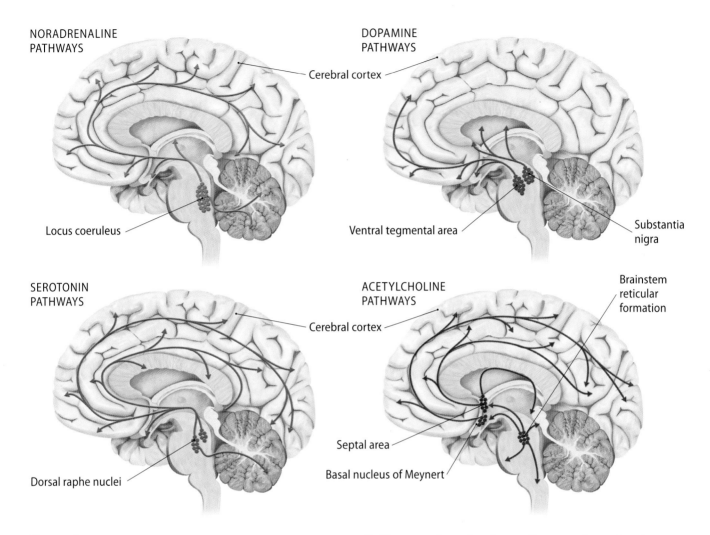

NORADRENALINE PATHWAYS

Cerebral cortex

Locus coeruleus

DOPAMINE PATHWAYS

Cerebral cortex

Ventral tegmental area

Substantia nigra

SEROTONIN PATHWAYS

Cerebral cortex

Dorsal raphe nuclei

ACETYLCHOLINE PATHWAYS

Brainstem reticular formation

Septal area

Basal nucleus of Meynert

Ketamine

The primary action of ketamine, a general anesthetic, is at the NMDA receptor, where it disrupts the brain's excitatory transmission in a way that strongly alters perceived reality, referred to as a dissociative state. For this reason it is abused, usually by injection into a muscle, but whether such abuse can develop into drug dependence is subject to debate.

Dextromethorphan

Some cough medicines contain dextromethorphan (e.g., Robitussin DM), which suppresses coughing by blocking irritating sensations from the throat. At far higher doses, dextromethorphan causes dissociation and halluci-nations (among other side effects), and is commonly abused for that reason. Although dextromethorphan is a chemical derivative of synthetic opioids, its action is more similar to ketamine than opioids.

↑ **Many psychoactive drugs affect emotion-related neurotransmitter systems—which have widespread effects on the cerebral cortex—involving serotonin, noradrenaline, dopamine, and acetylcholine.**

Anabolic steroids

Anabolic steroids are synthetic hormones that cause the body to build muscle, which is why they are often abused by athletes. In addition to their effects (and serious side effects) on the body, these steroids are fat soluble and cross the blood–brain barrier. Like normal sex hormones, they can affect behavior, and do so in a much more concentrated and noticeable way when taken in high doses. Chronic abuse is linked to aggression, violent behavior, and depression, although the personalities of people likely to abuse these drugs are also a factor in this link.

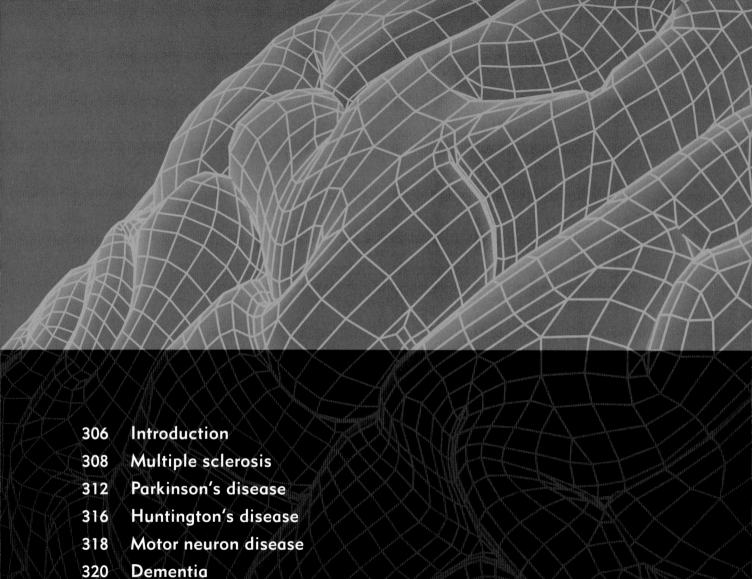

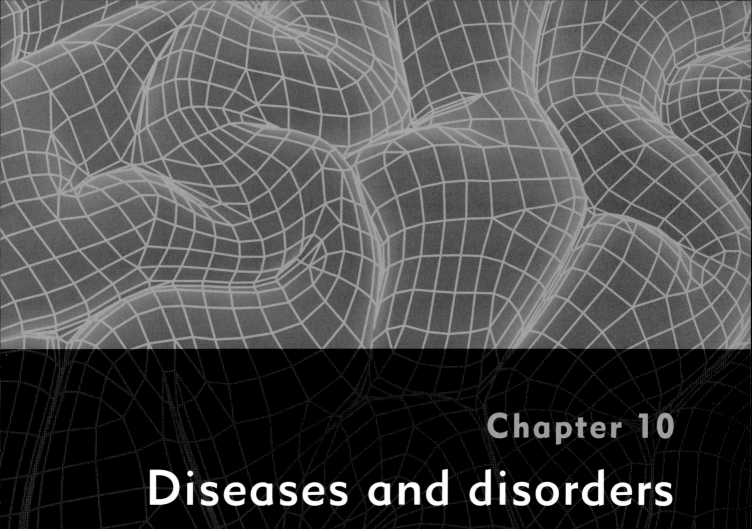

Chapter 10

Diseases and disorders

Introduction

Diseases and disorders of the brain may cause anything from mild intellectual disability, to gradual loss of function over many years, to sudden death. Those brain diseases arising from degenerative or inflammatory changes of the brain and its blood vessels, which get worse with increasing age, are a major cause of health costs and disability.

Diseases of the brain may be developmental or acquired. Developmental diseases arise from either abnormal developmental processes or damaging factors in the environment during uterine or early postnatal life. Acquired diseases are caused by adverse events during maturity. In fact, most brain diseases arise from a combination of causes including genes, lifestyle, and environmental factors.

Delirium

Abnormal brain function usually arises from internal abnormalities, but the brain is so dependent on the rest of the body for oxygen, nutrients, and hormonal support that anything that alters the function of the cardiovascular, respiratory, endocrine, and urinary systems can also have profound effects on brain function. This is particularly striking in delirium, a disordered mental state consisting of confusion, distorted sensations, disorientation, fears, hallucinations, excitement, and restlessness. It is often seen in fever, alcohol or drug withdrawal, head trauma, and in the elderly with cardiorespiratory problems.

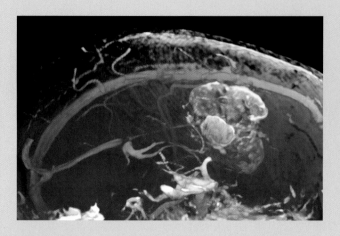

↑ **This colored 3-D MRI image shows a large glioma (orange), a type of central nervous system tumor that arises from glial cells. About half of all primary brain tumors are gliomas.**

Infection and autoimmune disease

The brain and spinal cord have such a delicate internal structure that they enjoy a privileged position behind a blood–brain barrier that makes it difficult for immune system cells and molecules to reach the brain interior. Sometimes invasive microorganisms from outside the body (viruses, bacteria, fungi, and parasites), or the abnormally hyperactive cells of the body's immune system, penetrate this barrier. A particularly devastating group of brain infections called the spongiform encephalopathies (including "mad cow disease" and Creutzfeldt–Jakob) is caused by a type of abnormal protein (prion) that may be ingested by eating meat from diseased animals, or introduced into the brain because of inadequate sterilization of neurosurgical instruments. When the body's own immune defenses damage the white matter of the brain and spinal cord, the result is the disabling disease called multiple sclerosis.

Strokes

A sudden loss of function due to changes in the blood supply to the brain is called a stroke. In developed countries, stroke affects 110 to 250 people per 100,000 each year and it causes between 12 and 14 percent of all deaths. The chance of stroke increases rapidly with advancing age, doubling for every decade of life after age 55. More than three quarters of stroke victims are over 65 years of age. Any one incident of stroke is a serious medical emergency: about a third of strokes result in death and about one fifth lead to permanent institutional care.

Degenerative brain diseases

Degenerative brain diseases have symptoms that develop slowly and progress continuously over months or years. Broadly, these diseases can be separated according to the main site affected: those affecting the cerebral cortex (primarily dementias like Alzheimer's disease and frontotemporal dementia); those affecting the basal ganglia and/or midbrain (Huntington's disease, progressive supranuclear palsy, Parkinson's disease); or those affecting the motor nerve cells of the brainstem and spinal cord (motor neuron disease).

Tumors

A tumor is simply a lump of cells, but we often use the word to mean either a benign growth or a malignant cancer. Malignant tumors that arise in the brain (primary brain cancers) are usually the result of glial cells dividing out of control and invading the surrounding brain tissue. The factors that cause these gliomas to develop are poorly understood. The rich blood supply to the brain means that any tumor cells circulating from cancer starting in other organs are likely to lodge in the brain and cause secondary cancers.

↓ **Age-related degenerative brain diseases are characterized by the accumulation of neurofibrillary tangles inside nerve cells; while outside, amyloid plaques can cause loss of nerve cells, degeneration of axons, and decay of their myelin sheaths.**

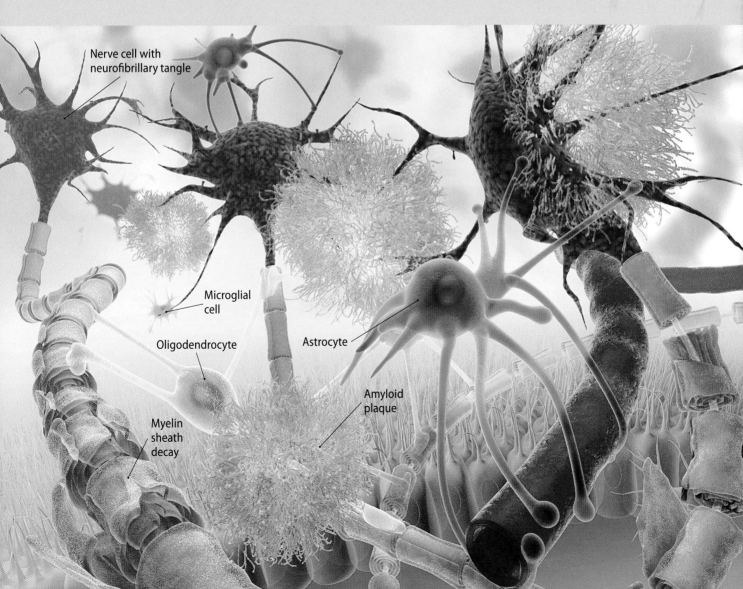

Nerve cell with neurofibrillary tangle

Microglial cell

Oligodendrocyte

Astrocyte

Amyloid plaque

Myelin sheath decay

Multiple sclerosis

Multiple sclerosis is an autoimmune condition, meaning that the body's own defense system attacks the central nervous system tissue. It involves the destruction of the myelin sheaths around nerve cells and the production of plaques. This interferes with the transmission of impulses by nerve cells, and disrupts signals sent throughout the central nervous system.

A common early feature of this disease is a problem with vision, which may be loss of vision in one eye, due to a plaque on the optic nerve (retrobulbar neuritis), or loss of vision in both eyes, if the plaque is on the optic chiasm. This may show up as problems seeing a red pinhead against a neutral background, before vision for other colors is lost. Tiredness and heaviness in one limb is also a common presenting symptom. Abnormal or poorly controlled movements sap energy and increased activity in deep tendon reflex circuits can cause limb stiffness.

Plaques on the white matter of the spinal cord cause abnormal sensation, like pins and needles in the limbs, or problems with the control of the voluntary muscles or urinary bladder. Plaques in the white matter of the brainstem may interfere with the command signals

↓ **This fluorescent light photograph shows a spinal cord affected by multiple sclerosis. Reactive astrocytes and glial progenitor cells are producing proteins (red and green) in an attempt to repair damage.**

→ **In this micrograph, microglial cells (round) are ingesting oligodendrocytes (branched). Microglia normally ingest cell debris as part of the immune response. In multiple sclerosis they attack oligodendrocytes and the myelin of axons.**

that coordinate eye movements, or if the plaque is in the white matter of the cerebellum, there will be difficulty in coordinating muscle activity in the trunk, limbs, or head, with a resulting tremor and overshooting when attempting to reach for objects. Sometimes plaques may form in the white matter of the cerebral hemispheres causing a variety of symptoms such as problems with any of the senses or even behavioral changes such as an unjustified euphoria. The latter symptom usually follows plaques in the white matter of the lower frontal lobe that interfere with output from the orbitofrontal cortex.

Attacks and remissions

A key feature of multiple sclerosis is that symptoms come and go in phases of attack, remission, and relapse. The actual symptoms that are due to loss of myelin are irreversible, but once the swelling of surrounding tissue is reduced about two to six weeks after the initial attack, the symptoms may subside to give a period of remission. Relapses are often associated with colds or chills, injuries, overwork, and exposure to bad weather, so it is important that susceptible people protect themselves from these. With each ensuing attack, the remissions are usually less complete, so overall condition progressively deteriorates.

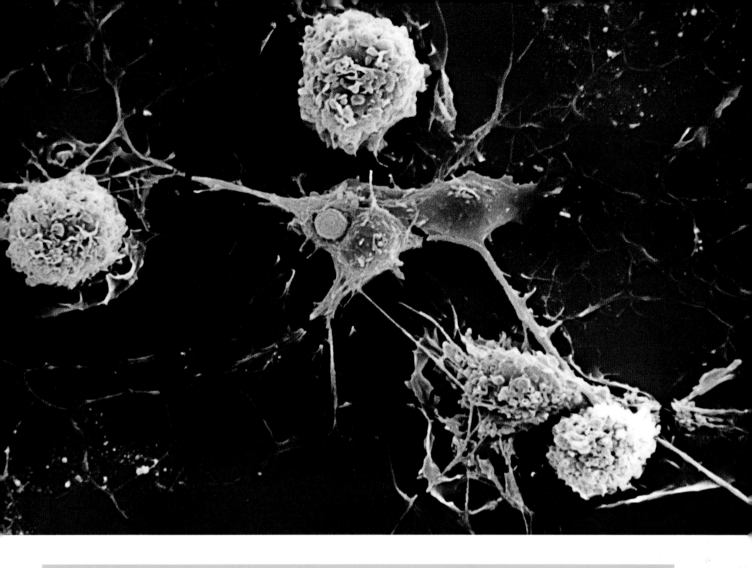

An autoimmune disease

Multiple sclerosis is a disease of the white matter of the brain, with patchy regions of the white matter becoming inflamed, losing their myelin, and hardening to form plaques (hence the term sclerosis, which means hardening). The underlying process is due to a type of white blood cell called the T lymphocyte incorrectly identifying the myelin of the central nervous system as a foreign protein and orchestrating an immune system attack. This process destroys the myelin around axons, causing abnormal nerve impulse transmission and "cross-talk" between damaged axons, leading to abnormal sensations. Attempts by oligodendrocytes to repair the damage often lead to the formation of scar tissue.

→ **Damage to the myelin sheaths of axons is the key change in multiple sclerosis, causing slow and abnormal transmission and cross-talk between axons that are in close contact.**

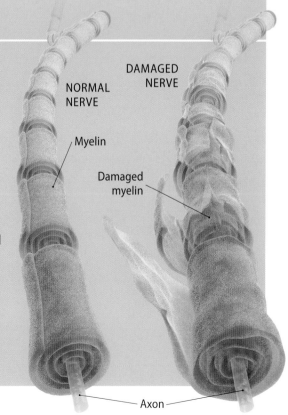

NORMAL NERVE

DAMAGED NERVE

Myelin

Damaged myelin

Axon

Geographic and racial distribution

Multiple sclerosis affects about 100 per 100,000 people in places populated mainly by Caucasians, but there are significant geographical factors involved. Prevalence of multiple sclerosis increases with distance from the equator, being much more common in temperate than tropical countries. On the other hand, genetic factors clearly have a major role to play. Having a parent with multiple sclerosis increases the risk of developing the disease by 30 fold and the risk is increased 300 times if one has an identical twin with the disease.

Some racial groups are at a much higher risk than others. The risk is lowest for black Africans and Asians (a relative risk of less than 0.001 and about 0.06, respectively), but highest for northern Europeans (relative risk of 1.3). There are also patches of the world where the disease is strikingly common. When a population migrates from a high- to low-risk area, the relative risk declines, suggesting that the disease is caused by a combination of genetic and environmental factors.

→ **The Orkney and Shetland islands off the north coast of mainland Scotland are thought to have the highest incidence of multiple sclerosis in the world. This may be due to a combination of low sunlight levels for much of the year and genetic factors in the population of Celtic and Scandinavian descent.**

Causes of multiple sclerosis

Modern theories on the causes of multiple sclerosis are centered on the potential role of viruses and Vitamin D deficiency. People who have been infected with the Epstein–Barr virus that causes infectious mononucleosis have a 23 times greater risk of developing multiple sclerosis in later life. It is thought that in some people, T lymphocytes that are activated during the Epstein–Barr virus infection cross into the brain and spinal cord from the blood and mistakenly activate an immune response. This involves the recruitment of other immune system cells like B lymphocytes and the native microglia of the brain that inflame and damage the axons and their myelin coats. Some scientists have suggested that prior infection with herpes viruses may also be responsible.

Vitamin D is known to play a significant role in regulation of the immune system. Vitamin D inhibits the cell division and activity of the T lymphocytes that attack the body's own tissues, so a deficiency of Vitamin D in the womb or in early childhood due to limited sun exposure or dietary intake could help an abnormal autoimmune attack to begin. This may explain the link between latitude and prevalence of the disease.

Treatment of multiple sclerosis

Treatment of multiple sclerosis is aimed at either providing symptomatic relief or reducing the over-activity of the immune system (see box opposite).

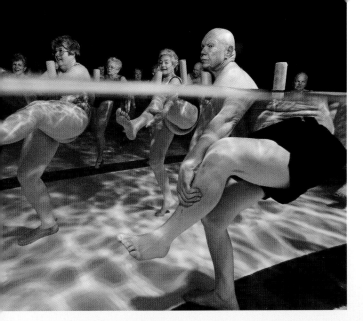

↑ **Gentle exercise like aqua aerobics can help maintain nervous system function in people with multiple sclerosis. It can be helpful in relieving pain, reducing muscle rigidity, and improving balance.**

Symptoms and treatment

Symptom	Treatment
Pain	Physiotherapy (exercise, heat, hydrotherapy)
Spasticity (rigid muscles)	Stretching, exercises to strengthen muscles, muscle relaxants, surgery
Fatigue	Conserving energy, adjusting the home environment to reduce exertion
Bladder problems	Anticholinergic drugs, catheterization, pelvic floor exercises
Bowel problems	Improved fluid and dietary fiber intake
Balance problems	Physiotherapy, exercise, anticonvulsant drugs
Cardiovascular dysfunction	Exercise under medical supervision
Tremor and unsteady gait	Drugs like propranolol, clonazepam, isoniazid Neurosurgery to relieve tremor Exercise, limb cooling

Medications such as interferon, glatiramer, monoclonal antibodies, and sphingosine-1-phosphate receptor modulator act against the immune system in a variety of ways. These reduce proliferation of the damaging T lymphocytes, inhibit the production of tumor necrosis factor that can damage the white matter, restore the role of T helper 2 suppressor cells which tone down the inflammation, and help to stabilize the blood–brain barrier so that white blood cells cannot so readily migrate into the brain and cause damage. Collectively these disease-modifying medications can reduce the frequency of attacks by as much as 70 percent. Unfortunately, side effects may include flulike symptoms, abnormal liver function, palpitations (heart fluttering or thumping), chest pain, respiratory tract infections, and local reactions at the injection site.

Parkinson's disease

First described in 1817 by the British physician James Parkinson, Parkinson's disease is an incurable disease of the central nervous system, characterized by gradual, progressive muscle rigidity, a masklike facial expression, shuffling walk, tremors, and clumsiness.

Parkinson's disease usually begins in the fifth or sixth decade and affects about 1 to 2 percent of people over 65, and about 6 percent of people over 85 years.

The most striking abnormality of Parkinson's disease is degeneration of dopamine-using nerve cells in the brainstem (substantia nigra and other regions). These nerve cells have axons that make contact with the nerve cells of the striatum, so when they are lost there is decreased activity in the basal ganglia loop circuits, hence the problems of reduced freedom of movement.

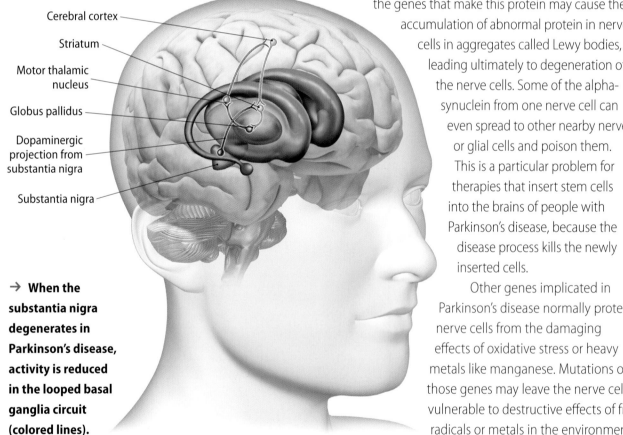

Cerebral cortex

Striatum

Motor thalamic nucleus

Globus pallidus

Dopaminergic projection from substantia nigra

Substantia nigra

→ **When the substantia nigra degenerates in Parkinson's disease, activity is reduced in the looped basal ganglia circuit (colored lines).**

What causes Parkinson's disease?

The disease process of Parkinson's disease probably arises from an interaction between genetic and environmental factors, but recent research is pointing most strongly to the importance of abnormal genes. Studies of families where Parkinson's disease appears to be inherited have led to the identification of as many as ten genes that may be responsible. The first of these to be identified were those associated with production of a protein called alpha-synuclein. This protein normally regulates the level of dopamine in nerve terminals. Abnormal versions of the genes that make this protein may cause the accumulation of abnormal protein in nerve cells in aggregates called Lewy bodies, leading ultimately to degeneration of the nerve cells. Some of the alpha-synuclein from one nerve cell can even spread to other nearby nerve or glial cells and poison them. This is a particular problem for therapies that insert stem cells into the brains of people with Parkinson's disease, because the disease process kills the newly inserted cells.

Other genes implicated in Parkinson's disease normally protect nerve cells from the damaging effects of oxidative stress or heavy metals like manganese. Mutations of those genes may leave the nerve cells vulnerable to destructive effects of free radicals or metals in the environment.

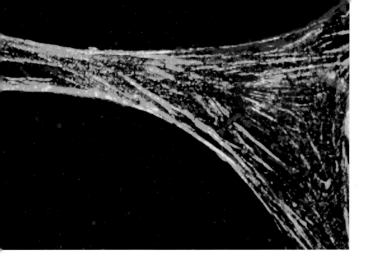

↑ **In this fluorescent micrograph of a glial cell, the nucleus is blue and the protein alpha-synuclein is red. The accumulation of this protein is thought to cause the neuron degeneration seen in Parkinson's disease.**

Progressive supranuclear palsy

This disease may have a similar initial presentation to Parkinson's disease and can often be confused with it. It has an age of onset between 40 and 65 years; more males are affected than females (2:1) and the survival time from the onset of symptoms is five to ten years. The clinical picture is of a progressive loss of eye movements, problems with the articulation of speech, and rigidity of muscles, particularly the neck. The abnormalities are mainly found in the substantia nigra of the midbrain and subthalamic nucleus of the diencephalon, but with frontal lobe abnormalities as well.

Nonmotor Parkinson's symptoms

Although the main symptoms and signs of Parkinson's disease involve abnormal movements, other disabling features of the disease involve changes in behavior and mood. Various forms of depression can affect as many as 40 percent of Parkinson's disease patients and anxiety disorders can affect between 20 and 50 percent. Apathy is a particular problem, affecting as many as 60 percent of all people with Parkinson's disease. Hallucinations (mainly visual, but also auditory) are also common in the disease, affecting as many as half of all people with the disease.

Many people with Parkinson's experience problems with control of their autonomic nervous system. This can cause difficulty in controlling blood pressure and maintaining the activity of the gut. They may feel faint when getting out of bed because the autonomic nervous system cannot adjust their blood pressure to the new posture.

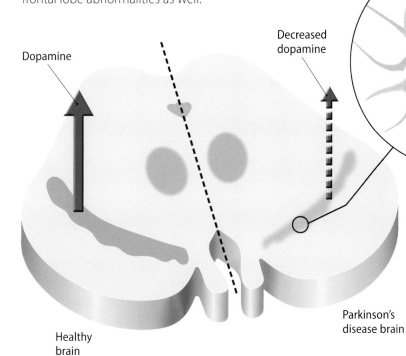

Dopamine

Decreased dopamine

Lewy body

Healthy brain

Parkinson's disease brain

← **In Parkinson's disease, the protein alpha-synuclein accumulates inside the nerve cell body as Lewy bodies, causing degeneration of the nerve cell and the loss of the dopamine-dependent connection with the striatum.**

Therapeutic tools for Parkinson's disease

Treatment	How it works
Dopaminergic medication	This type of treatment replaces the dopamine that is lost due to the degeneration of the dopamine-producing cells of the substantia nigra. Dopamine itself cannot cross the blood–brain barrier, so the oral medication uses chemicals like L-dopa that can cross the blood–brain barrier and are converted into dopamine within the brain. Dopaminergic medication improves the mood and motivation of patients.
Anticholinergic medication	Anticholinergics are important drugs, particularly in relieving the tremor. They block the receptors for acetylcholine in the brain and are believed to work by adjusting the balance between brain pathways that use dopamine and acetylcholine.
Antidepressant medication	Tricyclic antidepressants, selective serotonin reuptake inhibitors, and selective noradrenaline reuptake inhibitors have all been used to improve mood. They do this by making more serotonin and/or noradrenaline available in nerve pathways that control mood.
Cognitive behavioral therapy	This treatment is aimed at stimulating and training the patient, thereby reducing depressive symptoms and negative thoughts, and improving the patient's perception of social support.
Transcranial magnetic stimulation	This therapy uses strong magnetic fields outside the skull to stimulate nerve cells inside the brain. Magnetic fields are effective over only a very short range so this therapy is aimed at stimulating the superficial motor areas of the cortex. This stimulation can increase available dopamine in the striatum and relieve the patient's motor and psychiatric symptoms.
Deep brain stimulation (DBS)	DBS uses electrodes inserted deep inside the brain to stimulate the subthalamic nucleus. Activation of nerve cells in the subthalamic nucleus raises activity in the loop circuits that run through the basal ganglia, giving the patient more freedom of movement. Electrical stimulation of the inner part of the globus pallidus is also effective in relieving the motor symptoms experienced by people with Parkinson's disease.

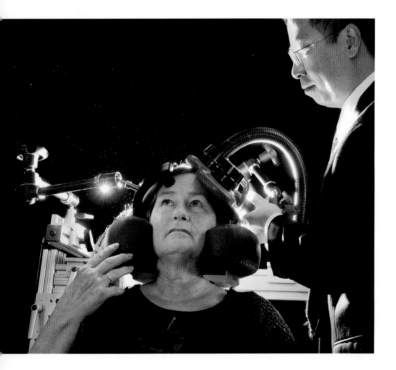

Treatment of Parkinson's disease

Parkinson's disease therapy is aimed at not just alleviating the movement problems, but also relieving the autonomic, behavioral, and psychiatric effects of the disease. Symptoms can be relieved or controlled by medications, which work by increasing levels of dopamine in the brain. Regular rest periods and avoidance of stress will help symptoms such as tremor. Physical therapy, speech therapy, occupational therapy, social work, and other counseling services help the affected person to function as normally as possible.

← **Magnetic stimulation of the superficial motor cortex is one treatment for Parkinson's disease. It increases the overall activity in the basal ganglia circuit, improving mobility and relieving psychiatric symptoms.**

Stem cell and growth factor therapy

An exciting prospect for future treatment of Parkinson's disease is to replace the lost dopamine-using cells of the substantia nigra with nerve cells grown from stem cells. Stem cells are cells that are able to mature into a variety of different adult cells. They include bone marrow stem cells, human embryonic stem cells, and skin-derived stem cells. Studies have shown that stem cells can differentiate into dopamine-producing nerve cells when grown in the laboratory under the appropriate conditions. These would have to be inserted as a graft into the patient's brain through a needle and must survive to grow axons to nerve cells of the striatum. Potential side effects of this sort of therapy include tumor formation when the stem cells grow out of control, immune system rejection of the grafted tissue, and abnormal movements because of contamination of the graft with other types of nerve cells.

Another avenue of treatment under research is the use of growth factors, like glial cell line-derived neurotrophic factor (GDNF), that promote nerve cell survival and outgrowth. One problem with this approach is that GDNF may stimulate overgrowth of other transmitter systems, resulting in abnormal movements.

↓ **Deep brain stimulation (DBS) therapy works via electrodes inserted in the brain (the dark lines in this X-ray). These electrodes send electrical impulses to specific motor areas of the brain, to improve overall activity in the motor circuitry.**

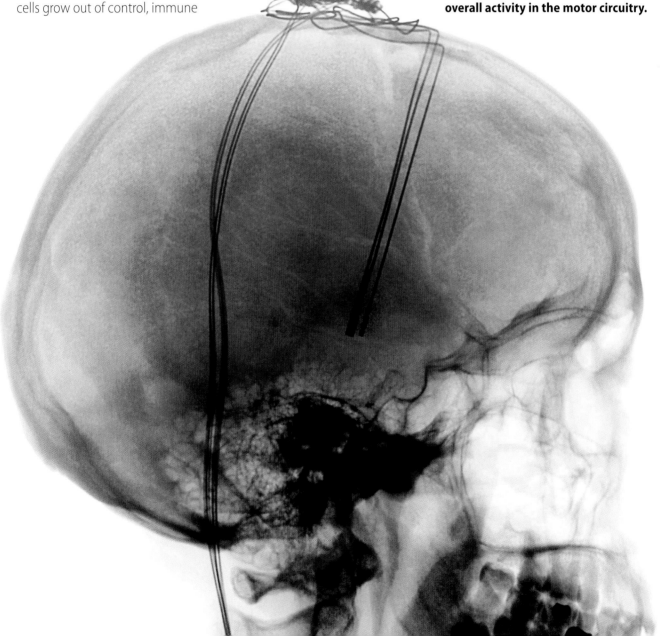

Huntington's disease

Unique among degenerative brain diseases, Huntington's disease is inherited, and environmental factors do not play any role. If a parent has the disease, each son or daughter in their family has a one in two chance of inheriting it. Huntington's disease is fatal within about 15 years of onset.

Huntington's is a rare disease—the incidence is only about 5 per 100,000—and both sexes are equally affected. It usually begins between the ages of 30 and 50 when the affected person notices the onset of involuntary, jerky, and contorted movements of the limbs. These dancelike movements are called chorea (Greek for "dance"). Other symptoms and signs include problems with articulate speech (dysarthria), abnormal eye movements, and stronger deep tendon reflexes. Mental deterioration and severe personality changes follow. Affected people may develop anxiety, obsessive-compulsive behavior, paranoia, and depression.

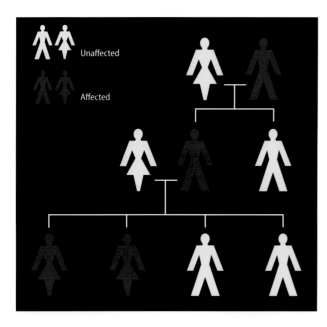

↑ **Huntington's disease is equally likely to occur in either sex and anyone with one copy of the gene will develop the disease. On average half the children of an affected person will also develop the disease.**

Pathological changes lag behind the symptoms and signs and 1 percent of affected people show no abnormalities at the time of death. There is an average 20 percent loss of brain volume at death and most of that loss is in the striatum. The cerebral cortex is also profoundly affected, with as many as 70 percent of nerve cells in some layers being lost.

Novel treatments for Huntington's disease

Research is aimed at finding ways to protect nerve cells in the striatum from the damaging effects of the huntingtin protein (see "The cause of Huntington's disease," opposite). One promising strategy is to use growth factors to arm the nerve cells with additional nutritional and survival support. Another approach is to use gene therapy to reduce or remove the mutant huntingtin protein, but these genes have to be inserted into the patient's DNA, a therapeutic technique that is in its infancy.

Growth factor strategies use brain-derived neuro-trophic factor (BDNF), ciliary neurotrophic factor (CNTF), or glial cell line-derived neurotrophic factors (GDNF). BDNF in the cerebral cortex has been shown to support the survival of nerve cells in the striatum. In Huntington's disease the mutant protein huntingtin reduces the levels of BDNF in the brain, and people with the genetic mutation that gives rise to huntingtin have lower BDNF levels. The rationale behind this approach is that restoring neurotrophic support may help nerve cells survive, but effective delivery of BDNF to the correct site in sufficient concentration has practical problems. Delivery is often by the use of viruses that must cross the blood–brain barrier.

The cause of Huntington's disease

Chromosome 4

CAG repeats

Huntingtin protein inclusions

Huntington's disease is caused by a defective gene which results in the gradual destruction of nerve cells. The gene for the disease is on chromosome 4. The mutation is a multiple repetition (between 38 and 121 repeats) of the base pairs C (cytosine), A (adenine), and G (guanine) in the patient's DNA, so they have long chains of CAGCAGCAGCAG… etc. The more repeats, the earlier the onset of the disease. Even unaffected people have some repeats (8 to 27), but when the number exceeds 35 symptoms and signs of Huntington's disease are seen.

This abnormal gene codes for an anomalous protein called huntingtin that accumulates in some nerve cells and causes them to degenerate.

→ **Huntington's disease is due to an abnormal gene on chromosome 4 with multiple repeats of the bases CAG. These excess repeats make a damaging protein called huntingtin.**

Degenerating nerve cell

Cortical degeneration

DEGENERATED BRAIN

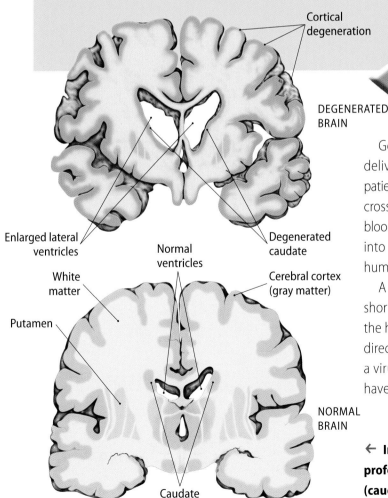

Enlarged lateral ventricles

Normal ventricles

Degenerated caudate

White matter

Cerebral cortex (gray matter)

Putamen

NORMAL BRAIN

Caudate nucleus

Gene therapy uses specially modified viruses to deliver a new gene into the genetic code of the patient's nerve cells. Modified adenoviruses are able to cross the blood–brain barrier when injected into the bloodstream of experimental animals and be taken up into nerve cells, but effective use of these agents in humans needs further study.

A final strategy being researched involves the use of short chains of RNA to interfere with the production of the huntingtin protein. These molecules must be either directly injected into the striatum or incorporated into a virus that can penetrate the blood–brain barrier to have an effect.

← **In the later stages of Huntington's disease, there is profound degeneration of nerve cells in the striatum (caudate and putamen) and cerebral cortex.**

Motor neuron disease

The primary site of this disease is the motor nerve cells of the spinal cord, brainstem, or cerebral cortex. There is no significant cognitive impairment and patients become progressively paralyzed by loss of motor control. Death is usually by pneumonia and paralysis of the respiratory muscles.

Motor neuron disease usually starts at age 55 to 60 and affects men more than women. The disease can feature one of three patterns: mainly involving the spinal cord motor nerve cells (progressive muscular atrophy); mainly involving descending motor pathways from the cerebral cortex to the spinal cord (amyotrophic lateral sclerosis); or mainly involving brainstem motor nerve cells (progressive bulbar palsy).

Clinical features depend on which pattern the disease follows. Progressive muscular atrophy is a gradual wasting and weakness of the muscles of the limbs and trunk. This may proceed for several years and people with this type can survive for much longer than those who have the amyotrophic lateral sclerosis type.

People with amyotrophic lateral sclerosis usually experience fatigue and muscle aches as early symptoms, leading on to weakness and wasting of their limb

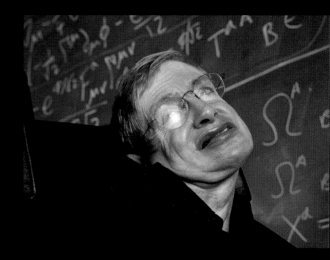

↑ **Motor neuron disease cripples the body, but leaves the personality and mind, including great minds like that of physicist Stephen Hawking, untouched.**

muscles. Muscles may be twitchy and deep tendon reflexes increased in strength. As the disease progresses, muscles controlled by the brainstem will eventually be involved, and swallowing can be affected, so the patient has difficulty controlling saliva and preventing its movement into the airway. The disease is relentlessly progressive, often leading to death from pneumonia four to five years after the onset of the disease.

Initial symptoms of progressive bulbar palsy include weakness of muscles of the tongue, chewing muscles, facial muscles, and muscles for swallowing. People with this form usually die within a year or two of diagnosis from pneumonia, because they are unable to control the flow of saliva and prevent its movement into the airway and lungs.

Future therapies

Potential treatments of this disease currently under research include protecting nerve cells from oxidative stress, providing nerve growth factors to help maintain the survival of motor nerve cells, gene therapy to prolong survival of nerve cells and delay the progression of symptoms, and injection of stem cells to replace lost motor nerve cells. Gene therapy is aimed at switching off some of the abnormal genes involved in the disease or delivering growth factors to promote survival of the remaining nerve cells.

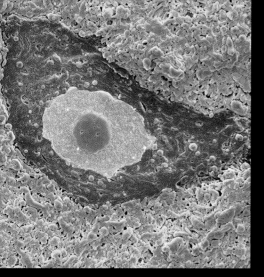

↑ **A healthy motor nerve cell is revealed in this micrograph. Motor neuron disease involves the gradual degeneration of such cells in the brain and spinal cord.**

→ **Motor nerve cells have cell bodies in the ventral horn of the spinal cord (shown in situ in red and isolated in green) and connect to muscles. In motor neuron disease, the motor nerve cells degenerate and are surrounded by astrocytes, the ventral horn shrinks, and the muscles waste away.**

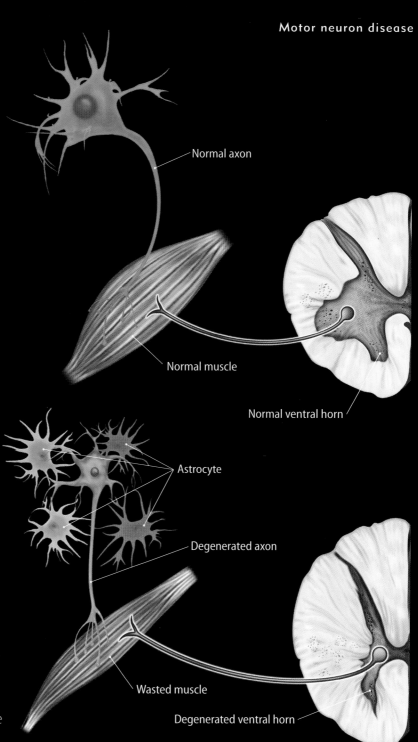

Normal axon

Normal muscle

Normal ventral horn

Astrocyte

Degenerated axon

Wasted muscle

Degenerated ventral horn

Causes

Most cases of motor neuron disease occur sporadically, in other words there is no pattern of inheritance, but about 5 to 10 percent of cases are a recurrent instance within a family. This has led to the identification of more than 18 defective genes that can cause the disease. Study of these genes has also provided clues to the common disease processes that cause the degeneration of the motor nerve cells.

Motor nerve cell death can be caused by many different mechanisms involving both the nerve cells themselves and the surrounding glial cells. These mechanisms include inflammation from the activity of astrocytes and microglia, abnormal function of the mitochondria that provide energy for nerve cells, oxidative stress from free radical molecules produced during the lifetime of the nerve cell, accumulation of damaging proteins as cells age, damaged transport of material along axons, and the release of the excitotoxic chemical glutamate from nearby dying cells. Nerve cells cannot be replenished, so even a very slow and gradual loss of motor nerve cells will eventually have profound effects on the person's ability to perform activities of daily living.

Dementia

Dementia is a deterioration or loss of intellectual function, reasoning ability, and memory, due to degeneration and death of brain tissue. People with dementia experience progressive confusion and disorientation over 5 to 15 years, usually culminating in complete dependence on carers.

Dementia generally occurs in elderly people. Forms of dementia include frontotemporal dementia; vascular dementia due to many tiny infarctions in the forebrain caused by widespread small artery disease; and those resulting from chronic alcoholism, degenerative diseases, and metabolic disorders. However, virtually all epidemiological surveys indicate that Alzheimer's disease is the single major cause of cortical dementia, accounting for about 55 percent of all cases on its own and contributing along with other cerebral diseases to a further 20 percent of cases of dementia.

Alzheimer's disease
The age of onset for Alzheimer's disease is from 30 onward, but it is most common after the age of 65 and affects more females than males. A few people have a genetic form with a mutation in the gene responsible for amyloid precursor protein (situated on chromosome 21), but most genetic cases involve mutations on chromo-

somes 14 and 1. The disease is clearly caused by many different genetic and nongenetic factors, many of them unknown, but affected people share a common pathology, implying that there is a single disease mechanism operating despite the diverse causes.

Clinically, people with Alzheimer's disease present with amnesia (forgetfulness), defects in spatial perception, and language abnormalities (aphasia) as the most common problems, but late problems include muscular rigidity and diminished movement. Memory of the most remote past is usually relatively preserved while declarative memory (memory for facts, events, and the meaning of words) is progressively diminished.

↓ **This colored micrograph of the brain of a person with Alzheimer's reveals a large plaque (yellow/black at lower left). This contains the abnormal amyloid protein. Also seen are several neurofibrillary tangles (smaller yellow/black areas) in thickened parts of nerve cells.**

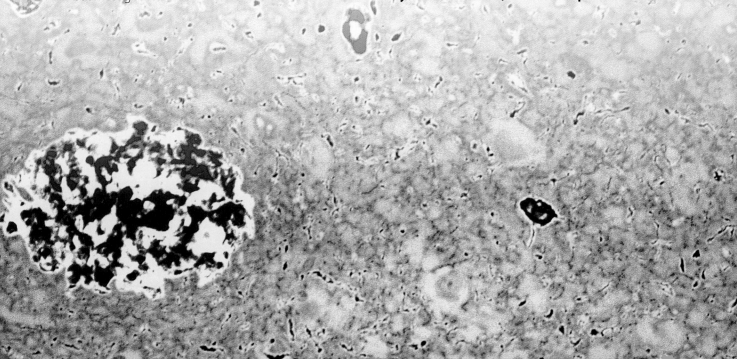

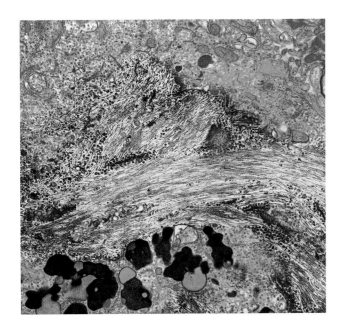

↑ **The yellow mass in this micrograph is a neurofibrillary tangle inside a brain cell (green). The tangle consists of abnormal aggregates of the protein tau.**

Brain changes in Alzheimer's disease

Alzheimer's disease is confirmed after death by the presence of numerous neurofibrillary tangles and "senile" plaques, which are degenerative changes within and outside nerve cells. The brains of dementia patients often show the external signs of loss of cerebral cortex volume, with narrowing of the gyral bumps on the brain surface as nerve cells degenerate and die. These degenerative changes are

→ **In the later stages of Alzheimer's disease, the gray matter areas of the cerebral cortex are so extensively degenerated that the brain tissue shrinks and the ventricles enlarge. The hippocampus and the frontal lobes are most affected.**

often found in the cerebral cortex and hippocampus. They damage nerve cells, give rise to abnormal cell function, and ultimately cause the death of the cell itself. The major noncellular component of senile plaques is the short protein called amyloid beta (Aβ), which is able to accumulate into large sheets. Neurofibrillary tangles are bands of abnormal filamentous material, which form and accumulate in the nerve cell bodies and often extend into the dendrites. The tangles are mainly composed of the microtubule-associated protein called tau. Excessive accumulation of this protein in the nerve cell body is undoubtedly damaging. The presence of many plaques and tangles is diagnostic for Alzheimer's disease, but does not predict the degree of clinical impairment. It seems that the best indicator of clinical change is the density of cortical nerve cells and synapses—the more of these that have been lost, the more severe the symptoms observed during life.

Alzheimer's disease almost invariably develops in all people with Down syndrome who survive to age 40. This is consistent with the observation that the gene that produces the precursor protein for amyloid beta is coded on the same chromosome (21) that is present as an extra copy in Down syndrome.

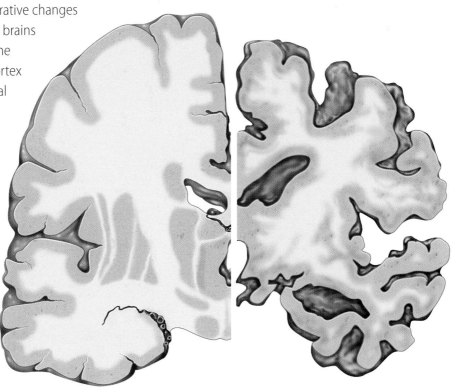

Normal brain   Alzheimer's brain

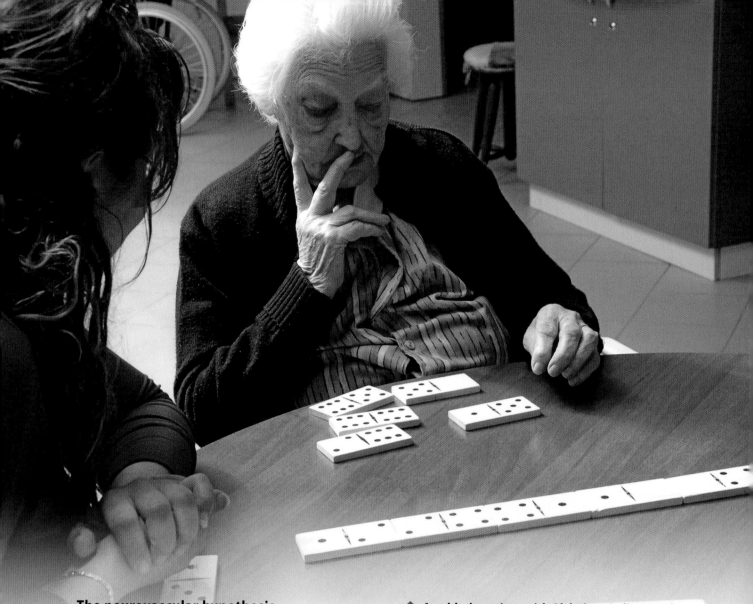

The neurovascular hypothesis for Alzheimer's disease

Studies have revealed a clear overlap between the risk factors for cerebral vessel disease and Alzheimer's disease, prompting researchers to suggest that damage to blood vessels in the brain is an important root cause for Alzheimer's disease. Midlife diabetes mellitus, high blood pressure, and obesity contribute to both Alzheimer's disease and vascular dementia. In addition, poor blood flow, silent strokes, and episodes of low blood oxygen all increase the risk of Alzheimer's disease.

The two-hit vascular hypothesis for Alzheimer's disease proposes that the initial predisposing factor (hit one) is due to vascular factors (damage to the blood–brain barrier and poor blood flow, due to elevated blood pressure, diabetes, heart disease, or stroke). The damage to the blood–brain barrier reduces the removal of amyloid beta from the brain and causes the accumulation of toxins in

↑ **An elderly patient with Alzheimer's disease plays dominoes to help preserve her memory, hand mobility, and dexterity. The progression of Alzheimer's disease can also be monitored in this way.**

the brain. Vascular injury also increases the production of amyloid beta in brain tissue from a naturally occurring precursor protein (hit two). Accumulating toxins, the build-up of amyloid beta, and poor blood flow in the brain converge to cause the death of nerve cells, resulting in cognitive decline and eventual dementia.

This hypothesis sounds an important warning for people living in developed countries. The current explosion of obesity in the Western world is likely to pose many serious public health problems in the future as the obese population ages into the dementia-susceptible age range.

Frontotemporal dementia

Frontotemporal dementia is the second most common form of early onset dementia after Alzheimer's disease. An early and prominent sign is social misconduct with indications of frontal lobe damage. Muscle rigidity and poor movement are relatively late occurrences. An EEG may be normal and the main pathological feature is marked degeneration of the frontal and temporal lobes. In some cases swollen nerve cells known as Pick cells are present, but in others the only change is the accumulation of tiny spaces (vacuoles) in the cortical tissue. In 50 percent of cases of frontotemporal dementia there is a clear family history. A gene on chromosome 17 has been linked to a number of families, while others seemed to be caused by an abnormal gene on chromosome 3.

Treatment of dementia

Current drug treatment for Alzheimer's disease and related forms of dementia is centered around the role of the neurotransmitter acetylcholine. One feature of these diseases is the degeneration of acetylcholine-producing cells in the base of the forebrain. These project to the cerebral cortex and hippocampus and may be important for maintaining memory function. Some drugs inhibit the cholinesterase enzyme that breaks down acetylcholine. This boosts the concentration of acetylcholine at cortical and hippocampal synapses resulting in a modest slowing of cognitive decline.

Another group of drugs (NMDA antagonists) acts on one of the receptors for the neurotransmitter glutamate. Unfortunately, both cholinesterase inhibitors and NMDA antagonists only alleviate the symptoms and do not alter the course of the disease.

Apart from drugs, other treatments are also important. Cognitive function can be enhanced and retained by training and stimulation. Computerized devices may be used for this, but the most effective treatments are those that require professional therapists and are labor-intensive.

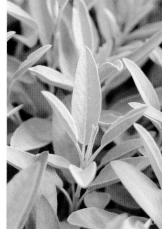

→ **The search continues for effective treatments for dementia, including therapies from natural sources like sage plants (pictured). The goal is to protect and preserve nerve cells and their connections from the disease process.**

Novel therapies for Alzheimer's disease

Two broad groups of novel therapies for Alzheimer's disease are currently under research: stem cell grafting and vaccine therapy.

Stem cell grafting is a process whereby young cells that have the ability to mature into a wide range of cell types are introduced into the brain. The goal is to replace some or all of the nerve cells lost during the disease process. This form of grafting could be most effective in parts of the brain where vulnerable nerve cells with key functions have been lost, e.g., the acetylcholine-producing cells of the basal forebrain, and the hippocampus. These grafts would have to be introduced by deep brain injection and would have to be capable of surviving and prospering in a brain environment that may be hostile because of the disease process.

The vaccine approach has been tested in animals, but is yet to be tried in humans. Animals have been genetically manipulated so that they accumulate amyloid beta in plaques and develop learning deficits early in life. When these animals are vaccinated with the abnormal protein during early life, they have better retention of learning ability and have fewer plaques in their ageing brains than unvaccinated siblings.

Vascular brain disease

The dependence of the brain on its rich vascular supply makes it particularly susceptible to disease processes that affect blood vessels. Vascular brain diseases may present as pain, a gradual decline in cognitive ability, or a sudden loss of brain function.

A rupture or leakage of blood from vessels inside the brain or in the meningeal compartments that surround the brain is known as a cerebral hemorrhage. This may be caused by external forces (see "Brain injury," pp. 268–71) or can result from disorders of the brain's vascular system. A severe narrowing or complete obstruction of the blood vessels that supply the brain is known as a cerebral infarction or, more commonly, a stroke.

Subarachnoid hemorrhage

Some patients have an intrinsic weakness of the cerebral arterial walls, particularly the arteries around the base of the brain (Circle of Willis). These weak spots stretch in response to pressure inside the artery, causing a balloonlike swelling known as an aneurysm. An aneurysm can damage surrounding nerve tissue by compressing it, or can rupture to cause a subarachnoid hemorrhage. In this last disorder, blood tracks rapidly through the subarachnoid space around the brain, irritating nervous tissue and the meninges. People with subarachnoid hemorrhage experience a sudden onset of severe headache and may die from the effects of the blood on cerebrospinal fluid flow and pressure inside the skull. Subarachnoid hemorrhage can be avoided by the surgical clipping of aneurysms before they rupture.

Intracerebral hemorrhage

Bleeding inside the brain itself most commonly arises from rupture of tiny thin-walled arteries that pass through the brain tissue. These vessels are particularly thin and vulnerable in the deep parts of the forebrain around the basal ganglia and white matter pathways. A major contributing factor in this type of hemorrhage is elevated blood pressure. Vessel rupture leads to blood forcing its way under pressure through the delicate brain tissue, with devastating effects.

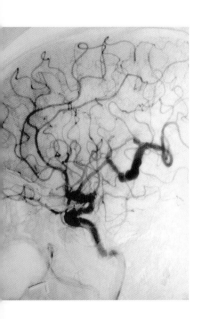

← **This cerebral angiogram performed following the injection of a contrast medium shows a serpentine aneurysm (gray) along the middle cerebral artery.**

→ **In this colored 3-D CT scan of the brain and skull of a person with an intracerebral hemorrhage, blood (red) is leaking into the ventricles of the brain, creating a solid mass known as a hematoma.**

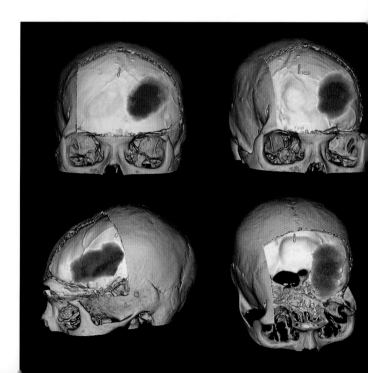

Preventing and managing stroke

The most important medical approach to stroke is prevention. Stopping smoking, keeping blood pressure within the optimal range, avoiding or properly treating diabetes mellitus, controlling body weight and blood fats, and engaging in regular physical exercise are important strategies for reducing your risk of stroke. Promptly seeking medical attention if you experience any of the symptoms of stroke (e.g., sudden numbness or vision loss, or problems moving a limb) is vital so that doctors can minimize the amount of damage from the stroke. Some people at risk of stroke may be prescribed aspirin to reduce the chance of blood coagulating on the lining of their arteries.

↓ **Obstruction of cerebral arteries to the brain often occurs when blood coagulates (forms a thrombus) on an arterial wall affected by atherosclerosis. The brain tissue will be deprived of oxygen and begin to die unless the obstruction is removed quickly.**

Atherosclerosis

Thrombus

CEREBRAL INFARCTION (STROKE)

Stroke

Loss or reduction of the blood supply to an organ is called ischemia. If the tissue of the organ begins to die because of this disordered blood supply, the process is called infarction. A cerebral infarction (better known as a stroke) usually results from blockage of the arteries that bring blood to the brain, but the veins that drain the brain may also become blocked, disrupting the flow through the capillary bed of the brain and causing tissue death.

Most adults in developed countries have a disease process called atherosclerosis affecting their arteries.

This involves the accumulation of fatty material and fibrous or calcified material in plaques within the arterial wall. These reduce the internal area of the vessel, obstructing flow to the brain and hardening the vessel wall (sclerosis). Sudden obstruction of a brain artery can occur when a plaque ruptures or when blood coagulates onto the damaged vessel lining. Adopting a healthy lifestyle that minimizes the possibility of developing atherosclerosis is the best approach for avoiding stroke.

Cellular and molecular stroke damage

The brain needs a steady supply of glucose and oxygen and even a few minutes of ischemia can trigger a cascade of events that damage nerve cells. As soon as the brain tissue is deprived of oxygen, it starts to rely on less effective anaerobic (oxygen-free) metabolism. The loss of usable energy causes the cellular pumps that maintain the balance of charged particles between the inside and outside of nerve cells to fail. The nerve cells fire wildly and sporadically because of this, worsening the electrical balance of their membranes. Failure of nerve and glial cell metabolism also raises the concentration of the amino acid glutamate in the tissue fluid around them. Glutamate is a neurotransmitter, so the release of glutamate excites surrounding nerve cells to death by flooding their interior with calcium, spreading the zone of tissue damage far beyond the initial site. Flow of calcium into the nerve cells in turn causes production and release

Stopping the cascade of stroke damage

A major goal of stroke management is to reduce the damage of the stroke cascade. This is achieved by firstly controlling blood pressure if hemorrhage is the cause and relieving arterial blockage if the obstruction is recent. Drugs that block the excitotoxic effects of glutamate (NMDA or AMPA receptor blockers), if given within a few hours of an ischemic episode, may be able to reduce or stop nerve cell damage.

↓ **Excessive release of glutamate causes an influx of calcium into nearby nerve cells, triggering damaging internal effects that include activation of degradative enzymes and destruction of cell membranes.**

Excessive glutamate release

Oxygen-starved nerve cell

Injured overexcited nerve cell

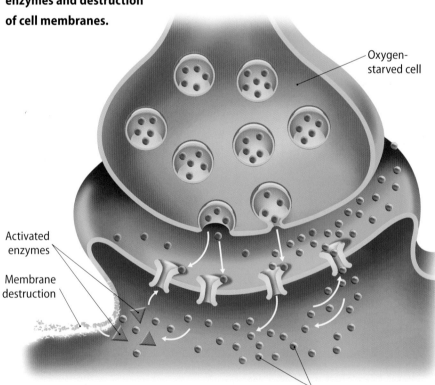

Oxygen-starved cell

Activated enzymes

Membrane destruction

Excess calcium

↑ **Damage to one nerve cell may cause excessive release of excitatory chemical glutamate onto other nerve cells, leading to a cascade of damaging effects in surrounding nerve cells.**

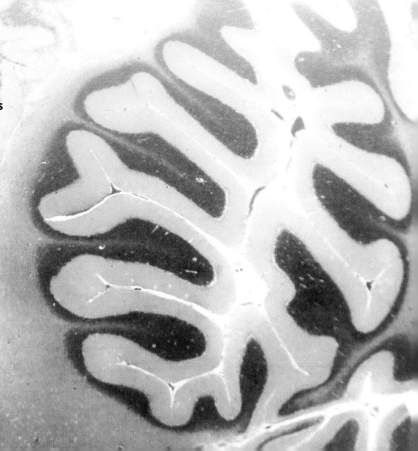

→ Physiotherapy can help stroke patients to recover mobility. The brain may eventually regain control over the paralyzed areas, or techniques can be learned to compensate for loss of mobility.

of other active molecules (like nitric oxide) and the activation of natural enzymes in the nerve cells that break up their internal structure.

So although the original region of damage from blood loss may be quite small (the umbral zone), the cascade of secondary effects due to the release of glutamate, nitric oxide, and highly reactive molecules made from water and oxygen (free radicals) causes a zone of damage (the penumbral zone) that is much larger than the initial region.

Recovery after a stroke

When a person has had a stroke, there is usually an initial phase of rapid improvement that lasts days to weeks. This is followed by a second phase of slower improvement that may proceed over months to years. The initial damage to tissue occurs in the central or umbral region, but secondary changes occur in the surrounding tissue

(penumbral region). Secondary effects in the penumbra are due to tissue swelling and disturbances of the brain's smallest blood vessels. If the swelling and vasculature disruption in the penumbra subside soon after the stroke, then function returns rapidly (the first phase of recovery). The effectiveness of the second phase of recovery depends on the brain's ability to redistribute function and adjust connections (plasticity), which is much greater in younger than older people.

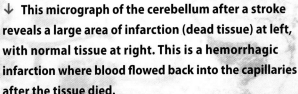
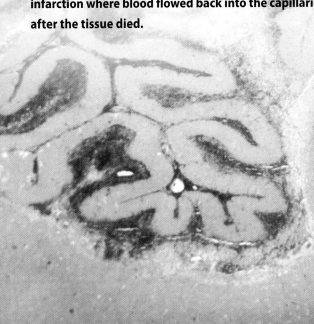

↓ This micrograph of the cerebellum after a stroke reveals a large area of infarction (dead tissue) at left, with normal tissue at right. This is a hemorrhagic infarction where blood flowed back into the capillaries after the tissue died.

Tumors of the nervous system

Tumors may arise in the brain and spinal cord itself (primary tumors) or enter the brain and spinal cord by spreading through the bloodstream from other parts of the body (secondary tumors).

A growing tumor may reveal itself when it raises pressure inside the skull cavity, causing severe headaches, nausea, and vomiting. Symptoms may also result from a tumor pressing on a nerve or damaging a certain area of the brain, resulting in changes in speech, vision, or hearing; changes in mood or personality; difficulties balancing or walking; or numbness in the limbs.

Factors that contribute to the development of a brain tumor include an inherited disease like neurofibromatosis, increasing age, previous exposure of the head to

radiation, occupational exposure to vinyl chloride, and a weakened immune system (from infection with the Epstein–Barr virus or HIV), but most brain tumors develop with no known cause.

Gliomas

Most primary brain tumors are gliomas, meaning that they arise from glia or their precursor cells. The commonest type of glioma is derived from astrocytes (astrocytoma) and may range in aggressiveness from

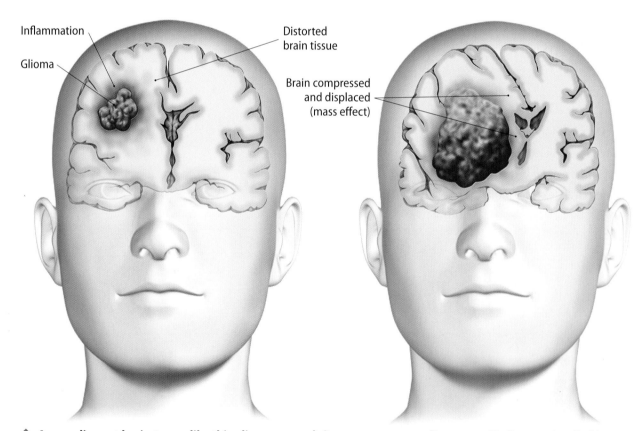

Inflammation

Glioma

Distorted brain tissue

Brain compressed and displaced (mass effect)

↑ **As a malignant brain tumor like this glioma expands it causes a surrounding area of inflammation (left), as well as compressing and shifting nearby brain tissue (left and right). The raised pressure inside the skull causes headaches and vomiting and the shifting brain tissue can damage delicate nerve cells.**

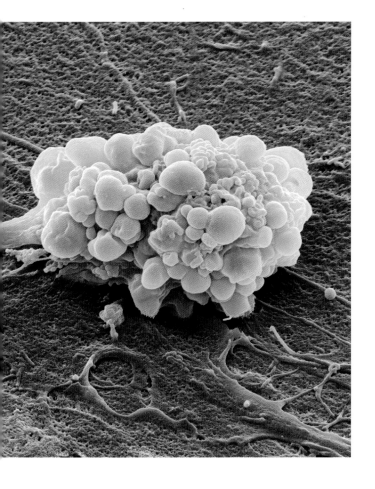

Do cellphones cause brain tumors?

This is a controversial area. Most studies at the time of writing do not find that radiation from cellphones is a cause of primary brain tumors. Nevertheless, there has not been sufficient time for the effects of long-term exposure of the developing brains of children and teenagers to this form of radiation to become apparent. Sound advice would be for all cellphone users to use earphones and a flexible cord to maintain a safe distance of at least 1.5 feet (0.5 meters) between the cellphone and their brain.

← **Gliomas are a type of tumor that arises from glial cells of the central nervous system. Gliomas can be very aggressive and spread quickly through surrounding healthy brain tissue.**

the less aggressive and relatively well-differentiated type that look much like normal astrocytes, through to a highly invasive type (glioblastoma) made up of cells that look almost embryonic. Glioblastomas enlarge rapidly and invade surrounding tissue so extensively that no precise boundaries to the tumor may be found, making it extremely difficult to remove them surgically. Rapidly growing tumors are supplied by a tangle of fine blood vessels that may easily rupture, causing sudden changes in the patient's condition. The symptoms of a malignant glioma include headaches (often worse in the morning), memory loss, drowsiness, convulsions, and a progressive loss of brain function over several weeks.

Other, less common types of glioma may arise from the oligodendrocytes (oligodendroglioma) or the ependymal cells that line the ventricles of the brain's interior (ependymoma). The second type is particularly significant because it can cause obstruction to the flow of cerebrospinal fluid through the brain.

Medulloblastoma

This type of brain tumor is seen in children and is different from gliomas in that it has the ability to produce primitive nerve cells. It is often found along the midline of the cerebellum, which it may damage, producing a wide-gaited walk with poor muscle coordination. It is susceptible to radiation treatment, but may spread along the spinal cord.

Meningioma

The connective tissue that makes up the membranes surrounding the brain may also be the site of tumors. These are often slowly growing but can have serious effects when they press on functional areas of the cerebral cortex. Many meningiomas arise from the web of dura mater that separates the two halves of the brain, so many symptoms and signs of meningiomas involve compression of midline cortical areas. A common symptom is gradually increasing weakness and loss of

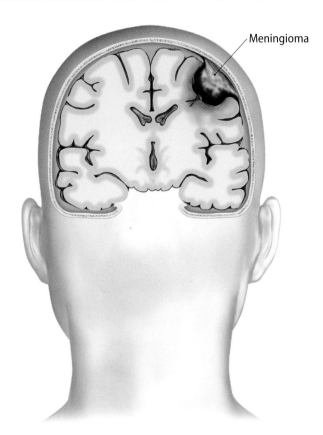

Meningioma

↑ **Meningiomas arise from the membranes that surround the brain. They are less aggressive than gliomas, but can cause serious damage by compressing functional areas of the cerebral cortex.**

feeling in the legs, due to compression of the primary motor and somatosensory areas that serve the lower limbs. Meningiomas around the olfactory nerve may cause loss of smell in one or both nostrils and a feeling of euphoria (due to damage to the orbitofrontal cortex). A meningioma around the optic and oculomotor nerves causes loss of vision, a droopy eyelid, and double vision.

Acoustic neuroma

This tumor grows from Schwann cells of the vestibulo-cochlear nerve. Occasionally a similar tumor may develop on the trigeminal nerve. This tumor type does not invade the brain, but produces symptoms and signs by compressing surrounding tissue. Patients initially experience loss of hearing and balance, followed by nausea, vertigo, and problems with eye coordination as the tumor grows against the cerebellum and brainstem.

Pituitary tumors

Pituitary tumors are not particularly aggressive, but the region they grow in is so important that these tumors have profound effects. They commonly arise from the endocrine cells of the pituitary gland and expand within the skull to destroy the surrounding gland. Symptoms develop slowly and may include loss of libido, reduction of body hair, cessation of menstrual cycles in women, increase in weight, and intolerance of cold. The pituitary sits below the optic chiasm where the visual pathways cross before entering the brain, so growth of the tumor often cuts through the visual axons. Patients may not notice that their vision is being lost from the side of the visual field for each eye and instead complain of headache and blurring of central vision. Treatment to spare the patient's vision is by surgery.

Sometimes a pituitary tumor produces hormones in excess (usually growth hormone), causing gigantism in children or adolescents, or acromegaly in adults. In acromegaly there is overgrowth of the bones of the skull, jaw, hands, and feet and thickening of the soft tissue of the face and tongue. This type of tumor rarely affects vision and is usually treated with targeted radiation.

Craniopharyngioma

Craniopharyngioma tumors develop in children from the remnants of the embryonic structure that forms the front of the pituitary gland. It expands to destroy the pituitary gland and the hypothalamus. Children with this tumor often complain of headache and poor vision. Surgical removal is a demanding procedure because of the involvement of surrounding vital structures like the internal carotid artery and the optic nerves from the eyes.

Secondary brain tumors

The brain is a common site for tumor cells from other parts of the body to lodge and grow. Common tumor types include those from the lung, breast, bowel, and pigment cells of the skin (melanoma). Secondary tumors are usually multiple because they are the result of simultaneously seeding the vessel bed of the entire brain with many tumor cells.

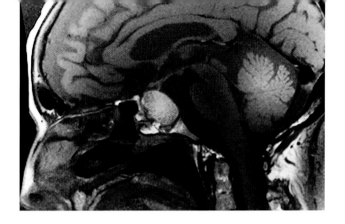

↑ **A pituitary tumor (pink, at center) is usually benign (not cancerous), and does not spread to other parts of the body, but it can lead to disturbances of vision and body growth, and changes in hormonal balance.**

↓ **Removal of brain tumors is extremely delicate surgery. Modern neurosurgical techniques use advanced 3-D imaging, fiber optic instruments, and even robotics to gain access to tiny spaces in the skull and brain and remove abnormal growths.**

Treatment of brain tumors

Slowly growing tumors that are not causing symptoms may not need any treatment. Where the tumor is neatly confined and easy to remove without damage to surrounding vital structures, surgery is the optimal treatment. Where the tumor is more diffuse and is spreading through nearby brain tissue, radiotherapy is the best option. This is given as a series of daily X-ray beam treatments over two to six weeks. Only a limited range of drugs are suitable for treating brain tumors. A major problem with drug therapy is the difficulty of getting the drug to cross the blood–brain barrier.

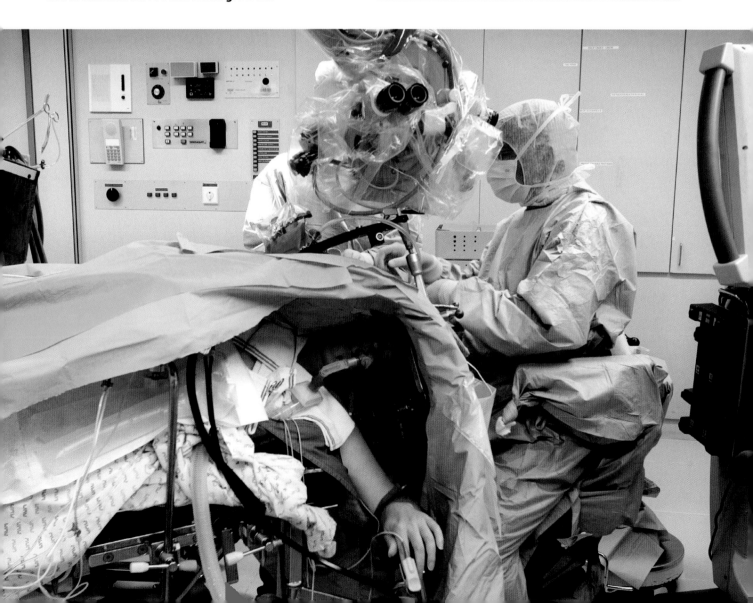

Disorders of brain development

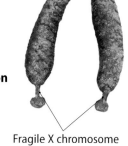

Abnormal brain development may result from defective genes (Kallmann syndrome), abnormal or extra chromosomes (Down syndrome and fragile X), or adverse environmental effects.

The brain is susceptible to developmental disorders at every stage of its growth: formation of the embryonic nervous system tube, production of nerve cells by cell division, migration of nerve cells, outgrowth of axons and dendrites, and formation of correct connections.

→ **Fragile X syndrome is a common cause of intellectual disability in males. It is due to an abnormal gene on the X chromosome.**

Fragile X chromosome

Neural tube defects

The embryonic brain develops by folding of a flat plate (the neural plate) into a tube (the neural tube) during the 19th to 25th days of development. If the closure is incomplete at the head end, the brain will not develop (anencephaly); if the closure is incomplete at the tail end, the spinal cord will not form properly (spina bifida). Anencephaly is incompatible with life after birth, but children with serious spina bifida can survive into adult life if treated surgically, albeit with lower limb paralysis and ongoing problems with bowel and bladder control. Ensuring that all women of reproductive age have adequate dietary folate intake *before* they become pregnant can reduce the incidence of neural tube defects by at least 30 percent.

Chromosomal abnormalities

People with Down syndrome have three copies of chromosome 21 instead of the usual two. Along with a range of physical abnormalities, the most significant feature of the condition is that mental development is retarded. Adults with Down syndrome have an average mental age of about eight years. Nearly all Down syndrome adults will develop Alzheimer's disease and become prematurely demented.

Fragile X syndrome is the most common cause of inherited intellectual disability and is due to a defect involving a gene called the FMR1 gene. The abnormality

occurs in the X chromosome, of which females have two and males only have one. Boys with the defective chromosome will be intellectually disabled; women with only one damaged X chromosome will be carriers of the disease.

Damaging environmental agents

Sites of nerve cell production are particularly vulnerable to damage by a variety of physical, chemical, and infective agents. These include ionizing radiation (e.g., fetal victims of the Hiroshima and Nagasaki atomic bombs), elevated maternal temperature, toxins (alcohol, anticancer drugs, methyl mercury), and viruses (measles, cytomegalovirus). Interruption of the process of nerve cell production leads to reduced nerve cell populations in the adult brain and a small brain size (micrencephaly).

Hydrocephalus

Obstruction of the ventricular system of the brain, particularly at narrow sites like the interventricular foramina between the lateral ventricles and third ventricle, or at the narrow cerebral aqueduct between the third and fourth ventricles, may occur during development. Cerebrospinal fluid production will usually continue, with the result that ventricles upstream of the blockage dilate, stretching and thinning the neural tissue in the wall of the brain. This stretching of developing brain tissue can tear the delicate growing axons, killing

Fetal alcohol spectrum disorders

Exposure of the developing brain and retina to alcohol in utero causes a range of effects with serious consequences for the future intellectual ability of the child. A baby with fetal alcohol syndrome will have an abnormal face (flat nasal bridge, thin upper lip, upturned nose, flat philtrum between the nose and upper lip), reduced size of frontal midline brain structures (septum and frontal lobes), small eyes, and a defective optic nerve.

→ **Children with fetal alcohol spectrum disorder may have a smaller and less developed brain, particularly the midline frontal region of the cerebral cortex, and a smaller corpus callosum and cerebellum.**

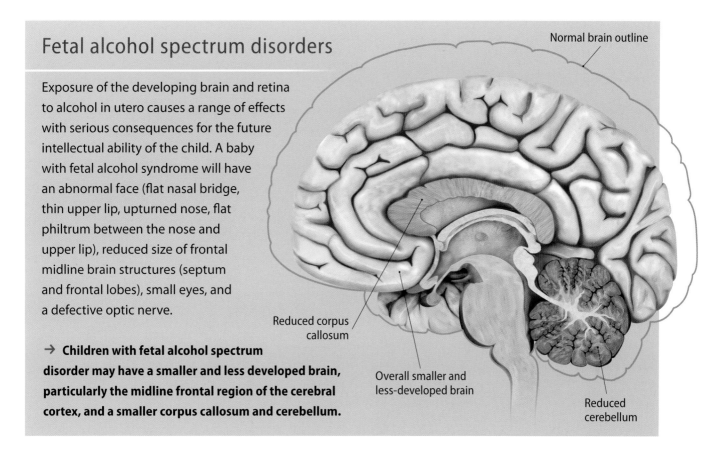

Normal brain outline

Reduced corpus callosum

Overall smaller and less-developed brain

Reduced cerebellum

nerve cells in the cortex before they have reached their mature shape. This swelling of the ventricular system is known as internal hydrocephalus and is often a cause of intellectual disability unless properly treated. If it arises before birth it may cause obstructed delivery because the infant's head will be too large to pass through the maternal pelvis. If it arises postnatally it may be detected by measurements of the infant's head. Draining the excess cerebrospinal fluid from the ventricle system of the brain to either the right atrium of the heart or the abdominal cavity can relieve the pressure and alleviate most of the adverse effects.

Kallmann syndrome

This syndrome is a disorder involving genes that regulate the growth of olfactory axons into the brain, as well as the migration of cells from the embryonic nose to the hypothalamus that will produce sex hormone regulatory factors. Affected people have no sense of smell, have small testes or ovaries, and are infertile.

← **The dark green shape in this colored MRI image is an enlarged lateral ventricle; a condition called hydrocephalus. This problem is treated by shunting fluid from the ventricles to the heart or abdomen.**

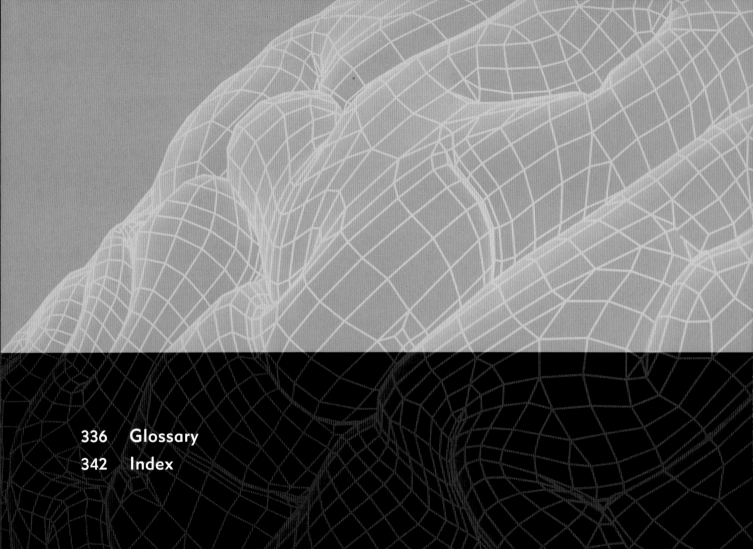

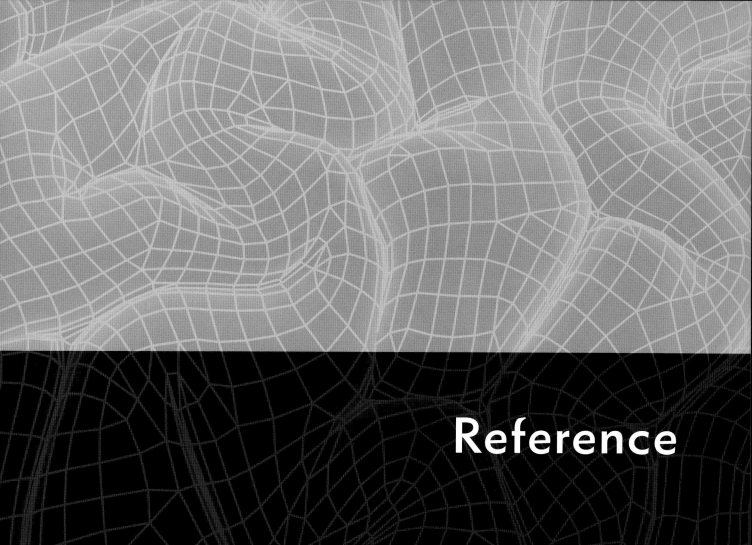

Reference

Glossary

A

acetylcholine A neurotransmitter chemical used in the brain, the autonomic nervous system, and when nerves contact skeletal muscles.

action potential A moving wave of electrical activity that usually travels from the nerve cell body to the axon terminal.

addiction Dependence on a substance that has gone beyond voluntary control.

adrenaline A hormone and neurotransmitter produced by the inner part (medulla) of the adrenal gland. It is released into the bloodstream in times of emergency to increase heart rate, force of heart contraction, airflow through the lung airways, and blood flow to muscles. It is also known as epinephrine.

afterpolarization The change in voltage across the axon membrane that occurs at the end of the action potential, returning the membrane to its original state.

Alzheimer's disease A progressive degenerative brain disease where nerve cells are lost from the cerebral cortex and brainstem and the patient gradually loses the ability to reason, remember events, and perform daily tasks.

amygdala An almond-shaped region in the temporal lobe that is concerned with emotions such as anger and fear.

anesthesia Literally, the loss of sensation. It may be general, in which case the patient is unconscious; or local, i.e., confined to a specific region of the body.

anterior The direction toward the front of the body.

aphasia Loss of the ability to understand or express spoken language, even though the motor control of articulation is intact.

apraxia Loss of the ability to perform complex motor tasks, e.g., construct a drawing, even though the control of individual muscles is intact.

arachnoid The delicate middle layer of the meninges. It is firmly attached to the inside of the dura mater.

arcuate fasciculus The arching bundle of axons that joins Wernicke's and Broca's areas, allowing two-way communication to control language.

association areas An area of cerebral cortex that does not perform a specific motor or sensory task, but is concerned with processing higher cortical functions, such as planning, social behavior, memory, and language.

astrocyte A star-shaped glial cell that supports nerve cells and maintains a constant internal environment in the brain.

ataxia Uncoordinated movement, usually due to damage to the cerebellum.

atherosclerosis A disease process where fatty, fibrous, and even calcified material accumulates in the wall of large and medium-sized arteries.

audition The process of perceiving sound. It depends on the inner ear, brainstem, thalamus, and auditory areas in the cerebral cortex.

auditory cortex The part of the cerebral cortex concerned with processing sound information. It lies on the upper surface of the temporal lobe.

autonomic nervous system The part of the nervous system concerned with control of automatic bodily functions, e.g., blood pressure, heart rate, gut movement.

axon The long process of a nerve cell. It is used by the nerve cell to communicate by action potentials with the dendrites or axons of other nerve cells.

axon reflex A mechanism by which pain-sensitive axons spread impulses to the areas surrounding an insect bite or abrasion, causing inflammation to spread.

B

basal ganglia A collection of nerve cells deep inside the brain that are concerned with control of motor function (e.g., caudate, putamen, globus pallidus, subthalamic nucleus).

bipolar cells Nerve cells with only two processes. Examples include the bipolar cells of the retina and the ganglion cells of the inner ear.

bipolar depression A type of mental illness where the patient experiences periods of depression and hypomania or mania (abnormally elevated mood and mental activity).

blood–brain barrier The barrier in the wall of cerebral blood vessels that prevents large molecules from entering the privileged environment of the brain.

bouton The buttonlike ending of an axon where contact is made with another nerve cell.

brainstem The part of the brain that lies between the thalamus and the spinal cord. It is divided into midbrain, pons, and medulla oblongata.

brainwaves Waves of electrical activity in the cortical surface of the brain which can be detected by an electroencephalogram (EEG).

Broca's area One of the language areas of the cerebral cortex. It lies in the left frontal cortex of most people and is concerned with expressive aspects of speech.

Brodmann areas A series of areas in the cerebral cortex, identified by neuroscientist Korbinian Brodmann on the basis of differences in nerve cell structure. Most Brodmann areas serve specific functions.

C

cardiovascular system The body system that pumps blood around the body. It consists of the heart, arteries, capillaries, and veins.

caudal Literally meaning the direction toward the tail of the animal. In humans it means a direction down the brainstem or spinal cord.

central nervous system The brain and spinal cord, as opposed to the peripheral nervous system, which is all the nerves and ganglia outside the brain and spinal cord.

cerebellum The part of the brain attached to the back of the brainstem. It is concerned with coordination of movement.

cerebral cortex The folded, outer layer of the cerebral hemispheres. The cortex is made up of an outer layer of gray matter and underlying white matter.

cerebral hemispheres The two prominent halves of the forebrain. Each hemisphere is covered with cortex and has basal ganglia in its depths.

cerebrospinal fluid The clear fluid that fills the ventricles within the brain and the subarachnoid space around the brain and spinal cord.

cerebrum The two halves of the cerebral hemispheres taken together. *See* cerebral hemispheres.

chemically gated channel Ion channels in the membrane of an axon that open in response to the presence of specific chemicals.

chorea Brisk, purposeless, dancelike movements made by some patients with diseases of the basal ganglia.

choroid plexus Special structures in the ventricles of the brain that produce most of the cerebrospinal fluid.

chromosome A tightly spiraled collection of DNA and accompanying proteins. Humans have 23 chromosomal pairs.

cingulate gyrus A band of cerebral cortex surrounding the corpus callosum on the medial surface of each cerebral hemisphere.

circadian rhythm Literally meaning "about a day." The natural daily cycle of nervous system activity that controls sleep and waking.

circuit A series of nerve cells connected together by synapses and serving a specific function.

cognition The process of thinking.

consciousness Being aware of oneself and of one's surroundings.

corpus callosum A large bundle of axons that connects the two cerebral hemispheres, allowing transfer of information between the two sides.

cranial nerves Nerves attached to the brain and mainly concerned with sensory or motor function in the head and neck. Twelve pairs of nerves are recognized in humans.

CT scan Computerized tomography. An imaging system where a computer constructs two- or three-dimensional images of the body based on the absorption of X-rays by body tissue.

cytoplasm The substance inside the cell that surrounds the nucleus. The cytoplasm includes structures called organelles (e.g., mitochondria) that perform cellular functions.

D

declarative memory Memory that can be consciously and verbally recalled.

dementia A progressive loss of intellectual function that accompanies degenerative brain diseases such as Alzheimer's.

dendrite The branching processes of nerve cells that receive synaptic contacts from the axons of other nerve cells.

depolarization The shift in the voltage across an axonal membrane that occurs during the action potential.

dermatome The strip of skin supplied by a single spinal nerve.

desynchronization The phase of EEG activity during sleep when there are no obvious cortical waves and the thalamus and cortex are acting independently.

diencephalon The central part of the brain that is traditionally defined as including the thalamus, hypothalamus, subthalamus, and epithalamus (including the pineal gland).

dopamine A neurotransmitter chemical used by the nerve cells of the substantia nigra of the midbrain to regulate motor activity.

dorsal The direction toward the back in the brainstem and spinal cord.

dorsal horn The part of the gray matter of the spinal cord that processes sensory information from the skin, joints, muscles, and internal organs.

dorsal root ganglion cells Sensory ganglion cells that lie alongside the spinal cord and carry information about pain, touch, temperature, and joint position to the dorsal horn.

dream sleep Usually synonymous with rapid eye movement (REM) sleep, a type of sleep where the sleeper experiences vivid dreams while all the muscles in the body, apart from those moving the eyes, are inactive.

dura mater The tough outer layer of the meninges.

E

EEG Electroencephalography. A technique for recording electrical activity arising from the cerebral cortex. This technique produces an electroencephalogram (also called an EEG).

endocrine system A system of ductless glands that secrete hormones into the blood to regulate the internal function of the body.

endoplasmic reticulum Complex folded membranes inside the cell that manufacture proteins.

enteric nervous system The nerve cell network within the wall of the gut. It controls gut movement and gland secretion.

epilepsy Abnormal electrical discharges in the cerebral cortex that may cause episodes of lost consciousness or jerking fits.

excitotoxicity The release of glutamate from damaged nerve cells causing abnormal excitation and further damage to surrounding nerve cells.

F

facial nucleus A group of nerve cells in the pons that control the muscles of facial expression.

flexion reflex *See* withdrawal reflex.

forebrain The front region of the brain that includes the cerebral hemispheres and the diencephalon.

fornix An arching bundle of fibers that connects structures in the temporal lobe with the septal region and hypothalamus.

frontal lobe The front part of the cerebral cortex. It contains areas concerned with planning and motor function.

G

GABA An abbreviation of gamma aminobutyric acid, a neurotransmitter used at inhibitory synapses.

ganglia Collections of nerve cell bodies outside the central nervous system. They may be sensory or autonomic in function.

ganglion cells Cells lying within ganglia. They may be sensory or autonomic in function.

genome The sum total of the genetic code that regulates the development and function of the cells of the body.

glia Cells that support and defend the central nervous system. They include astrocytes, oligodendrocytes, and microglia.

globus pallidus Part of the basal ganglia.

glutamate An amino acid that is also used as an excitatory neurotransmitter in the brain.

Golgi apparatus A type of structure inside the cell that packages substances for transport.

gray matter The part of brain and spinal cord tissue that has an abundance of nerve cell bodies, making it look gray in its fresh state.

growth factors Natural chemicals that regulate the growth of nerve cells and their axons. They are usually most active during development when connections are being formed.

gustation The sense of taste. It relies on taste receptors (taste buds) on the tongue and soft palate.

gyrus (pl. gyri) The elevations on the surface of the cerebral cortex. Gyri are separated by grooves (sulci).

H

hallucination A complex false sensory perception, e.g., a disembodied voice or a smell.

hippocampus The folded structure in the temporal lobe that plays a critical role in laying down new memories.

homeostasis The process by which the autonomic nervous system maintains a constant internal body environment.

hormone A chemical secreted from endocrine glands into the bloodstream to act on distant organs.

Huntington's disease A genetic disease where degeneration of nerve cells in the caudate nucleus and cerebral cortex causes abnormal movements and progressive dementia.

hypothalamus The part of the brain that lies below the thalamus and above the pituitary gland. It controls the autonomic nervous system and pituitary gland.

I

insula A region of cerebral cortex hidden between the frontal and temporal lobes.

interneuron A nerve cell that is interposed between long pathway nerve cells and has a short axon. Groups of interneurons process information locally.

ion A charged atom. Important ions for nerve cell function include sodium, potassium, chloride, and calcium.

ion channel A special protein embedded in the nerve cell membrane that selectively allows movement of ions across the membrane.

L

lateral The direction toward the side of the head or body.

lateral geniculate nucleus A group of nerve cells in the thalamus that process visual information before passing it to the visual cortex.

ligand-gated channel An ion channel that opens when a very specific neurotransmitter molecule binds to a site (receptor) on the channel.

limbic system The part of the forebrain that is concerned with emotions and memory. It lies at the medial rim or edge of the cerebral cortex.

lobe A region of the cerebral cortex. Five are recognized: frontal, parietal, temporal, occipital, and insula.

locus coeruleus A group of nerve cells in the brainstem that use noradrenaline in their connections with much of the brain.

long-term memory Memory that lasts for more than a few minutes. It requires the storage of memorized information in diverse parts of the cerebral cortex.

M

macula Literally meaning a "spot." It is used for the macula lutea (yellow spot) in the retina, which has pigment that reduces scattering of blue light. It is also used for two sensory regions of the inner ear (maculae of the utricle and saccule).

mechanically gated channel An ion channel that opens when hair processes of the receptor cells in the inner ear are bent by fluid movement.

medial The direction toward the midline of the body.

medulla oblongata The lower part of the brainstem, situated between the pons and the spinal cord.

melatonin A hormone produced in the pineal gland to regulate circadian rhythms.

meninges The membranes (dura mater, arachnoid, and pia mater) that surround and protect the brain.

metabolism The biochemical processes by which a cell produces energy and manufactures essential chemicals.

microglia The type of glial cell that provides defense against foreign invaders.

midbrain The upper part of the brainstem. It has nerve cells for controlling muscles in and around the eye.

mind The understanding, reasoning, and intellectual faculties of the conscious person considered as a whole.

mitral cell A type of nerve cell in the olfactory bulb that carries information about odors into the olfactory areas of the brain.

motor cortex The part of the cerebral cortex that directly or indirectly controls movement.

motor nerve cell The nerve cells that either directly contact muscles, or directly control the nerve cells that contact muscles.

MRI scan Magnetic resonance imaging. A type of brain imaging that uses strong magnetic fields to map the distribution and state of hydrogen atoms in the brain.

multiple sclerosis A disease in which the myelin coating of axons in the brain and spinal cord is attacked by the patient's immune system.

myelin sheath The fatty coating around axons that increases the speed and reliability of nerve impulse transmission.

myotome The collection of muscles supplied by a particular spinal nerve.

N

neglect syndrome A clinical condition arising from damage to the right parietal lobe, where the patient ignores the left side of their body.

nerve A collection of axons and their connective tissue coatings that connect the central nervous system with muscles, skin, joints, or internal organs.

nerve cell A cell type adapted for the processing and transmission of information. Also called a neuron.

nerve fiber An axon and its connective tissue coating.

nervous system The collection of nerve cells and their supporting tissues that are concerned with processing sensory information, making decisions, and performing motor actions.

neurodegenerative disease A group of brain diseases (e.g., Alzheimer's, Parkinson's, Huntington's) in which nerve cells slowly die off, with accompanying loss of function.

neurotransmitter A chemical released at a synapse to act on receptors in the membrane of another nerve cell.

neurotrophic factors Secreted chemical factors that attract and support axon growth during development and repair.

nociceptor A pain-sensitive nerve fiber.

node of Ranvier A tiny gap between the myelin coatings of an axon, where the axon membrane is exposed. The action potential jumps between successive nodes.

noradrenaline A neurotransmitter used by the locus coeruleus of the brainstem. It is also known as norepinephrine.

nucleus The structure within the cell that contains the DNA and regulates cell function.

nucleus of the solitary tract A group of nerve cells in the brainstem that receive sensory information about taste and input from internal organs of the chest and abdomen. It is important in appetite control.

O

obsessive–compulsive disorder A psychiatric disorder characterized by obsessive thoughts (e.g., about germs) and compulsions to perform rituals (e.g., wash hands repetitively).

occipital lobe The part of the cerebral cortex at the back of the brain.

olfaction The sense of smell.

oligodendrocyte A type of glial cell that makes the myelin coating of axons in the central nervous system.

opiate An opioid drug such as codeine, morphine, or heroin made from the sap of the opium poppy *Papaver somniferum*.

opioid Any neurotransmitter or drug that activates opioid receptors, usually producing analgesia and sometimes pleasure.

optic chiasm The place where axons from retinal ganglion cells in the medial part of the retina cross to the opposite side of the brain.

optic nerve The cranial nerve that carries visual information from the retina to the brain.

orbital cortex The part of the frontal lobe that lies over the orbits (eye sockets).

P

Papez circuit A brain circuit that connects components of the limbic system. It plays a key role in laying down new declarative memories.

parallel processing The simultaneous processing of different aspects of sensory information (e.g., color, visual texture, movement, and visual contrast).

paralysis An inability to move a part, a side, or the whole of the body.

parasympathetic nervous system The part of the autonomic nervous system that is concerned with restoring energy reserves and returning the body to rest.

parietal lobe The part of the cerebral cortex between the frontal and occipital lobes.

Parkinson's disease A disease caused by degeneration of dopaminergic nerve cells in the substantia nigra.

pathway A collection of axons running in parallel and serving a similar function.

peripheral nervous system The nerves and ganglia outside the brain and spinal cord.

PET scan Positron emission tomography. A type of imaging that maps the position of radioactively labeled chemicals in the brain.

phobia An unreasoned or irrational fear of everyday objects or situations.

pia mater The innermost and most delicate layer of the meninges. It is in direct contact with the brain surface.

pineal gland A gland at the back of the diencephalon. It secretes melatonin and is involved in daily rhythms.

pituitary gland The master gland of the endocrine system that controls diverse functions and glands throughout the body by its hormones. It is directly influenced by the hypothalamus.

plaque Hardening of tissue from a disease process. Plaques may form in gray matter in Alzheimer's disease, in white matter in multiple sclerosis, or in arterial walls during atherosclerosis.

plasticity The ability of the nervous system to change its connections in response to environmental influences, particularly during early life.

pons The bridgelike part of the brainstem that contains nerve cells that project to the cerebellar hemispheres.

posterior The direction toward the back of the body.

postganglionic fiber The second in a chain of nerve cells in the autonomic nervous system.

prefrontal cortex The part of the frontal lobe that is important for planning and social behavior.

preganglionic fiber The first in a chain of nerve cells in the autonomic nervous system.

premotor cortex The part of the motor cortex that directs complex motor actions.

primary visual cortex The part of the visual cortex that receives direct connections from the lateral geniculate nucleus. It is the first cortical site of visual information processing.

process Any extension from the body of a nerve cell. It includes axons and dendrites.

proprioception The sense of joint position and muscle length and tension. It is used in muscle coordination.

Purkinje cell Large nerve cells in the cerebellar cortex that provide the only output from the cerebellar cortex to the deep cerebellar nuclei.

R

raphe nuclei Groups of nerve cells arranged down the midline of the brainstem. Many use serotonin as their neurotransmitter.

referred pain Pain arising from disease in an organ that is felt in a different body region from the organ.

reflex An automatic stereotyped response to a sensory stimulus.

REM sleep Rapid eye movement sleep. The type of sleep during which vivid dreams are experienced.

reticular formation A network of nerve cells in the brainstem that perform diverse automatic functions.

retina The part of the nervous system at the back of the eye that processes visual information from the light that falls on it.

reuptake The recycling of a neurotransmitter at some synapses by the reabsorption of a neurotransmitter into the axon after each impulse.

S

sagittal A plane through the body that divides it into left and right parts.

schizophrenia A mental illness characterized by delusions, hallucinations, and a blunting of emotional responses.

Schwann cell A type of cell that makes the myelin coating around the axons of the peripheral nervous system.

sensory axon An axon that serves a sensory function (e.g., touch, pain, temperature, or vibration).

sensory cortex Those parts of the cerebral cortex that serve a sensory function (e.g., touch, vision, or hearing).

serotonin A neurotransmitter that is used by nerve cells of the raphe nuclei of the brainstem to control sleep/waking cycles, mood, and pain perception.

short-term memory Memory that lasts for only a few minutes and is used to perform short-term tasks.

somatotosensory cortex The part of the cerebral cortex that processes sensory information from the body surface, muscles, and joints.

spinal cord The lower part of the central nervous system. It is protected by the vertebral column and has 31 spinal nerves attached to it.

spinal nerve One of 31 pairs of nerves that attach to the spinal cord. There are 8 in the neck, 12 in the chest, 5 in the lower back, 5 in the sacral area, and 1 in the tail (coccygeal) region.

stem cell A type of primitive cell that has the ability to transform into many different types of mature cells.

striatum Part of the basal ganglia. It can be divided into the dorsal striatum (caudate and putamen) and the ventral striatum (nucleus accumbens).

stroke A sudden loss of brain function as a result of cerebral infarction (lack of oxygen and death of tissue in some part of the brain) as a consequence of interruption of the blood supply to the brain or cerebral hemorrhage.

substantia nigra Literally "the black stuff." A group of nerve cells in the midbrain that use dopamine to regulate motor activity.

subthalamic nucleus One of the nerve cell groups in the basal ganglia. It regulates motor activity through connections with the globus pallidus.

subventricular zone A region of the embryonic brain where cell division produces small nerve cells and some glia.

sulcus (pl. sulci) A groove between two elevations on the brain surface.

superior The direction toward the top of the body.

sympathetic nervous system The part of the autonomic nervous system that is most active during emergency situations (fight or flight).

synapse The contact between the axon of one nerve cell and the dendrite or axon of another nerve cell.

synaptic cleft The narrow space where neurotransmitters are released from the presynaptic membrane and make contact with receptor molecules on the postsynaptic membrane.

T

temporal lobe The part of the cerebral cortex above and in front of the ear.

thalamus The large group of nerve cells in the center of the brain that relays information between the cerebral cortex and the brainstem and spinal cord.

T lymphocyte A type of white blood cell that helps the body fight certain infections as well as cancer.

transduction The process of converting one form of energy or chemical stimulus into another.

tremor A shaking form of abnormal movement. Tremor may occur either at rest or when an action is being performed.

U

umami One of the five basic flavors (the others being sweet, salt, sour, and bitter). It is is the perception of "savoriness" from the flavor-enhancing effects of the amino acid glutamate.

V

vagus nerve One of the cranial nerves that wanders through the neck, chest, and upper abdomen, supplying many internal organs.

ventral The direction toward the front of the spinal cord and brainstem or the underside of the forebrain.

ventricle A fluid-filled space within the brain. The ventricles contain cerebrospinal fluid and are remnants of the embryonic tubular brain.

vestibular apparatus The sensory structure in the inner ear that detects balance and acceleration.

vestibulocochlear nerve The cranial nerve that carries information about sound, balance, and acceleration from the inner ear to the brainstem.

visual cortex The part of the cerebral cortex that processes sight information from the retina.

voltage-gated channel A type of ion channel that opens in response to nearby electrical fields.

W

Wernicke's area A language area on the back of the left upper temporal lobe and extending into the parietal lobe. It is important for the comprehension of language and applying grammatical rules.

white matter The type of central nervous system tissue that is almost exclusively made up of axons and their myelin coats.

withdrawal reflex The spinal reflex that withdraws a body part from a dangerously hot or painful object.

working memory Short-term memory that is used over a period of a few minutes to complete immediate motor tasks.

Index

References to major subject areas
are in **bold** type.

H

habenular nuclei 32
hallucinations **159**, 313 *see also* illusions and
    hallucinations
hallucinogens 302
hangovers 294–5
Hawking, Stephen 318
head and neck reflexes **174–5**
    airway protection 175
    ear protection 175
    eye protection 174–5
    reflex pathways 174
hearing 21, **130–3** *see also* ears
    auditory pathway 132
    cochlea 131
    coding and transmitting sound
        information 132–3
    detecting direction of sound 133
    ear structure 130
    organ of Corti 132
    pressure waves to nerve impulses 131–2
    sound waves 130
    stereocilia 132
hemiballismus 28, 32, 179
hemiplegia 100
hemispheres, left and right **26–7**
    functions of each hemisphere 26
    language 26–7
    spatial perception 27
herbal medicines 291
hippocampus 18, 35
    brain-derived neurotrophic factor (BDNF)
        in 104, 316
    memory and 35, 229, 232
    olfactory pathways 144
histones 92, 93
Hockett, Charles 190
homeostasis 33, 39
hormones 36, 37, 86
    brain development and 99
    menopause and brain function 111
    stressful events and 248
Human Immunodeficiency Virus Type 1
    (HIV-1) 79
hunger 245, 293
Huntington's disease 179, 307, **316–17**
    cause 317
    duration 316
    gene therapy 317
    genes 316
    inherited degenerative disease 316
    later stages 317
    onset 316
    treatments 316–17

hydrocephalus 67, 332–3
hyperalgesia 155
hyperkinetic disorders 28
hypnotics 288–9
hypoglossal nerve 43
hypokinetic disorders 28
hypothalamo-hypophyseal portal
    system 36
hypothalamus 16, 30, 32–3
    addiction 292
    body systems and 33
    damage to 227
    emotions and 242, 247
    gender differences 33, 120–1
    olfactory pathways 144
    pituitary gland and 36
    regulation of appetite 33
    role 32–3
    sleep and 235–6, 237

I

illusions **158–9**
    blind spot 159
    tactile 158
    visual 158
imaging the brain **24–5**
    computerized tomography (CT) 24
    electroencephalography (EEG) *see* EEG
        (electroencephalogram)
    endoscopy of cerebrospinal fluid
        pathways 25
    magnetic resonance imaging (MRI) 24
    positron emission tomography (PET) 25
    safety of brain scans 25
infection and autoimmune disease 306
    multiple sclerosis *see* multiple sclerosis
insomnia 236–7
insula 18, 141
    gustation 21
insulin 33
intention tremor 47
internal senses **150–1**
interneurons 124
intracerebral hemorrhage 324
ischemia 325, 326
isocortex 18

J

Jennett, Bryan 239

K

Kallmann syndrome 332, 333
Kanisza triangle 158
ketamine 303
knee-jerk reflex 55

L

lactic acid 152
language 13, 20, 21, 186, **188–91**
    animal communication 190–1
    areas of brain **192–5**
    brain disease/injury and speech 192–3,
        194
    Broca's and Wernicke's areas 26–7, 229
    click languages 189–90
    displacement 191
    emotion in speech 27
    function beyond the cortex 194–5
    history of 188, 189
    Indo-European 189
    lateralization of language function 193
    left hemisphere function 26, 193
    listening 195, **196–9**
    productivity 191
    prosody 27, 193, 197
    reading, writing, and mathematical
        calculation **200–3**
    scanning speech 47
    sign 194
    singing 199
    speaking and listening **196–9**
    written 194
larynx 198
lateral fissure 18
lateral geniculate nucleus 30
left and right hemispheres **26–7**
    functions of each hemisphere 26
    language 26–7
    spatial perception 27
leptin 33
Lewy bodies 312, 313
lies and liars 211
limbic system 31, **34–5**, 242
    components 34
    damage to 35
    emotions and the amygdala 34
liver 295
locked-in syndrome 241
locus coeruleus 48, 49
long-term potentiation (LTP) 232
lumbar puncture 52, 67

Picture credits

b = bottom, c = center, l = left, r = right, t = top

AL = Alamy
CB = Corbis Images
DT = Dreamstime
GI = Getty Images
IS = iStockphoto
MEPL = Mary Evans Picture Library
SPL = Science Photo Library
SS = Shutterstock

1, 2–3 (background) CB, **6** IS, **10–11** CB, **12**t GI/SPL, **12**b GI/SPL, **13** GI/SPL, **15** GI/SPL, **17** GI, **19** SPL, **22** GI/SPL, **24** CB, **25**t GI/SPL, **25**c CB, **27** GI/SPL, **28** SPL, **31** GI/SPL, **35**t GI/SPL, **35**b GI/SPL, **37** GI/SPL, **38** GI, **41** GI/SPL, **44–5**c GI/SPL, **47**t IS, **47**b GI/SPL, **49** IS, **51** GI/SPL, **52** GI/SPL, **54** GI/SPL, **55** CB, **60** GI/SPL, **61** DT, **63** GI/SPL, **67** GI/SPL, **68** SPL, **70–1** CB, **75** GI/SPL, **76** SPL, **77**t GI/SPL, **77**b GI/SPL, **78** GI/SPL, **79**t GI/SPL, **79**b GI/SPL, **81** GI/SPL, **85** GI/SPL, **86** GI/SPL, **88–9** CB, **91** GI/SPL, **95** CB, **97** SPL, **98** GI/SPL, **100** GI/SPL, **101** DT, **102**l GI/SPL, **102–3**t IS, **104** GI/SPL, **105**t DT, **105**b GI/SPL, **107** DT, **108** GI, **109** IS, **110** CB, **111** IS, **112** IS, **115** IS, **116** GI/SPL, **118** IS, **119** IS, **121**tl IS, **121**tr IS, **122–3** CB, **124** GI/SPL , **125**t GI, **125**b GI, **129** IS, **132** GI/SPL, **134** IS, **136** GI, **139** GI/SPL, **143**t GI/SPL, **143**b GI/SPL, **145**t GI, **145**b IS, **147**t GI/SPL, **147**b IS, **149** CB, **152**t DT, **152**b GI/SPL, **155**t GI, **155**b GI, **159** Public Domain, **160–1** CB, **162** IS, **163** IS, **165** IS, **166**l GI, **166**r GI, **167**t IS, **167**b IS, **169** IS, **171** GI, **172**t GI/SPL, **172–3**b GI, **174** GI, **175**t CB, **175**b GI, **178** GI, **179** MEPL, **182**l GI/SPL, **182**r GI/SPL, **183** GI, **184–5** CB, **186–7**t GI, **186**b GI/SPL, **188** GI, **190**tl GI, **190–1** GI, **193**t AL, **193**c GI, **194**t GI, **194**b IS, **195** CB, **196**t GI, **196**c GI/SPL, **196**b GI/SPL, **198**t GI, **199** IS, **200** GI, **201**l SPL, **201**r GI, **202** GI, **203**t GI/SPL, **203**b DT, **204**l GI, **204**r GI, **205** GI, **206–7** IS, **207**b GI, **208** DT, **210**t IS, **210**b CB, **211** GI, **213**t GI/SPL, **213**b GI/SPL, **214**cl GI/SPL, **214**b CB, **215** GI, **216**t GI, **217** GI/SPL, **218** GI, **219**b IS, **220–1** CB, **222** GI/SPL, **223**l GI, **223**r IS, **224–5** CB, **226**t Figure provided by Daniel Simons. Simons, D.J., & Chabris, C.F. (1999). "Gorillas in our midst: Sustained inattentional blindness for dynamic events." *Perception*, 28, 1059–1074, **226**b IS, **227** GI/SPL, **228** CB, **229**t GI/SPL, **229**b GI, **230–1**t GI, **231**br GI, **234**t IS, **234**b CB, **236**b GI, **239** GI/SPL, **240** GI, **241**l CB, **241**r SPL, **243** Gross, L. (2006). "Evolution of neonatal imitation." PLoS Biol 4(9): e311 © 2006 Public Library of Science. doi:10.1371/journal.pbio.0040311, **245** GI, **246**t IS, **246**b SS, **247** CB, **248** CB, **249** GI, **250** GI/SPL, **252** GI, **253** GI, **254** GI/SPL, **254–5**t CB, **255**cr Image provided by Dr. Daniel R. Weinberger, Clinical Brain Disorders Branch, National Institute of Mental Health, **256** IS, **258**t GI, **258**b SPL, **259** CB, **260–1** CB, **262** GI, **263** IS, **265** CB, **266** IS, **269** CB, **271**t GI/SPL, **271**b GI/SPL, **273**t AL, **273**b IS, **275** GI, **276** GI/SPL, **278** GI/SPL, **280–1** CB, **282** CB, **283** CB, **284** GI, **286** IS, **287** CB, **288** IS, **289** IS, **290**t SS, **290–1**b SPL, **291** IS, **293**t GI, **293**b IS, **294–5** SS, **295**c CB, **295**bl GI/SPL, **295**br GI/SPL, **296**t SS, **296**b GI, **297** GI/SPL, **298** DT, **299**t GI, **299**b GI, **300**t GI/SPL, **300**b GI, **302**l GI/SPL, **302**r IS, **304–5** CB, **306** GI/SPL, **308** GI, **309** GI/SPL, **310–11**b GI, **311**t GI, **313** GI/SPL, **314** GI, **315** GI/SPL, **318** CB, **319** GI/SPL, **320** GI/SPL, **321** GI/SPL, **322** GI/SPL **323** IS, **324**l GI, **324**r GI, **327**t GI/SPL, **327**b GI/SPL, **329** GI/SPL, **331**t GI, **331**b GI/SPL, **333** GI

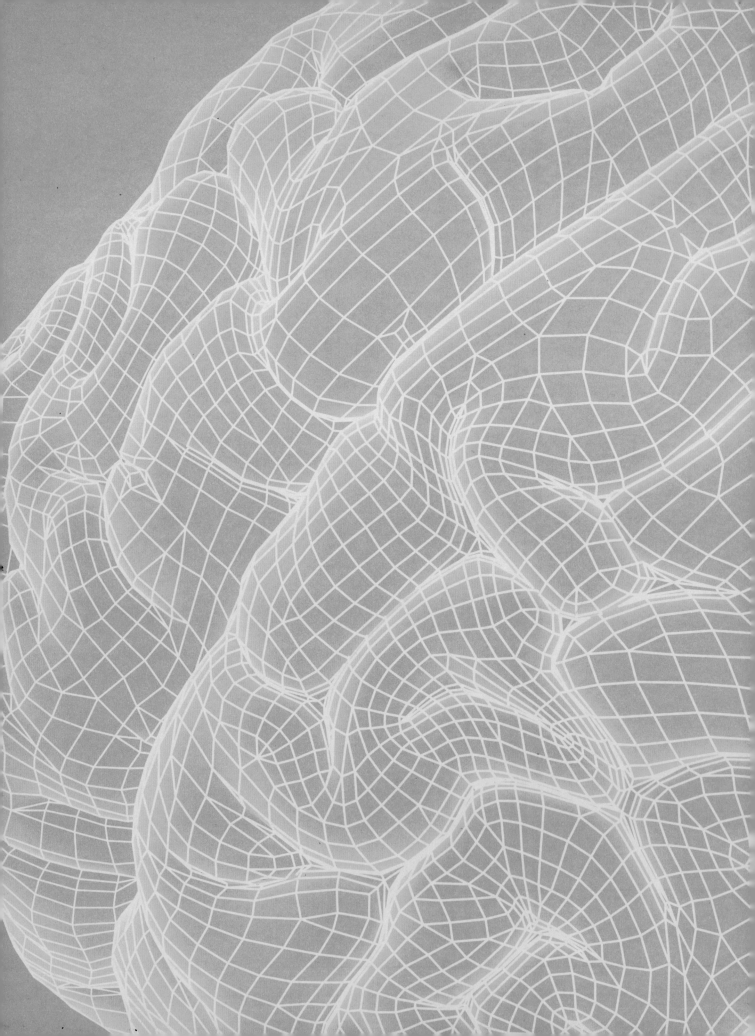